Sinonasal and Ventral Skull Base Malignancies

Editors

JEAN ANDERSON ELOY
MICHAEL SETZEN
JAMES K. LIU

OTOLARYNGOLOGIC CLINICS OF NORTH AMERICA

www.oto.theclinics.com

Consulting Editor
SUJANA S. CHANDRASEKHAR

April 2017 • Volume 50 • Number 2

ELSEVIER

1600 John F. Kennedy Boulevard • Suite 1800 • Philadelphia, Pennsylvania, 19103-2899

http://www.oto.theclinics.com

OTOLARYNGOLOGIC CLINICS OF NORTH AMERICA Volume 50, Number 2
April 2017 ISSN 0030-6665, ISBN-13: 978-0-323-52419-3

Editor: Jessica McCool
Developmental Editor: Alison Swety

Otolaryngologic Clinics of North America (ISSN 0030-6665) is published bimonthly by Elsevier, Inc., 360 Park Avenue South, New York, NY 10010-1710. Months of issue are February, April, June, August, October, and December. Business and Editorial Offices: 1600 John F. Kennedy Blvd., Suite 1800, Philadelphia, PA 19103-2899. Customer Service Office: 6277 Sea Harbor Drive, Orlando, FL 32887-4800. Periodicals postage paid at New York, NY and additional mailing offices. Subscription prices are $381.00 per year (US individuals), $803.00 per year (US institutions), $100.00 per year (US student/resident), $500.00 per year (Canadian individuals), $1017.00 per year (Canadian institutions), $556.00 per year (international individuals), $1017.00 per year (international institutions), $270.00 per year (international & Canadian student/resident). Foreign air speed delivery is included in all *Clinics'* subscription prices. All prices are subject to change without notice. **POSTMASTER:** Send address changes to *Otolaryngologic Clinics of North America*, Elsevier Health Sciences Division, Subscription Customer Service, 3251 Riverport Lane, Maryland Heights, MO 63043. **Telephone: 1-800-654-2452 (U.S. and Canada); 314-447-8871 (outside U.S. and Canada). Fax: 314-447-8029. E-mail: journalscustomerservice-usa@elsevier.com (for print support); journalsonlinesupport-usa@elsevier.com (for online support).**

Reprints. For copies of 100 or more of articles in this publication, please contact the Commercial Reprints Department, Elsevier Inc., 360 Park Avenue South, New York, NY 10010-1710. Tel.: 212-633-3874; Fax: 212-633-3820; E-mail: reprints@elsevier.com.

Otolaryngologic Clinics of North America is also published in Spanish by McGraw-Hill Interamericana Editores S.A., P.O. Box 5-237, 06500 Mexico D.F., Mexico.

Otolaryngologic Clinics of North America is covered in *MEDLINE/PubMed (Index Medicus), Current Contents/Clinical Medicine, Excerpta Medica, BIOSIS, Science Citation Index,* and *ISI/BIOMED.*

PROGRAM OBJECTIVE

The goal of the *Otolaryngologic Clinics of North America* is to provide information on the latest trends in patient management, the newest advances; and provide a sound basis for choosing treatment options in the field of otolaryngology.

LEARNING OBJECTIVES

Upon completion of this activity, participants will be able to:
1. Review the management of sinonasal and ventral skull base malignancies.
2. Discuss the evaluation and staging of sinonasal and ventral skull base malignancies.
3. Recognize endoscopic and open approaches in the treatment of sinonasal and ventral skull base malignancies.

ACCREDITATION

DISCLOSURE OF CONFLICTS OF INTEREST

UNAPPROVED/OFF-LABEL USE DISCLOSURE

and is not intended to promote off-label use of these medications. If you have any questions, contact the medical affairs department of the manufacturer for the most recent prescribing information.

TO ENROLL

To enroll in the *Otolaryngologic Clinics of North America* Continuing Medical Education program, call customer service at 1-800-654-2452 or sign up online at http://www.theclinics.com/home/cme. The CME program is available to subscribers for an additional annual fee of USD 260.

METHOD OF PARTICIPATION

In order to claim credit, participants must complete the following:
1. Complete enrolment as indicated above.
2. Read the activity.
3. Complete the CME Test and Evaluation. Participants must achieve a score of 70% on the test. All CME Tests and Evaluations must be completed online.

CME INQUIRIES/SPECIAL NEEDS

For all CME inquiries or special needs, please contact elsevierCME@elsevier.com.

Contributors

CONSULTING EDITOR

SUJANA S. CHANDRASEKHAR, MD
Director, New York Otology, Clinical Professor of Otolaryngology–Head and Neck Surgery, Hofstra-Northwell School of Medicine, Clinical Associate Professor of Otolaryngology–Head and Neck Surgery, Icahn School of Medicine at Mount Sinai, Past President, American Academy of Otolaryngology–Head and Neck Surgery, New York, New York

EDITORS

JEAN ANDERSON ELOY, MD, FACS
Professor and Vice Chairman, Director, Rhinology and Sinus Surgery, Director, Otolaryngology Research, Co-Director, Endoscopic Skull Base Surgery Program, Department of Otolaryngology–Head and Neck Surgery, Center for Skull Base and Pituitary Surgery, Neurological Institute of New Jersey, Professor, Department of Neurological Surgery, Professor of Ophthalmology and Visual Science, Departments of Neurological Surgery and Ophthalmology and Visual Science, Neurological Institute of New Jersey, Rutgers New Jersey Medical School, Newark, New Jersey

MICHAEL SETZEN, MD, FACS, FAAP
Chief, Rhinology Section, North Shore University Hospital, Manhasset, New York; Clinical Associate Professor, Department of Otolaryngology, NYU School of Medicine, Adjunct Clinical Assistant Professor Otolaryngology, Weill Cornell University College of Medicine, New York, New York

JAMES K. LIU, MD, FACS, FAANS
Departments of Neurological Surgery, Ophthalmology and Visual Science, and Otolaryngology–Head and Neck Surgery, Director, Center for Skull Base and Pituitary Surgery, Neurological Institute of New Jersey, Rutgers New Jersey Medical School, Newark, New Jersey

AUTHORS

RAMI ABDOU, MD
Resident, Department of Otolaryngology–Head and Neck Surgery, Neurological Institute of New Jersey, Rutgers New Jersey Medical School, Newark, New Jersey

GHASSAN ALOKBY, MD
Division of Rhinology and Endoscopic Skull Base Surgery, Department of Otolaryngology–Head and Neck Surgery, Prince Sultan Military Medical City, Riyadh, Saudi Arabia

SOLY BAREDES, MD, FACS
Professor and Chair, Department of Otolaryngology–Head and Neck Surgery, Center for
Skull Base and Pituitary Surgery, Neurological Institute of New Jersey, Rutgers New
Jersey Medical School, Newark, New Jersey

ANDRE BEER-FURLAN, MD
Clinical Fellow in Skull Base Surgery, Department of Neurological Surgery, The Ohio State
University Wexner Medical Center, Columbus, Ohio

BRYAN M. BRANDON, MD
Resident Physician, Department of Otolaryngology–Head and Neck Surgery, University of
North Carolina at Chapel Hill, Chapel Hill, North Carolina

RICARDO L. CARRAU, MD
Professor, Departments of Neurological Surgery and Otolaryngology–Head and Neck
Surgery, Director of the Comprehensive Skull Base Surgery Program, The Ohio State
University Wexner Medical Center, Columbus, Ohio

ROY R. CASIANO, MD, FACS
Professor and Vice Chairman, Director, Rhinology and Endoscopic Skull Base Program,
Department of Otolaryngology, Miller School of Medicine, University of Miami, Miami,
Florida

BHISHAMJIT S. CHERA, MD
Associate Professor, Director of Patient Safety and Quality, Department of Radiation
Oncology, University of North Carolina Hospitals, Chapel Hill, North Carolina

ALEXANDER G. CHIU, MD
Chair, Department of Otolaryngology–Head and Neck Surgery, University of Kansas
School of Medicine, Kansas City, Kansas

WILLIAM T. COULDWELL, MD, PhD
Department of Neurosurgery, Clinical Neurosciences Center, University of Utah, Salt Lake
City, Utah

DIPAN D. DESAI, BS
Department of Otolaryngology–Head and Neck Surgery, University of North Carolina at
Chapel Hill, Chapel Hill, North Carolina

CHARLES S. EBERT, MD, MPH
Associate Professor, Department of Otolaryngology–Head and Neck Surgery, University
of North Carolina at Chapel Hill, Chapel Hill, North Carolina

JEAN ANDERSON ELOY, MD, FACS
Professor and Vice Chairman, Director, Rhinology and Sinus Surgery, Director,
Otolaryngology Research, Co-Director, Endoscopic Skull Base Surgery Program,
Department of Otolaryngology–Head and Neck Surgery, Center for Skull Base and
Pituitary Surgery, Neurological Institute of New Jersey, Professor, Department of
Neurological Surgery, Professor of Ophthalmology and Visual Science, Departments of
Neurological Surgery and Ophthalmology and Visual Science, Neurological Institute of
New Jersey, Rutgers New Jersey Medical School, Newark, New Jersey

JUAN C. FERNANDEZ-MIRANDA, MD
Associate Professor, Departments of Otolaryngology and Neurological Surgery, UPMC
Presbyterian, University of Pittsburgh Medical Center, University of Pittsburgh School of
Medicine, Associate Director, UPMC Center for Cranial Base Surgery, Pittsburgh,
Pennsylvania

ADAM J. FOLBE, MD
Departments of Otolaryngology–Head and Neck Surgery and Neurosurgery, Wayne State University School of Medicine, Detroit, Michigan

PAUL A. GARDNER, MD
Associate Professor, Departments of Otolaryngology and Neurological Surgery, University of Pittsburgh School of Medicine, Co-Director, UPMC Center for Cranial Base Surgery, Pittsburgh, Pennsylvania

SATISH GOVINDARAJ, MD
Associate Professor and Vice Chair for Clinical Affairs, Department of Otolaryngology–Head and Neck Surgery, Associate Professor of Neurosurgery, Icahn School of Medicine at Mount Sinai, New York, New York

RALPH ABI HACHEM, MD
Clinical Fellow in Skull Base Surgery, Department of Otolaryngology–Head and Neck Surgery, The Ohio State University Wexner Medical Center, Columbus, Ohio

RICHARD J. HARVEY, MD, PhD
Rhinology and Skull Base Research Group, Applied Medical Research Centre, University of New South Wales, Faculty of Medicine and Health Sciences, Macquarie University, Sydney, New South Wales, Australia

JUAN C. HERNANDEZ-PRERA, MD
Assistant Professor, Department of Pathology, Mount Sinai Beth Israel, Icahn School of Medicine at Mount Sinai, New York, New York

JOSEPH M. HOXWORTH, MD
Consultant, Section of Neuroradiology, Assistant Professor, Department of Radiology, Mayo Clinic College of Medicine, Mayo Clinic, Phoenix, Arizona

ALFRED M. ILORETA, MD
Assistant Professor, Department of Otolaryngology–Head and Neck Surgery, Icahn School of Medicine at Mount Sinai, New York, New York

LAWRENCE KASHAT, MD, MSc
Resident, Department of Otolaryngology, University of Connecticut, Farmington, Connecticut

SARAH S. KILIC, MA
Department of Radiation Oncology, Rutgers New Jersey Medical School, Newark, New Jersey

SUAT KILIC, BA
Department of Otolaryngology–Head and Neck Surgery, Rutgers New Jersey Medical School, Newark, New Jersey

DEVYANI LAL, MD
Consultant, Department of Otolaryngology–Head and Neck Surgery, Consultant, Department of Neurological Surgery, Associate Professor, Mayo Clinic College of Medicine, Mayo Clinic, Phoenix, Arizona

CHRISTOPHER H. LE, MD
Assistant Professor, Department of Otolaryngology, University of Arizona, Tucson, Arizona

STEFAN LIEBER, MD
Department of Neurological Surgery, UPMC Presbyterian, University of Pittsburgh
Medical Center, Pittsburgh, Pennsylvania

DERRICK T. LIN, MD, FACS
Director, Division of Head and Neck Oncology, Daniel Miller Chair of Otology and
Laryngology, Massachusetts Eye and Ear Infirmary, Massachusetts General Hospital,
Associate Professor, Harvard Medical School, Boston, Massachusetts

JAMES K. LIU, MD, FACS, FAANS
Departments of Neurological Surgery, Ophthalmology and Visual Science, and
Otolaryngology–Head and Neck Surgery, Director, Center for Skull Base and Pituitary
Surgery, Neurological Institute of New Jersey, Rutgers New Jersey Medical School,
Newark, New Jersey

LEILA J. MADY, MD, PhD, MPH
Resident, Department of Otolaryngology–Head and Neck Surgery, University of
Pittsburgh Medical Center, Pittsburgh, Pennsylvania

EMILY MARCHIANO, MD
Resident, Department of Otolaryngology–Head and Neck Surgery, University of
Michigan Health System, University of Michigan Medical School, Ann Arbor, Michigan

THOMAS H. NAGEL, MD
Assistant Professor, Department of Otolaryngology–Head and Neck Surgery, Mayo
Clinic, Phoenix, Arizona

GREGORY S. NEEL, MD
Resident, Department of Otolaryngology–Head and Neck Surgery, Mayo Clinic, Phoenix,
Arizona

CRISTIAN FERRAREZE NUNES, MD
Department of Neurological Surgery, UPMC Presbyterian, University of Pittsburgh
Medical Center, Pittsburgh, Pennsylvania

GRETCHEN M. OAKLEY, MD
Department of Otolaryngology–Head and Neck Surgery, University of California
San Francisco, San Francisco, California; Rhinology and Skull Base Research Group,
Applied Medical Research Centre, University of New South Wales, Sydney, New South
Wales, Australia

ENVER OZER, MD
Professor, Department of Otolaryngology–Head and Neck Surgery, The Ohio State
University Wexner Medical Center, Columbus, Ohio

ELIZABETH L. PERKINS, MD
Resident Physician, Department of Otolaryngology–Head and Neck Surgery, University of
North Carolina at Chapel Hill, Chapel Hill, North Carolina

MICHAEL J. PFISTERER, MD
Rhinology and Endoscopic Skull Base Surgery Fellow, Department of
Otolaryngology–Head and Neck Surgery, Neurological Institute of New Jersey,
Rutgers New Jersey Medical School, Newark, New Jersey

DANIEL PREVEDELLO, MD
Associate Professor, Departments of Neurological Surgery and Otolaryngology–Head
and Neck Surgery, The Ohio State University Wexner Medical Center, Columbus, Ohio

AMOL RAHEJA, MBBS, MCH
Department of Neurosurgery, Clinical Neurosciences Center, University of Utah, Salt Lake City, Utah

SANJEET RANGARAJAN, MD
Chief Resident, Department of Otolaryngology–Head and Neck Surgery, The Ohio State University Wexner Medical Center, Columbus, Ohio

GEORGE A. SCANGAS, MD
Department of Otolaryngology, Massachusetts Eye and Ear Infirmary, Harvard Medical School, Boston, Massachusetts

MICHAEL SETZEN, MD, FACS, FAAP
Chief, Rhinology Section, North Shore University Hospital, Manhasset, New York; Clinical Associate Professor, Department of Otolaryngology, NYU School of Medicine, Adjunct Clinical Assistant Professor Otolaryngology, Weill Cornell University College of Medicine, New York, New York

CARL H. SNYDERMAN, MD, MBA
Professor, Departments of Otolaryngology and Neurological Surgery, University of Pittsburgh School of Medicine, Co-Director, UPMC Center for Cranial Base Surgery, Pittsburgh, Pennsylvania

SATYAN B. SREENATH, MD
Department of Otolaryngology–Head and Neck Surgery, University of North Carolina at Chapel Hill, Chapel Hill, North Carolina

PETER F. SVIDER, MD
Resident, Department of Otolaryngology–Head and Neck Surgery, Wayne State University School of Medicine, Detroit, Michigan

BRIAN D. THORP, MD
Assistant Professor, Department of Otolaryngology–Head and Neck Surgery, University of North Carolina at Chapel Hill, Chapel Hill, North Carolina

CHARLES C.L. TONG, MD
Resident, Department of Otolaryngology–Head and Neck Surgery, Icahn School of Medicine at Mount Sinai, New York, New York

ALEJANDRO VÁZQUEZ, MD
Department of Otolaryngology–Head and Neck Surgery, Neurological Institute of New Jersey, Rutgers New Jersey Medical School, Newark, New Jersey

ERIC W. WANG, MD
Associate Professor, Departments of Otolaryngology–Head and Neck Surgery and Neurological Surgery, UPMC Eye and Ear Institute, University of Pittsburgh Medical Center, University of Pittsburgh School of Medicine, Director of Education, UPMC Center for Cranial Base Surgery, Pittsburgh, Pennsylvania

KYLE WANG, MD
Department of Radiation Oncology, University of North Carolina Hospitals, Chapel Hill, North Carolina

THOMAS J. WILLSON, MD
Department of Otolaryngology–Head and Neck Surgery, UPMC Eye and Ear Institute, University of Pittsburgh Medical Center, Pittsburgh, Pennsylvania

ANNI WONG, MS
Departments of Neurological Surgery and Otolaryngology–Head and Neck Surgery, Neurological Institute of New Jersey, Rutgers New Jersey Medical School, Newark, New Jersey

ADAM M. ZANATION, MD
Associate Professor, Division of Head and Neck Surgery, Department of Otolaryngology–Head and Neck Surgery, Department of Neurosurgery, University of North Carolina Hospitals, University of North Carolina at Chapel Hill, Chapel Hill, North Carolina

Contents

> Significant technological advances have fostered a movement toward minimally invasive surgical interventions for the management of ventral skull base malignancies. The care of patients with these lesions ideally involves an interdisciplinary skull base team that includes otolaryngologists, neurologic surgeons, radiation oncologists, and medical oncologists. This article describes considerations essential for diagnosis, prognosis, and preoperative evaluation. Furthermore, surgical nuances, strategies for skull base reconstruction, and nonsurgical options are briefly discussed. This overview may be useful as an up-to-date description of the challenging clinical scenarios associated with these lesions.

> A wide variety of tumors present in the sinonasal and ventral skull base. Patients often have nonspecific symptoms initially and present with advanced tumors, affecting the orbit and other adjacent structures. Evaluation of these malignancies with modern imaging techniques can define tumor invasion, but biopsy is often required to establish a diagnosis because most have a nonspecific appearance. A thorough understanding of the anatomy is the key to treatment planning, and a multidisciplinary approach determines the optimal strategy.

> Malignancies of the sinonasal region and ventral skull base include a varied group of uncommon tumors that are a challenge to treat. These malignancies, with few exceptions, often present late because of their insidious growth and bland symptomatology. As with malignancies of other sites, the primary goal in surgical management is complete resection with negative margins. This presents a unique surgical challenge in that these lesions lie within a region of densely populated anatomic real estate. This fact reinforces the importance of complete preoperative work-up and a sound anatomic understanding. This article discusses key anatomic regions and their importance from an endonasal perspective.

approach morbidity, endoscopic endonasal surgery allows an easier re-covery and earlier transition to adjuvant radiotherapy. The endoscopic approach is minimal access but rarely minimally invasive. Surgeons should not hesitate to gain wide surgical exposure of the pterygopalatine, infra-temporal fossa, and petrocavernous carotid artery to ensure comfortable maneuverability and easy visualization of the tumor and its normal tissue margins. This method maximizes the chances of complete resection and effective postoperative surveillance.

Surgical management of clival lesions presents numerous therapeutic chal-lenges because of the close proximity of surrounding critical structures. With a detailed understanding of the endoscopic endonasal approach and relevant considerations, appropriate lesions can be removed in a safe and minimally invasive manner. Use of this technique as a primary approach represents the standard of care for many lesions at leading skull base centers, although adjunct techniques may be necessary in extensive lesions and those with significant lateral extension.

Combined transcranial and endoscopic endonasal approaches remain useful in the treatment of ventral skull base malignancies. The extended bifrontal transbasal approach provides wide access to the anterior ventral skull base and paranasal sinuses without transfacial incisions. In more extensive lesions, the bifrontal transbasal approach can then be combined with an endoscopic endonasal approach (EEA) from below. This article reviews the indications, surgical technique, and operative nuances of combined trans-basal and EEA (cranionasal) approaches for the surgical management of ventral skull base malignancies.

 Video content accompanies this article at http://www.oto.theclinics. com.

The orbit may be frequently involved by sinonasal or ventral skull base ma-lignancy. This involvement bodes a poorer prognosis for survival. Multimo-dality therapy with surgery and radiation therapy is usually attempted to optimize local control and overall survival. Oncologic surgical resection with negative margins is critical to local control and survival. In the past, any involvement of the orbit was deemed to necessitate orbital sacrifice. However, contemporary studies show that in carefully selected cases, orbital preservation does not adversely impact survival. In addition, novel reconstructive techniques can help minimize complications and optimize functional and aesthetic outcomes.

Sinonasal and ventral skull base malignancies are rare tumors that arise in
a complex anatomic location juxtaposed with critically important normal
tissues. The standard treatment paradigm for most histologies has been
surgery followed by postoperative radiation therapy. Because of their propensity to present at an advanced stage and the presence of nearby critical structures, patients are at risk for severe radiation-induced long-term
toxicity. Recent advances in radiotherapy technique have improved the
therapeutic ratio between tumor control and normal tissue toxicity. This
article reviews issues pertinent to the use of radiotherapy in the management of these tumors.

In most cases of advanced sinonasal and ventral skull base cancer, a
multimodal treatment approach provides the best chance for improved
outcomes. Depending on the tumor type and extent of disease, systemic
chemotherapy has been shown to play an important role in neoadjuvant,
concomitant, and adjuvant settings. The lack of randomized trials continues to limit its indications. Further high-quality studies are needed to understand ideal chemotherapeutic regimens and their role and sequential
timing in sinonasal and ventral skull base cancer.

Cancers develop secondary to genetic and epigenetic changes that provide the cell with a survival advantage that promotes cellular immortality.
Malignancy arises when tumors use mechanisms to evade detection
and destruction by the immune system. Many malignancies seem to elicit
an immune response, yet somehow manage to avoid destruction by the
cells of the immune system. Cancers may evade this immune response
by numerous mechanisms. Several targeted immune therapies are available that block some of these inhibitory signals and enhance the cell-
mediated immune response. Many of these agents hold significant promise for future treatment of sinonasal and ventral skull base malignancies.

The management of sinonasal and ventral skull base malignancies is best
performed by a team. Although the composition of the team may vary, it is
important to have multidisciplinary representation. There are multiple obstacles, both individual and institutional, that must be overcome to

develop a highly functioning team. Adequate training is an important part of team-building and can be fostered with surgical telementoring. A quality improvement program should be incorporated into the activities of a skull base team.

Sinonasal and ventral skull base malignancies are a rare, heterogeneous group of cancers. Although prognosis usually depends on many factors, long-term survival rates remain low despite recent advances. Population-based databases are powerful resources for studying survival outcomes. However, institutional retrospective chart-review studies have been able to provide more insight on recurrence patterns, morbidity, and quality-of-life metrics, as well as more details of the treatment information that may affect outcomes. This article discusses general considerations for understanding reported outcome data, summarizes the overall outcomes and their determinants, and provides histology-specific outcomes reported in the literature.

Population-based cancer registries allow for data collection on the scale of large populations, outside the limits of a single institution, and facilitate study of rare entities. The SEER database has been used to study more than 7000 cases encompassing a wide variety of relatively rare sinonasal malignant histologies. Clinically useful parameters have been gleaned from these analyses. Important limitations, such as omission of chemotherapy data, surgical approach used, type of radiation administered, and selection and confounding bias, should be considered. Nevertheless, population-based analyses yield readily generalizable and clinically relevant information regarding the management of sinonasal malignancies for the practicing clinician.

OTOLARYNGOLOGIC CLINICS
OF NORTH AMERICA

RELATED INTEREST

Neurosurgery Clinics of North America
July 2015 (Vol. 26, Issue 3)
Endoscopic Endonasal Skull Base Surgery
Daniel M. Prevedello, *Editor*
Available at: http://www.neurosurgery.theclinics.com

THE CLINICS ARE AVAILABLE ONLINE!
Access your subscription at:
www.theclinics.com

Foreword

Anterior Skull Base Malignancies—The Otolaryngologist's Contribution

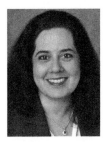

Sujana S. Chandrasekhar, MD
Consulting Editor

The anterior skull base represents a challenging space necessitating surgical collaboration between Otolaryngology, Neurosurgery, and Ophthalmology. The input of those specialties as well as from Medical and Radiation Oncology, Radiology, Nuclear Medicine and Imaging, and affiliated Allied Healthcare Specialists is vital. It enables optimal patient outcome, from a tumor removal and disease-free survival perspective as well as in how it pertains to quality of life.

Otolaryngologists, whether or not they incorporate anterior skull base surgery into their practices, should be aware of techniques for early and accurate evaluation, anatomical considerations, particularly with relation to the structures of the orbit and the nerves and vessels near the cavernous sinus, and the various surgical approaches for tumor resection. It is not enough to resect; these tumors affect the appearance of the patient's face, the first thing that is presented to the world around them. Reconstruction techniques to manage the defect to minimize cosmetic deformity must be understood as this is often a primary concern of the patient and their family. Extirpative and reconstructive surgery, targeted chemotherapy and radiotherapy, and incorporating a multidisciplinary team for analysis, treatment, and outcome assessment keep the patient in the center of the care paradigm. When the treating team understands and conveys the individual and population-based outcomes, the patient and their family can fully participate in a shared decision-making process.

Drs Jean Anderson Eloy, Michael Setzen, and James K. Liu have compiled a comprehensive review of anterior skull base malignancies in this issue of *Otolaryngologic Clinics of North America*. The reader will be left with a thorough understanding of the state-of-the-art and -science in diagnosing, determining etiology, and offering targeted medical, surgical, and adjuvant therapies to the patient who presents with a sinonasal or ventral skull base cancer. I congratulate the authors of each article on their

Otolaryngol Clin N Am 50 (2017) xix–xx
http://dx.doi.org/10.1016/j.otc.2017.01.002
0030-6665/17/© 2017 Published by Elsevier Inc.

oto.theclinics.com

far-ranging exploration of each subject, and the guest editors on presenting a thorough exposition of this complex topic and making it accessible to the reader.

Sujana S. Chandrasekhar, MD
Department of Otolaryngology–
Head and Neck Surgery
Hofstra-Northwell School of Medicine
Icahn School of Medicine at Mount Sinai
1421 Third Avenue, 4th Floor
New York, NY 10028, USA

E-mail address:
ssc@nyotology.com

Preface

Sinonasal and Ventral Skull Base Malignancies

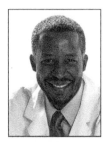 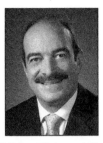 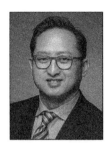

Jean Anderson Eloy, MD, FACS

Michael Setzen, MD, FACS, FAAP

James K. Liu, MD, FACS, FAANS

Editors

Over the last decades, management of sinonasal and ventral skull base malignancies has evolved significantly as a result of new advances in surgical instrumentations and optical devices, newer endoscopic and open techniques, better understanding of the sinonasal and ventral skull base anatomy, and improvement in radiotherapeutic, chemotherapeutic, and targeted treatment of these lesions. In addition, emphasis on multidisciplinary approach and closer collaborations between surgical teams has improved the ability to resect these lesions with less morbidity.

In this issue of *Otolaryngologic Clinics of North America* dedicated to sinonasal and ventral skull base malignancies, we discuss the epidemiology and recent progress in our understanding of these lesions and their management. It is with great honor that we guest-edit this important issue on "Sinonasal and Ventral Skull Base Malignancies." We hope that this issue will be valuable to the otolaryngologists, neurosurgeons, ophthalmologists, radiation and medical oncologists, and allied health care workers involved in the care of patients with these complex malignancies.

Jean Anderson Eloy, MD, FACS
Rhinology and Sinus Surgery
Otolaryngology Research
Endoscopic Skull Base Surgery Program
Department of Otolaryngology–Head and Neck Surgery
Neurological Institute of New Jersey
Rutgers New Jersey Medical School
90 Bergen Street, Suite 8100
Newark, NJ 07103, USA

Otolaryngol Clin N Am 50 (2017) xxi–xxii
http://dx.doi.org/10.1016/j.otc.2017.01.001
0030-6665/17/© 2017 Published by Elsevier Inc.

Michael Setzen, MD, FACS, FAAP
North Shore University Hospital
Manhasset, NY, USA

NYU School of Medicine
Weill Cornell University College of Medicine
600 Northern Boulevard, Suite 312
Great Neck, NY 11021, USA

James K. Liu, MD, FACS, FAANS
Center for Skull Base and Pituitary Surgery
Department of Neurological Surgery
Neurological Institute of New Jersey
Rutgers New Jersey Medical School
90 Bergen Street, Suite 8100
Newark, NJ 07103, USA

E-mail addresses:
jean.anderson.eloy@gmail.com (J.A. Eloy)
michaelsetzen@gmail.com (M. Setzen)
liuj10@njms.rutgers.edu (J.K. Liu)

Overview of Sinonasal and Ventral Skull Base Malignancy Management

 CrossMark

Peter F. Svider, MD[a], Michael Setzen, MD[b,c,d,1], Soly Baredes, MD[e,f], James K. Liu, MD[e,f,g], Jean Anderson Eloy, MD[e,f,g,h,*]

KEYWORDS

- Skull base malignancy • Skull base • Skull base defect • Skull base surgery
- Sinonasal malignancy • Radiotherapy • Chemotherapy • Cerebrospinal fluid leakage

KEY POINTS

- Due to the close proximity of critical structures, initial evaluation should include assessment of visual complaints (eg, diplopia) and extraocular movements, unilateral middle ear effusion suggesting Eustachian tube obstruction, as well as thorough endoscopic examination of the nasal cavity. Additionally, evaluation of the neck should be performed to rule out any lymphadenopathy.

Continued

Financial Disclosures: None.
Conflicts of Interest: Speaker for MEDA on their Speakers Bureau for Dymista (not related to current subject) (M. Setzen).
[a] Department of Otolaryngology – Head and Neck Surgery, Wayne State University School of Medicine, 4201 Saint Antoine, 5E-UHC, Detroit, MI 4201, USA; [b] Rhinology Section, North Shore University Hospital, Manhasset, NY, USA; [c] Department of Otolaryngology, New York University School of Medicine, New York, NY, USA; [d] Weill Cornell University College of Medicine, New York, NY, USA; [e] Department of Otolaryngology – Head and Neck Surgery, Center for Skull Base and Pituitary Surgery, Neurological Institute of New Jersey, Rutgers New Jersey Medical School, 90 Bergen Street, Suite 8100, Newark, NJ 07103, USA; [f] Endoscopic Skull Base Surgery Program, Department of Otolaryngology – Head and Neck Surgery, Rhinology and Sinus Surgery, Otolaryngology Research, Center for Skull Base and Pituitary Surgery, Neurological Institute of New Jersey, Rutgers New Jersey Medical School, 90 Bergen Street, Suite 8100, Newark, NJ 07103, USA; [g] Department of Neurological Surgery, Rutgers New Jersey Medical School, 90 Bergen Street, Suite 8100, Newark, NJ 07103, USA; [h] Department of Ophthalmology and Visual Science, Rutgers New Jersey Medical School, 90 Bergen Street, Suite 8100, Newark, NJ 07103, USA
[1] Present address: 600 Northern Boulevard, Suite 312, Great Neck, NY, 11021.
* Corresponding author. Endoscopic Skull Base Surgery Program, Department of Otolaryngology – Head and Neck Surgery, Rhinology and Sinus Surgery, Otolaryngology Research, Neurological Institute of New Jersey, Rutgers New Jersey Medical School, 90 Bergen Street, Suite 8100, Newark, NJ 07103.
E-mail address: jean.anderson.eloy@gmail.com

Otolaryngol Clin N Am 50 (2017) 205–219
http://dx.doi.org/10.1016/j.otc.2016.12.001
0030-6665/17/© 2016 Elsevier Inc. All rights reserved.

Continued

- Orbital involvement may be suspected from history, physical examination, and imaging. Nonetheless, the gold standard for determining orbital involvement, is intraoperative frozen section and permanent pathology, as it may be difficult to ascertain whether imaging is showing periorbital edema, orbital content displacement, or frank invasion.
- In lesions involving the cavernous sinus, avoidance of internal carotid artery resection lowers the risk of cerebrovascular accident and hemorrhage, although resection is sometimes necessary with extensive tumor involvement. In cases in which the internal carotid artery must be sacrificed, revascularization procedures should be considered.

Abbreviations

CN	Cranial Nerve
CT	Computed Tomography
ITF	Infratemporal Fossa
MR	Magnetic Resonance
PPF	Pterygopalatine Fossa

INTRODUCTION

The therapeutic repertoire for management of sinonasal and ventral skull base malignancies has expanded significantly in recent decades. A variety of considerations are responsible for these advances, including innovative surgical and optical technologies, increased understanding of endoscopic endonasal anatomy, and the increasingly targeted nature of nonsurgical therapies. As a result, the management of ventral skull base malignancies has evolved from extensive resection with potentially devastating and disfiguring sequelae to a largely minimally invasive endeavor. Advances in the care of patients with these malignancies have facilitated the formation of interdisciplinary skull base teams, with otolaryngologists, neurosurgeons, radiation oncologists, and medical oncologists all playing a critical role. Despite these developments, advanced lesions still present significant clinical challenges due to the close proximity of critical structures. This overview presents an up-to-date survey of novel therapies and surgical approaches that may be of use in the challenging clinical scenarios typically associated with sinonasal and ventral skull base malignancies.

DIAGNOSIS

Initial diagnosis of sinonasal and ventral skull base malignancies can be difficult, as presenting signs and symptoms may be nonspecific. Patients often present with nasal congestion, facial pain, facial discomfort, or rhinorrhea indistinguishable from chronic rhinosinusitis. Deciding which patients warrant more rigorous diagnostic workup can be a difficult undertaking. Additional aspects of the history that may support obtaining further workup include unilateral symptoms of acute onset, as well as complaints associated with cranial neuropathies. Due to the close proximity of critical structures, initial evaluation should include assessment of visual complaints (eg, diplopia) and extraocular movements, unilateral middle ear effusion suggesting Eustachian tube obstruction, as well as thorough endoscopic examination of the nasal cavity

(**Fig. 1**). Additionally, evaluation of the neck should be performed to rule out lymphade-nopathy. Although uncommon with most sinonasal and ventral skull base malig-nancies, lymph node metastasis may be present with nasal cavity tumors and nasopharyngeal carcinoma; in fact, this is the most common presentation among pa-tients with the latter.[1–6]

In addition to a thorough examination that includes endoscopic evaluation, patients with worrisome clinical signs and symptoms, particularly those with paresthesias, diplopia, unilateral symptoms, and cranial neuropathies, should undergo imaging evaluation. Computed tomography (CT) scans with 2- to 4-mm cuts are the "work-horse" imaging modality for initial evaluation of sinonasal pathologies, as this provides detailed information regarding bone, ventral skull base, and orbital involve-ment (**Fig. 2**A). Magnetic resonance (MR) imaging further delineates soft tissue involvement, and is helpful in assessing the extent of dural invasion in ventral skull base malignancies (**Fig. 2**B–D); the use of postcontrast gadolinium-enhanced MR is critical (see **Fig. 2**B–D).[7] These modalities are also used for intraoperative neurona-vigation purposes in patients who are surgical candidates. Although conventional MR and CT provide valuable information and can allow the operating surgeon to formu-late a detailed surgical plan, evaluation with angiography may also be necessary depending on the extent of the lesion and concern for involvement of vascular struc-tures. CT (**Fig. 3**) and MR angiography are noninvasive alternatives to conventional angiography, and can be helpful for evaluating the integrity of major vessels. For example, these modalities can usually determine the extent of tumor involvement around the internal carotid artery, helping determine whether a purely endoscopic approach is appropriate or whether a combined approach is warranted. Conventional angiography can also provide additional information if there is significant tumor encasement, particularly with regard to the extent of collateral circulation. PET and PET-CT imaging is also valuable for evaluating regional and distal metastases (**Figs. 4** and **5**).[8]

In addition to obtaining appropriate imaging, there are several other critical aspects of initial and preoperative evaluation. For sinonasal and ventral skull base lesions involving the sella, many surgeons advocate obtaining baseline levels of hormones produced by the pituitary gland, and close collaboration with endocrinology

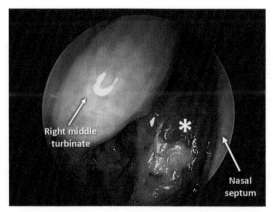

Fig. 1. Nasal endoscopy of a patient who presented with recurrent epistaxis and was diag-nosed with a large right-sided sinonasal and ventral skull base hemangiopericytoma; *asterisk* depicts lesion.

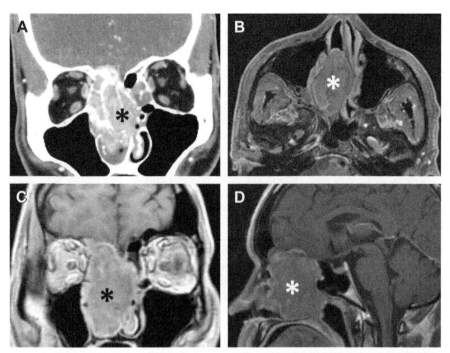

Fig. 2. Coronal (*A*) CT scan with intravenous contrast of a large right-sided sinonasal and ventral skull base olfactory neuroblastoma (esthesioneuroblastoma). Axial (*B*), coronal (*C*), and sagittal (*D*) T1-weighted gadolinium-enhanced MR imaging of the same patient; *asterisk* depicts lesion.

colleagues. Just as importantly, there should be comprehensive discussion of obtaining a biopsy when feasible. Biopsy of undiagnosed nasal lesions in the office without first obtaining imaging is discouraged in most situations, as imaging can provide information about intracranial connection and the vascular nature of a lesion. Some lesions with the potential to be vascular in origin are more safely biopsied in the operating room.

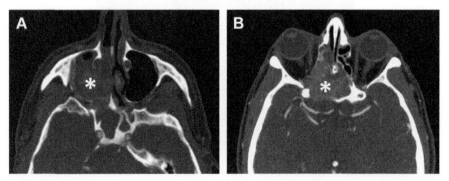

Fig. 3. Axial (*A* and *B*) CT angiography scan of a patient with a large sinonasal and ventral skull base moderately differentiated invasive squamous cell carcinoma; *asterisk* depicts lesion.

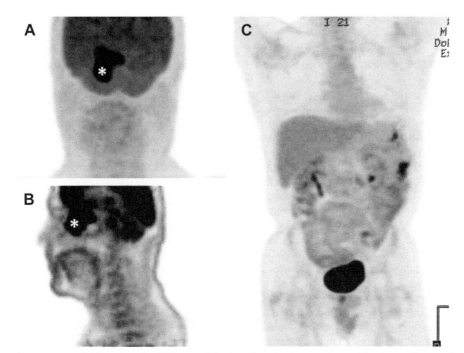

Fig. 4. Coronal (*A*) and sagittal (*B*) PET of the head region in a patient with a large sinonasal and ventral skull base moderately differentiated invasive squamous cell carcinoma. Coronal (*C*) PET of the body in the same patient; asterisk depicts lesion.

ANATOMIC CONSIDERATIONS IN ENDOSCOPIC APPROACHES

There are numerous anatomic variants that should be noted on preoperative imaging. Although these are many of the same structures essential for success in endoscopic sinus surgery, there are additional considerations in more advanced lesions involving the sinonasal and ventral skull base. A comprehensive review of individual structures

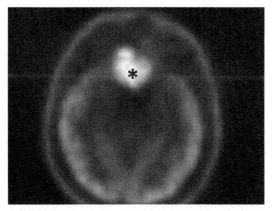

Fig. 5. Axial PET-CT scan of the head region of a patient with a large sinonasal and ventral skull base moderately differentiated invasive squamous cell carcinoma; *asterisk* depicts lesion.

relevant to specific lesions is discussed (see Satish Govindaraj and colleagues article, "Evaluation of Patients with Sinonasal and Ventral Skull Base Malignancies," and Thomas J. Willson and colleagues article, "Anatomic Consideration in Sinonasal and Ventral Skull Base Malignancy Surgery," and specific chapters focusing on pterygopalatine, infratemporal, clival, and orbital lesions).

The depth of the olfactory fossa should be noted on preoperative CT. The Keros classification organizes this value into 3 different types: a type 1 Keros lamina lateralis (1–3 mm) is relatively "safe" compared with a type 3 lamina (8–16 mm), as the latter is more easily disrupted intraoperatively.[9–11]

There are several relevant structures associated with the sphenoid sinus. The presence of an Onodi cell may be important, as these may encompass the optic nerve.[10,12] In general, knowing the location of the optic nerve and internal carotid artery is important, as there can be bony dehiscence over these structures in a significant proportion of patients.[13] Deviation of the sphenoid intersinus septum should be noted as well, particularly in relation to the internal carotid artery. Finally, involvement of the cavernous sinus and associated structures should be noted.

Several structures should be evaluated in preoperative imaging to prevent orbital complications. Failure to recognize variants in the medial orbital wall can result in injury to the extraocular muscles.[10,14] Furthermore, the preoperative CT should be evaluated for the uncinate attachment to avoid violation of the lamina papyracea. Other key structures of which to note the location are the ethmoidal vessels; in particular, damage to an anterior ethmoid artery located within the ethmoid sinus can cause this structure to retract into the orbit, causing a retro-orbital hematoma. If this artery needs to be divided (as is typically performed in endoscopic anterior ventral skull base resections), it should be done closer to the cribriform plate to prevent this complication. With regard to tumor involvement of orbital structures, CT can help delineate involvement of orbital bone, superior orbital fissure, inferior orbital fissure, and optic foramen. Expansion of these foramina suggest tumor involvement. As detailed previously, MR can further evaluate soft tissue involvement, including neural involvement; importantly, secretions located in the lacrimal sac can sometimes be distinguished from tumor invasion.[15] In a significant proportion of cases, however, it may be difficult even for MR imaging to distinguish edema from invasion of soft tissues.

Several structures related to the frontal sinus are readily identified on preoperative imaging. The operating surgeon should be cognizant of suprabullar cells, frontal cells, and the extent of an agger nasi cell.[16,17] When present, the agger nasi cell is located anteriorly, with suprabullar cells and the fovea ethmoidalis posteriorly. A discussion of extended frontal sinusotomy procedures, such as a Draf III, is beyond the scope of this analysis; however, performance of these may need to be considered depending on the location and extent of the lesion. With regard to an endoscopic anterior ventral skull base resection, the posterior table of the frontal sinus is the anterosuperior limit whereas the planum sphenoidale is the posteroinferior limit of tumor resection. These can both be identified on preoperative imaging.

A variety of lesions have been noted to involve the clivus, the bony structure separating the nasopharynx and the posterior cranial fossa. Clival anatomy can be evaluated on fine cut CT. The upper portion of the clivus is behind the sphenoid sinus and sellar structures, although inferiorly the clivus is behind the posterior sphenoid body and basiocciput.[18] Most clival lesions originate at the midline and are chordomas, whereas paramedian lesions should raise the index of suspicion for other etiologies such as chondrosarcomas. CT can help evaluate the impact on surrounding structures; lesions that elevate the pituitary gland are likely clival or nasopharyngeal in origin, rather than being an invasive pituitary lesion with inferior extension.[19]

Considerations related to open and combined approaches are comprehensively detailed (see Elizabeth Perkins and colleagues article, "Transfacial and Craniofacial Approaches for Resection of Sinonasal and Ventral Skull Base Malignancies," and James K. Liu and colleagues article, "Combined Endoscopic and Open Approaches in the Management of Sinonasal and Ventral Skull Base Malignancies," in this issue).

OUTCOMES

Until recently, craniofacial resection and other open techniques were predominantly used in the management of sinonasal and ventral skull base malignancies. With the shift toward endoscopic endonasal and combined approaches in a significant proportion of cases, questions have arisen regarding the efficacy of such minimally invasive approaches. One theoretic concern with endoscopic approaches stems from the traditional oncologic principle of en bloc resection, which is not followed with endoscopic techniques. In one retrospective analysis comparing open and closed approaches, transnasal endoscopic skull base resection was noted to be associated with a shorter hospital stay and lower recurrence rate; no differences were noted in survival or metastasis rates.[20] A later and larger study by the same group had similar findings.[21] Another intra-institutional series noted that there was not an increased risk of positive margins with the use of endoscopic approaches.[22] The literature on this topic is almost entirely composed of small single-institution series, and further larger-scale analysis may be needed. Nonetheless, initial investigations into this question do not reveal any consensus regarding decreased efficacy by use of minimally invasive endoscopic techniques. These findings should still be viewed carefully, as selection bias typically caused smaller ventral skull base malignancies to be generally treated with the endoscopic approach, and much larger lesions with inherently poorer prognosis to be treated with the open approaches.

Malignancies involving the sinonasal and ventral skull base are typically discovered at advanced stages, thus harboring a poor prognosis. There are numerous specific staging systems based on histology, and the American Joint Committee on Cancer (AJCC) also offers a staging system for all sinonasal cancers.[23] Going by the AJCC staging classification, 5-year survival drops from 63% for stage I disease down to 35% for stage IV malignancies.[23] These figures may vary widely by specific structures and pathology encountered. In general, squamous cell carcinoma is the most common histology encountered among sinonasal and ventral skull base malignancies.[24] The 5-year disease-specific survival is generally highest for nasal cavity tumors when compared to other paranasal sinus sites.[24] Further staging and specific figures for outcomes and survival rates are discussed in greater detail (see Dipan D. Desai and colleagues article, "Staging of Sinonasal and Ventral Skull Base Malignancies," and Rami Abdou and Soly Baredes's article, "Population-Based Results in the Management of Sinonasal and Ventral Skull Base Malignancies," in this issue).

ENDOSCOPIC ENDONASAL RESECTION

Surgical nuances vary based on training, experience, surgeon preference (both neurosurgeon and otolaryngologist), as well as the specific location of a lesion. There are, however, several general principles that should be well understood by practitioners involved in these surgical procedures. Performing a complete endoscopic resection of a ventral skull base lesion near the cribriform region (anterior skull base lesion) involves resection of the cribriform plates, any involved dura, and olfactory bulbs. The specific structures involved with a malignancy guide the extent of further resection.

There are many variations based on surgical preferences, and the steps listed later in this article simply represent the techniques used at our own institutions. Many of these steps are discussed in further detail in other articles in this issue and are only briefly described here. After appropriate preoperative surgical planning, the intranasal component of a lesion is debulked with powered instrumentation. Ideally, the nasal septum and lateral nasal wall structures are visualized all the way posteriorly to the choanae before progressing further. Care should be taken to preserve the nasal septal mucosa during cases in which a nasoseptal flap may be used. However, it is preferable to use the nasoseptal flap on the unaffected side to prevent the possibility of repairing a created ventral skull base defect with a flap invaded by malignant cells. Bilateral total ethmoidectomies, maxillary antrostomies, followed by an extended sphenoid sinusotomy[25] are performed. Care is taken to avoid damage to the nasoseptal flap pedicle. Identification of the sphenopalatine foramen area is an important surgical step. In cases in which a pedicled nasoseptal flap is used, the sphenopalatine artery is cauterized only on the side contralateral to the flap. At this point we also identify critical structures adjacent to the sphenoid sinus, including the optic nerve (cranial nerve II) and the internal carotid arteries.

When necessary, a Draf III frontal sinusotomy is performed to further expand access in lesions abutting the frontal sinuses. If the lesion involves the ethmoid sinuses and medial maxilla, an endoscopic modified medial maxillectomy is typically performed. More detailed steps to remove the crista galli, resect the dural margins, and to address other ventral skull base structures are described (see Ghassan Alokby and Roy R. Casiano's article, "Endoscopic Resection of Sinonasal and Ventral Skull Base Malignancies," in this issue).

ORBITAL INVOLVEMENT

Direct tumor extension involving the orbit is associated with significantly decreased survival, with one analysis noting it decreased survival among patients with ethmoid cancers by nearly half to 44.4%.[26] Furthermore, the prognosis this portends suggests the need for multimodality therapy, including surgery, radiotherapy, and chemotherapy. Traditionally, orbital exenteration is performed for orbital extension, although contemporary literature suggests that there are select cases in which preservation may not impact survival. In nasal cavity tumors, approximately half of patients present at an advanced stage involving orbital extension, with this proportion growing for tumors involving and originating from the sinuses (**Fig. 6**).[26,27] Orbital involvement may be suspected from history and physical examination, as well as from CT and MR imaging. The gold standard for determining whether there is orbital involvement, however, is intraoperative frozen section and permanent pathology, as it may be difficult to distinguish periorbital edema from invasion in imaging.

Surgical resection plays an important role in lesions with orbital involvement. There are several findings associated with orbital involvement considered unresectable by most surgeons, including lesions with encasement of the internal carotid artery, significant intracranial parenchymal involvement, and any lesion in which it is not feasible to obtain negative margins. Detailed principles and nuances of surgical technique are discussed (see Gregory S. Neel and colleagues article, "Management of Orbital Involvement in Sinonasal and Ventral Skull base Malignancies," in this issue).

For lesions that only abut but do not involve the orbital bony boundaries, resection of only involved bone can be attempted, with frozen sections taken from the orbital periosteum (periorbita). This approach provides an opportunity to proceed with more orbital resection if necessary. For further orbital extension involving the

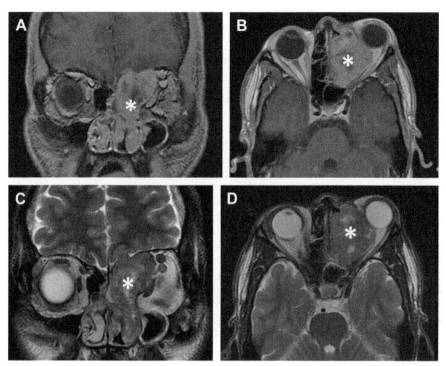

Fig. 6. Coronal (*A*) and axial (*B*) T1-weighted gadolinium-enhanced MR imaging of a patient with a large left-sided sinonasal and ventral skull base adenoid cystic carcinoma with marked intraorbital extension. Coronal (*C*) and axial (*D*) T2-weighted MR imaging of the same patient; *asterisk* depicts lesion.

periorbita, one can attempt to gently remove disease from the periorbita; in more advanced cases, if resection of the periorbita and a portion of underlying extraconal fat yields negative margins, then the remaining orbital structures can be preserved. There is not definitive consensus regarding this issue, as some surgeons feel that involvement of the periorbita is an indication for orbital exenteration; the reasoning behind this belief is that the periorbita acts as a barrier, and if tumor breaches this barrier, performing orbital exenteration is necessary to maximize survival.

CAVERNOUS SINUS INVOLVEMENT

Ventral skull base malignancies sometimes extend to and involve the cavernous sinus and adjacent structures. Direct spread is the mechanism in more than 80% of cases, whereas the remainder of cases involve extension via the various foramina and fissures located nearby.[28] Infrequently, some lesions represent metastases to the cavernous sinus. Although traditionally these lesions have been approached through an open transcranial technique, there has recently been increased popularity of endoscopic endonasal and transmaxillary approaches at select centers. An important decision on encountering these lesions is the question of how to address the intracavernous portion of the internal carotid artery. Avoiding carotid resection lowers the risk of cerebrovascular accidents and hemorrhage,[29] although sometimes resection is necessary based on the extent of tumor involvement with the carotid artery. In cases in which the internal carotid artery must be sacrificed, many surgeons perform revascularization procedures as feasible.[30,31]

PTERYGOPALATINE FOSSA AND INFRATEMPORAL FOSSA LESIONS

Pterygopalatine fossa (PPF) and infratemporal fossa (ITF) lesions traditionally have been managed through extensive open approaches. Recently, however, there has been an increase in the popularity of the endoscopic approach for select lesions.[32] One sizable series of cases managed via a transnasal endoscopic approach noted that 36 of 37 patients achieved radical resection solely through the use of endoscopic techniques, and that no local recurrences were observed for malignant lesions (median follow-up 38.5 months).[33] Other cadaveric studies evaluating the anatomy of such approaches noted that the inferior orbital nerve complex should be identifiable in cases in which this anatomy was not distorted, thus being a useful landmark for other critical structures including the foramen rotundum and anterolateral skull base.[34] Another analysis examining CT scans of the PPF noted several valuable anatomic pearls, including that the posterior PPF was closely associated with the middle lowest point of the sellar floor.[35] Endoscopic approaches to the ITF have also been explored. A cadaveric study comparing the endoscopic transpterygoid approach to an open preauricular approach noted that the former allowed for greater visualization and exposure of the nasopharynx, Eustachian tube, sella, and clivus.[36] Endoscopic approaches both to the PPF and ITF are further discussed (see Gretchen M. Oakley and Richard J. Harvey's article, "Endoscopic Resection of Pterygopalatine Fossa and Infratemporal Fossa Malignancies," in this issue).

CLIVAL LESIONS

As with other portions of the ventral skull base, management of clival lesions presents numerous surgical challenges due to the intimate proximity of critical structures, in this case being the basilar artery, brain stem, optic nerve, and internal carotid arteries. Over the past 2 decades, there has been a movement toward minimally invasive techniques for these lesions, and endoscopic endonasal approaches are considered the standard for most clival lesions.

As noted previously, the clivus is the portion of bone separating the posterior cranial fossa structures from the nasopharynx, sphenoid sinus, and parasellar structures. Most of these lesions are chordomas and chondrosarcomas, although the differential diagnosis is broader. Importantly, it is important to rule out a clival metastasis from another primary site. Intraoperatively, identification of the vidian nerve can be very helpful, as cognizance of this nerve may keep the surgeon below the horizontal internal carotid artery.[37]

ROBOTIC SKULL BASE SURGERY

Although not in widespread use at this time, robotic surgery may play an increasing role in the management of sinonasal and ventral skull base malignancies in the near future. Several cadaveric feasibility studies have been published. Carrau and colleagues[38] combined transoral robotic surgery (TORS) with an endoscopic endonasal approach, noting that using TORS allows for further dissection of the parapharyngeal space, ITF, and lower nasopharynx. Their findings reinforced that the use of TORS as a complementary technique to endoscopic approaches may provide a minimally invasive approach toward resection of lesions of the craniovertebral junction and ITF. Applications of this approach are further discussed (see Ralph Abi Hachem and colleagues article, "The Role of Robotic Surgery in Sinonasal and Ventral Skull Base Malignancy," in this issue).

VENTRAL SKULL BASE RECONSTRUCTION

A detailed survey of the various options for reconstruction of ventral skull base defects is included in the article on skull base reconstruction. There are many available techniques for ventral skull base reconstruction; the optimal method is dependent on the extent of resection, surgical approach (open vs endoscopic), pathology, and surgical preference. Despite the variety of reconstruction options, the main objective is to obliterate any communication between the intracranial space and the sinonasal cavity. When feasible, vascularized grafts are ideal, as there may be fewer postoperative problems with these and a greater degree of uptake.[39,40] In open techniques, the workhorse flaps for reconstruction include a pericranial flap and temporoparietal fascia flap. In endoscopic techniques, the vascularized pedicled nasoseptal flap (PNSF) has become the mainstay for reconstruction of large ventral skull base defects.[41]

Numerous nuances and variations of the PNSFs have been proposed in recent years.[42–47] The techniques of raising these flaps are described in further detail elsewhere, but the general steps are discussed here. The PNSF is placed over the ventral skull base defect and supported with additional packing; importantly, the mucoperichondrial side of the flap should be the one in contact with the defect. After applying the PNSF, Surgicel, gelfoam, and Merocel packing are typically used to bolster the repair in our institutions. For further nuances and variations, including mucosal sparing techniques, see Jean Anderson Eloy and colleagues article, "Management of Skull Base Defects after Surgical Resection of Sinonasal and Ventral Skull Base Malignancies," in this issue).

RADIOTHERAPY

Due to their infrequent nature relative to other cancers, there is a paucity of inquiry evaluating the use of nonsurgical therapies for sinonasal and ventral skull base malignancies. Specifically, few randomized controlled trials exist focusing on chemotherapy and radiotherapy for these lesions. Therefore, most regimens have been borrowed from management approaches for other malignancies as well as small series.

In general, adjuvant radiotherapy, with or without chemotherapy, is used in a substantial proportion of patients due to the significant potential for local recurrence. Radiotherapy is used only as the primary therapy when patients have too many comorbidities to allow for safe surgical resection, for cases with unresectable lesions, and for histologies known to be very radiosensitive. Conventional radiotherapy has been largely replaced with intensity-modulated radiotherapy (IMRT) in recent decades, particularly in sinonasal and skull base malignancies in which there is a close proximity to critical intracranial and orbital structures. Patients undergoing IMRT have a smaller risk of adverse sequelae associated with ocular and intracranial structure involvement.[48] Furthermore, studies have noted potentially enhanced survival, and importantly, a lesser incidence of dermatitis and xerostomia.[49] Other developments, including charged particle therapy and stereotactic techniques, have shown further promise in reducing complications and improving outcomes; these are further discussed (see Kyle Wang and colleagues article, "The Role of Radiation Therapy in the Management of Sinonasal and Ventral Skull Base Malignancies," in this issue). It is important to note that in addition to specific anatomic structures involved, techniques and regimens differ based on the tumor pathology identified.

CHEMOTHERAPY AND BIOLOGIC AGENTS

Chemotherapeutic agents have evolved considerably in the 7 decades since Sidney Farber demonstrated the impact of folate derivatives in suppressing the proliferation of malignant cells.[50] Nonetheless, there have been far fewer agents showing efficacy for head and neck cancers relative to those developed for other malignancies, and there are even fewer trials evaluating agents specifically for sinonasal and ventral skull base malignancies. As a result, improvement of survival for sinonasal cancers with chemotherapy remains disappointing, with a 5-year survival rate for advanced lesions approaching 30%.[51] Consequently, developing newer agents remains an unmet clinical necessity.

Systemic chemotherapy can be used for several different approaches, most commonly as part of concomitant chemoradiotherapy or adjuvant therapy. Most accepted protocols currently used involve platinum-based agents.[52–54] Prospective trials are lacking, and there have not been any significant analyses comparing different regimens. Notably, the development of biologic agents over the past decade, including cetuximab and other monoclonal antibodies, harbors significant potential for targeted therapy. Myriad pathways have been described as additional targets for future potential chemotherapeutic agents, including PD-1 inhibitors, other immune-altering therapies, and activators of the unfolded protein response.[55–62] Systemic therapies are discussed in greater detail (see George A. Scangas and colleagues article, "The Role of Chemotherapy in the Management of Sinonasal and Ventral Skull Base Malignancies," and L. Kashat and colleagues article, "The Role of Targeted Therapy in the Management of Sinonasal and Ventral Skull Base Malignancies," in this issue).

SUMMARY

Significant technological advances have fostered a movement toward minimally invasive surgical intervention for the management of sinonasal and ventral skull base malignancies. The care of patients with these lesions ideally involves an interdisciplinary skull base team composed of neurologic surgeons, otolaryngologists, radiation oncologists, and medical oncologists. This overview describes considerations essential for diagnosis, prognosis, and preoperative evaluation. Furthermore, surgical nuances, strategies for ventral skull base reconstruction, and nonsurgical options are also discussed. Our hope is that this overview may be useful as an up-to-date description of the challenging clinical scenarios associated with these lesions.

REFERENCES

1. Ho FC, Tham IW, Earnest A, et al. Patterns of regional lymph node metastasis of nasopharyngeal carcinoma: a meta-analysis of clinical evidence. BMC Cancer 2012;12:98.
2. Wang X, Hu C, Ying H, et al. Patterns of lymph node metastasis from nasopharyngeal carcinoma based on the 2013 updated consensus guidelines for neck node levels. Radiother Oncol 2015;115:41–5.
3. Unsal AA, Dubal PM, Patel TD, et al. Squamous cell carcinoma of the nasal cavity: a population-based analysis. Laryngoscope 2016;126:560–5.
4. Dubal PM, Bhojwani A, Patel TD, et al. Squamous cell carcinoma of the maxillary sinus: a population-based analysis. Laryngoscope 2016;126:399–404.
5. Bhojwani A, Unsal A, Dubal PM, et al. Frontal sinus malignancies: a population-based analysis of incidence and survival. Otolaryngol Head Neck Surg 2016; 154:735–41.

6. Ghosh R, Dubal PM, Chin OY, et al. Sphenoid sinus malignancies: a population-based comprehensive analysis. Int Forum Allergy Rhinol 2016;6:752–9.
7. McIntyre JB, Perez C, Penta M, et al. Patterns of dural involvement in sinonasal tumors: prospective correlation of magnetic resonance imaging and histopathologic findings. Int Forum Allergy Rhinol 2012;2:336–41.
8. Gil Z, Even-Sapir E, Margalit N, et al. Integrated PET/CT system for staging and surveillance of skull base tumors. Head Neck 2007;29:537–45.
9. Gauba V, Saleh GM, Dua G, et al. Radiological classification of anterior skull base anatomy prior to performing medial orbital wall decompression. Orbit 2006;25:93–6.
10. Svider PF, Baredes S, Eloy JA. Pitfalls in sinus surgery: an overview of complications. Otolaryngol Clin North Am 2015;48(5):725–37.
11. Eloy JA, Svider PF, Setzen M. Clinical pearls in endoscopic sinus surgery: key steps in preventing and dealing with complications. Am J Otolaryngol 2014;35:324–8.
12. Tomovic S, Esmaeili A, Chan NJ, et al. High-resolution computed tomography analysis of the prevalence of Onodi cells. Laryngoscope 2012;122:1470–3.
13. Tomovic S, Esmaeili A, Chan NJ, et al. High-resolution computed tomography analysis of variations of the sphenoid sinus. J Neurol Surg B Skull Base 2013;74:82–90.
14. Han JK, Higgins TS. Management of orbital complications in endoscopic sinus surgery. Curr Opin Otolaryngol Head Neck Surg 2010;18:32–6.
15. Eisen MD, Yousem DM, Loevner LA, et al. Preoperative imaging to predict orbital invasion by tumor. Head Neck 2000;22:456–62.
16. Casiano RR. "Frontal sinusotomy" in endoscopic sinus surgery dissection manual. New York: Marcel Dekker, Inc; 2002.
17. Folbe AJ, Svider PF, Eloy JA. Advances in endoscopic frontal sinus surgery. Oper Tech Otolaryngol Head Neck Surg 25.180–6.
18. Stamm AC, Pignatari SS, Vellutini E. Transnasal endoscopic surgical approaches to the clivus. Otolaryngol Clin North Am 2006;39:639–56, xi.
19. Neelakantan A, Rana AK. Benign and malignant diseases of the clivus. Clin Radiol 2014;69:1295–303.
20. Eloy JA, Vivero RJ, Hoang K, et al. Comparison of transnasal endoscopic and open craniofacial resection for malignant tumors of the anterior skull base. Laryngoscope 2009;119:834–40.
21. Wood JW, Eloy JA, Vivero RJ, et al. Efficacy of transnasal endoscopic resection for malignant anterior skull-base tumors. Int Forum Allergy Rhinol 2012;2:487–95.
22. Cohen MA, Liang J, Cohen IJ, et al. Endoscopic resection of advanced anterior skull base lesions: oncologically safe? ORL J Otorhinolaryngol Relat Spec 2009;71:123–8.
23. Cuccurullo V, Mansi L. AJCC cancer staging handbook: from the AJCC cancer staging manual (7th edition). Eur J Nucl Med Mol Imaging 2010;38(2):408.
24. Dutta R, Dubal PM, Svider PF, et al. Sinonasal malignancies: a population-based analysis of site-specific incidence and survival. Laryngoscope 2015;125:2491–7.
25. Eloy JA, Marchiano E, Vázquez A. Extended endoscopic and open sinus surgery for refractory chronic rhinosinusitis. Otolaryngol Clin North Am 2017;50(1):165–82.
26. Ganly I, Patel SG, Singh B, et al. Craniofacial resection for malignant paranasal sinus tumors: report of an International Collaborative Study. Head Neck 2005;27:575–84.

27. Lund VJ, Howard DJ, Wei WI, et al. Craniofacial resection for tumors of the nasal cavity and paranasal sinuses–a 17-year experience. Head Neck 1998;20:97–105.

28. Han J, Zhang Q, Kong F, et al. The incidence of invasion and metastasis of nasopharyngeal carcinoma at different anatomic sites in the skull base. Anat Rec (Hoboken) 2012;295:1252–9.

29. Brisman MH, Sen C, Catalano P. Results of surgery for head and neck tumors that involve the carotid artery at the skull base. J Neurosurg 1997;86:787–92.

30. Couldwell WT, MacDonald JD, Taussky P. Complete resection of the cavernous sinus-indications and technique. World Neurosurg 2014;82:1264–70.

31. Saito K, Fukuta K, Takahashi M, et al. Management of the cavernous sinus in en bloc resections of malignant skull base tumors. Head Neck 1999;21:734–42.

32. Eloy JA, Murray KP, Friedel ME, et al. Graduated endoscopic multiangle approach for access to the infratemporal fossa: a cadaveric study with clinical correlates. Otolaryngol Head Neck Surg 2012;147:369–78.

33. Battaglia P, Turri-Zanoni M, Lepera D, et al. Endoscopic transnasal approaches to pterygopalatine fossa tumors. Head Neck 2016;38(Suppl 1):E214–20.

34. Elhadi AM, Zaidi HA, Yagmurlu K, et al. Infraorbital nerve: a surgically relevant landmark for the pterygopalatine fossa, cavernous sinus, and anterolateral skull base in endoscopic transmaxillary approaches. J Neurosurg 2016;125(6): 1460–8.

35. Cheng Y, Xu H, Chen Y, et al. Location of pterygopalatine fossa and its relationships to the structures in sellar region. J Craniofac Surg 2015;26:1979–82.

36. Youssef A, Carrau RL, Tantawy A, et al. Endoscopic versus open approach to the infratemporal fossa: a cadaver study. J Neurol Surg B Skull Base 2015;76: 358–64.

37. Moussazadeh N, Kulwin C, Anand VK, et al. Endoscopic endonasal resection of skull base chondrosarcomas: technique and early results. J Neurosurg 2015;122: 735–42.

38. Carrau RL, Prevedello DM, de Lara D, et al. Combined transoral robotic surgery and endoscopic endonasal approach for the resection of extensive malignancies of the skull base. Head Neck 2013;35:E351–8.

39. Hachem RA, Elkhatib A, Beer-Furlan A, et al. Reconstructive techniques in skull base surgery after resection of malignant lesions: a wide array of choices. Curr Opin Otolaryngol Head Neck Surg 2016;24:91–7.

40. Harvey RJ, Parmar P, Sacks R, et al. Endoscopic skull base reconstruction of large dural defects: a systematic review of published evidence. Laryngoscope 2012;122:452–9.

41. Hadad G, Bassagasteguy L, Carrau RL, et al. A novel reconstructive technique after endoscopic expanded endonasal approaches: vascular pedicle nasoseptal flap. Laryngoscope 2006;116:1882–6.

42. Eloy JA, Choudhry OJ, Friedel ME, et al. Endoscopic nasoseptal flap repair of skull base defects: is addition of a dural sealant necessary? Otolaryngol Head Neck Surg 2012;147:161–6.

43. Eloy JA, Choudhry OJ, Shukla PA, et al. Nasoseptal flap repair after endoscopic transsellar versus expanded endonasal approaches: is there an increased risk of postoperative cerebrospinal fluid leak? Laryngoscope 2012;122:1219–25.

44. Eloy JA, Kalyoussef E, Choudhry OJ, et al. Salvage endoscopic nasoseptal flap repair of persistent cerebrospinal fluid leak after open skull base surgery. Am J Otolaryngol 2012;33:735–40.

45. Eloy JA, Kuperan AB, Choudhry OJ, et al. Efficacy of the pedicled nasoseptal flap without cerebrospinal fluid (CSF) diversion for repair of skull base defects: incidence of postoperative CSF leaks. Int Forum Allergy Rhinol 2012;2:397–401.
46. Eloy JA, Vazquez A, Mady LJ, et al. Mucosal-sparing posterior septectomy for endoscopic endonasal approach to the craniocervical junction. Am J Otolaryngol 2015;36:342–6.
47. Eloy JA, Vazquez A, Marchiano E, et al. Variations of mucosal-sparing septectomy for endonasal approach to the craniocervical junction. Laryngoscope 2016;126(10):2220–5.
48. Huang D, Xia P, Akazawa P, et al. Comparison of treatment plans using intensity-modulated radiotherapy and three-dimensional conformal radiotherapy for paranasal sinus carcinoma. Int J Radiat Oncol Biol Phys 2003;56:158–68.
49. Dirix P, Vanstraelen B, Jorissen M, et al. Intensity-modulated radiotherapy for sinonasal cancer: improved outcome compared to conventional radiotherapy. Int J Radiat Oncol Biol Phys 2010;78:998–1004.
50. Burchhardt DM, Sukari A. Chemotherapy in head and neck squamous cell cancer. In: Fribley A, editor. Targeting oral cancer. New York: Springer International Publishing; 2016. p. 53–69.
51. Bossi P, Saba NF, Vermorken JB, et al. The role of systemic therapy in the management of sinonasal cancer: a critical review. Cancer Treat Rev 2015;41:836–43.
52. Hoppe BS, Nelson CJ, Gomez DR, et al. Unresectable carcinoma of the paranasal sinuses: outcomes and toxicities. Int J Radiat Oncol Biol Phys 2008;72:763–9.
53. Lee MM, Vokes EE, Rosen A, et al. Multimodality therapy in advanced paranasal sinus carcinoma: superior long-term results. Cancer J Sci Am 1999;5:219–23.
54. Rosen A, Vokes EE, Scher N, et al. Locoregionally advanced paranasal sinus carcinoma. Favorable survival with multimodality therapy. Arch Otolaryngol Head Neck Surg 1993;119:743–6.
55. Feldman R, Gatalica Z, Knezetic J, et al. Molecular profiling of head and neck squamous cell carcinoma. Head Neck 2016;38(Suppl 1):E1625–38.
56. Fribley A, Zeng Q, Wang CY. Proteasome inhibitor PS-341 induces apoptosis through induction of endoplasmic reticulum stress-reactive oxygen species in head and neck squamous cell carcinoma cells. Mol Cell Biol 2004;24:9695–704.
57. Fribley AM, Miller JR, Brownell AL, et al. Celastrol induces unfolded protein response-dependent cell death in head and neck cancer. Exp Cell Res 2015;330:412–22.
58. Gentzler R, Hall R, Kunk PR, et al. Beyond melanoma: inhibiting the PD-1/PD-L1 pathway in solid tumors. Immunotherapy 2016;8:583–600.
59. Jayaraman P, Alfarano MG, Svider PF, et al. iNOS expression in CD4+ T cells limits Treg induction by repressing TGFbeta1: combined iNOS inhibition and Treg depletion unmask endogenous antitumor immunity. Clin Cancer Res 2014;20:6439–51.
60. Kim HS, Lee JY, Lim SH, et al. Association between PD-L1 and HPV status and the prognostic value of PD-L1 in oropharyngeal squamous cell carcinoma. Cancer Res Treat 2016;48:527–36.
61. Parikh F, Duluc D, Imai N, et al. Chemoradiotherapy-induced upregulation of PD-1 antagonizes immunity to HPV-related oropharyngeal cancer. Cancer Res 2014;74:7205–16.
62. Sidhu A, Miller JR, Tripathi A, et al. Borrelidin induces the unfolded protein response in oral cancer cells and chop-dependent apoptosis. ACS Med Chem Lett 2015;6:1122–7.

Evaluation of Patients with Sinonasal and Ventral Skull Base Malignancies

 CrossMark

Satish Govindaraj, MD[a],*, Alfred M. Iloreta, MD[a],
Charles C.L. Tong, MD[a], Juan C. Hernandez-Prera, MD[b]

KEYWORDS

- Skull base • Tumors • Imaging • Histology • Pathology • Office examination

KEY POINTS

- Work-up of sinonasal and ventral skull base malignances requires thorough history and physical examination, augmented by modern imaging techniques and histological evaluation.
- Lesions of the paranasal sinuses and ventral skull base often present in advanced stages, involving adjacent structures. Optimal treatment planning requires a multidisciplinary approach involving otolaryngology, ophthalmology, neurosurgery, plastic and reconstructive surgery, and oncology teams.
- The wide variety of cell types gives rise to an uncommon group of pathology. Definitive treatment requires an understanding of their etiologies and pattern of spread.

INTRODUCTION

The paranasal sinuses are a complex framework of air cavities with a wide range of tissue types. They give rise to both benign and malignant tumors that present with variable signs and symptoms, depending on their origin and spread. This article provides a summary of the clinical presentation of sinonasal and ventral skull base lesions, establishment of diagnosis, modern imaging technology, and histopathology of the most common tumors.

Disclosure Statement: The authors hereby declare no commercial or financial conflicts of interest.
[a] Department of Otolaryngology-Head and Neck Surgery, Icahn School of Medicine at Mount Sinai, One Gustave. L. Levy Place, Box 1189, New York, NY 10029, USA; [b] Department of Pathology, Mount Sinai Beth Israel, Icahn School of Medicine at Mount Sinai, First Avenue at 16th Street, New York, NY 10003, USA
* Corresponding author.
E-mail address: satish.govindaraj@mountsinai.org

Otolaryngol Clin N Am 50 (2017) 221–244
http://dx.doi.org/10.1016/j.otc.2016.12.002
0030-6665/17/© 2016 Elsevier Inc. All rights reserved.

EPIDEMIOLOGY

Although the incidence of overall sinonasal lesions is low, approximately 3% of computed tomography (CT) scans of the paranasal sinuses obtained reveal an osteoma.[1] Malignancies also account for only 3% to 6% of total head and neck neoplasms. There are known variations, however, across gender (2:1 male-to-female predilection), occupational exposure (woodwork dust, chrome, and nickel), and geography (higher incidence in Japan and Africa).[2] As for site of origin, the maxillary sinus is the most commonly involved followed by the ethmoids. Tumors arising in the paranasal sinuses have space to grow, and signs and symptoms are nonspecific, resulting in advanced staging at presentation. Unilateral nasal obstruction is the most common complaint.

CLINICAL PRESENTATION

Thorough history and physical examination, aided by high-definition endoscopic procedures, are the cornerstones of head and neck tumor diagnosis. For the general practitioner, early sinonasal tumors may only present with nasal obstruction, epistaxis, or obstructive pansinusitis. Unilateral complaints should raise the index of suspicion, as with signs and symptoms of adjacent structures (**Table 1**). A comprehensive list of common presenting symptoms and history is in **Box 1**.

PHYSICAL EXAMINATION

Tumors of the nasal cavity and paranasal sinuses are often the most challenging to examine. Both flexible and rigid endoscopy require adequate topical anesthesia and patient reassurance. Patients are prepped with application of atomized 4% lidocaine and oxymetazoline (or equivalent decongestant). Flexible nasolaryngoscopy provides adequate visualization of most intranasal lesions, with the extended capability of evaluating for nasopharyngeal and oropharyngeal extension. Rigid telescopes are generally preferred for high-definition characterization of lesions, office procedures, and video recording for pretreatment and post-treatment evaluation. A well-equipped examination room should be fitted with 2 monitors, with 1 facing the patient to provide reassurance, video recording, and storage console; a set of 0°, 30°, and 70° Hopkins rod telescopes (Karl Storz, Germany); and instruments for suctioning and débridement (**Fig. 1**). Adult rigid endoscopes are typically 4 mm in diameter and can be substituted with pediatric 2.7-mm endoscopes for patient comfort.

Table 1 Suspicious symptoms	
Early	**Advanced**
Unilateral epistaxis, sinusitis, obstruction	Anesthesia of the skin of the cheek and upper lip (V2 distribution)
Swelling of the upper gingiva or loose dentition	Diplopia
Headache	Proptosis
Hyposmia	Recurrent epistaxis
	Nasal obstruction refractory to medical therapy
	Palatal mass
	Trismus (invasion into the pteryoids)
	Cranial palsy (III, IV, and VI)
	Anosmia

Box 1
Rhinology and skull base–specific history

Facial pain or pressure

Nasal obstruction

Anterior or posterior purulent drainage

Hyposmia or anosmia

Fever

Headache

Halitosis

Dental pain

Fatigue

Cough

Ear pain

Vision changes

Epistaxis

Current sinonasal medications

Number of sinus infections per year requiring antibiotics

Prior sinonasal surgery

Known history of polyps

History of allergy testing and immunotherapy

Environmental allergies

Aspirin sensitivity

Occupation

Asthma

Smoking history

History of autoimmune disease

History of immune deficiency

Due to ventral skull base lesions' proximity to cranial nerves, orbits, and important vasculature, a complete head and neck examination is advocated. An overall survey should note gross facial deformity, and, if present, in-office photography is performed with base view, profile view, three-quarter view, and frontal view. Any facial incisions, external resection, flaps and grafts, and possible orbital exenteration should be discussed in conjunction with the neurosurgical and facial plastics team. As the number of tumors amenable to endoscopic resection grows, a patient-oriented approach and setting-appropriate expectations are the hallmarks of a rhinology practice.

In addition to the directed endoscopic view of the lesion, a systematic neurological examination of the cranial nerves is often warranted. Proptosis from mass effect and cranial nerves III, IV and VI palsies are frequent orbital complications of sinonasal tumors. Intraocular pressures, visual field testing, visual acuity, and afferent visual defect should be performed with a consultation with an ophthalmologist prior to treatment. Assessment of cranial nerve V should include light and sharp discrimination in all 3 divisions.

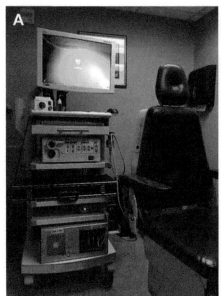
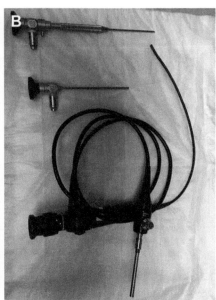

Fig. 1. Picture of endoscopy suite. (*A*) Endoscopy tower with video recording capabilities. (*B*) Flexible and rigid endoscopes.

A detailed review of system may also direct physical findings that warrant consultations. It is not uncommon for patients to complain of unilateral hearing loss, possibly from the obstruction of the eustachian tube orifice leading to middle ear effusion and conductive hearing loss. For advanced tumors involving the maxillary sinus floor, loose teeth and palatal swelling can lead to malfitting dentures. Symptoms from metastasis may also precede any from the primary tumor. Sinonasal tumor spread is seen with high cervical lymph nodes and occasionally to the node of Rouvière, the highest retropharyngeal lymph node in the neck.

DIAGNOSTIC PROCEDURES

The skull base represents a bony partition between intracranial contents and the nasal cavity, paranasal sinuses, and the orbit. It also contains foramina and fissures that transmit vessels and nerves that serve as pathways for tumor extension. Tumor involvement of such structures can only be assessed indirectly prior to surgery, and modern imaging techniques allow accurate assessment of tumor location, origin, extent of involvement, relationship to vessels and nerves, and adjacent organs.

Imaging Techniques: Computed Tomography

CT is the method of choice for assessment of osseous structures. CT is a widely available technique and is carried out using 5-mm sections during a single acquisition. Thinner sections are often required to provide the high anatomic detail of the skull base, and typically 1-mm sections are used to provide reconstructions into axial, sagittal, and coronal planes. The advantages and disadvantages of the technique are summarized in **Table 2**.

Imaging Techniques: MRI

MRI is the method of choice for assessment of soft tissues (dura, meninges, and brain) and tumor, after introduction of gadolinium contrast agent. MRI is often performed

Table 2 CT	
Advantages	**Disadvantages**
Excellent for bony structures, foramina, fissures, carotid canal, and calcification within the tumor	Inadequate for dura, meninges, and brain
	Ionizing radiation (especially for children)
	Allergy (iodinated contrast)
Widely available	Artifacts from dental restorations
Fast	Difficult to differentiate obstructed secretions from tumor without contrast

using 3-mm sections, and T1-weighted and T2-weighted sequences are used for evaluation of the anatomy (T1-weighted images) and lesion characterization (T2-weighted images). Magnetic resonance angiography is also used to define vascular anatomy and vascularity of lesions.

Cortical bone of the skull base is typically indicated by a signal void, with fatty marrow demonstrating signal intensity in T1-weighted images. Irregular signal void of the bony cortex often suggests invasion by the tumor (**Fig. 2**). Although the tumor is hyperintense in postcontrast T1-weighted sequences, comparison to precontrast images is important to differentiate fat from lesion. For this reason, fat-suppression technique has been developed to define intracranial extension and differentiation between cystic and solid lesions. It has also helped define perineural spread into the foramina because perineural invasion obliterates the fat at the extracranial openings. On T2-weighted images, MRI is used to evaluate the cavernous sinus, with loss of hyperintensity of the cerebrospinal fluid–containing Meckel cave. The carotid artery is well seen as a signal void passing through the skull base, with narrowing of the

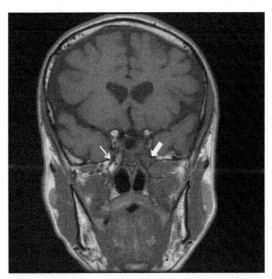

Fig. 2. Nasopharyngeal carcinoma invading the skull base. Coronal T1-weighted image shows the tumor arising in the nasopharynx on the left side. The tumor invades into the pterygoid process obliterating the bone marrow, with a signal void of the cortex of the bone (compare the *large white arrow* with *small white arrow*). (*From* radiopaedia.org.)

lumen suggesting invasion. Comparison with CT images for bony dehiscence is mandatory for preoperative planning.

PARANASAL AND VENTRAL SKULL BASE LESIONS

The skull base is composed of 5 bones: ethmoid, sphenoid, occipital, paired temporal, and paired frontal bones. The anterior part of the ventral skull base separates the anterior cranial fossa from the paranasal sinuses and orbits (**Fig. 3**). The anterior border is formed by the posterior wall of the frontal sinus and the posterior border is formed by the planum sphenoidale and anterior clinoid processes. The frontal bone forms the lateral limit, with the ethmoid bone forming the central part of the floor. The center is the cribriform plate, which has small perforations for the olfactory nerves to pass. The lateral wall is formed by the fovea ethmoidalis, or the roof of the ethmoid cavity.

A variety of lesions are encountered in the ventral skull base, and the pterygopalatine fossa serves as a portal for perineural spread and intracranial involvement. Posteriorly it contains foramen rotundum and the vidian canal; anteriorly it contains the inferior orbital fissure; medially it contains the sphenopalatine foramen, laterally it contains the pterygomaxillary fissure to communicate with the masticator space; and inferiorly it contains the greater and lesser palatine foramina.

TUMOR TYPES: EPITHELIAL TUMORS
Inverted Papilloma

All sinonasal papillomas derived from the surface mucosa of the sinonasal tract (also known as schneiderian membrane) and there are 3 different histological subtypes.[3] Exophytic or septal-type papillomas consist of broad-based papillary projections with well-developed fibrovascular cores. The papillae are lined by stratified squamoid to transitional epithelium with scattered mucocytes as well as rare ciliated columnar cells.[4] On the other hand, inverted papillomas arise on the lateral nasal wall and are characterized by variably thickened stratified squamoid to transitional epithelium growing downward into the underlying stroma (**Fig. 4**). The identification of mucocytes, intraepithelial mucous cysts, and mixed acute and chronic inflammation is

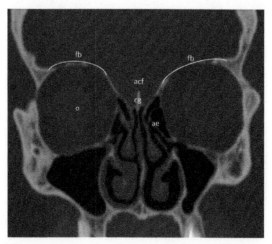

Fig. 3. Ventral skull base anatomy. acf, anterior cranial fossa; ae, anterior ethmoid; cg, crista galli; fb, frontal bone; o, orbit. (*From* radiopaedia.org.)

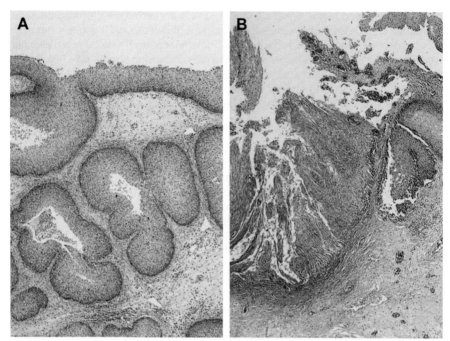

Fig. 4. (*A*) Hematoxylin-eosin slide of sinonasal inverted papilloma. (*B*) malignant transformation. Verrucous carcinoma arising in an inverted papilloma.

characteristic.[5] Oncocytic or cylindrical papillomas also arise on the lateral nasal wall but are composed of stratified columnar cells with abundant eosinophilic to granular cytoplasm. These lesions can show endophytic and/or exophytic growth, and cysts limited to the epithelium containing neutrophils are typically seen.[6] Transformation to carcinoma has been reported in inverted (approximately 10%) and oncocytic (4%–17%) types and rarely in exophytic papillomas.[7] Conventional keratinizing squamous cell carcinoma (SCC) is the most common carcinoma arising in sinonasal papillomas and most commonly it occurs synchronically; consequently, the presence of extensive keratinization in a sinonasal papilloma should prompt thorough histological examination.[8]

An etiological association between human papillomavirus (HPV) and sinonasal papillomas has been proposed. According to different series, HPV DNA, most commonly types 6 and 11, has been detected in approximately half and one-third of exophytic and inverted papillomas, respectively.[4,9] No link between HPV and oncocytic papillomas, however, has been established. Recently, the role of HPV in sinonasal papillomas has been challenged by a study that identified recurrent activating EGFR mutations in approximately 90% of inverted papillomas. A majority of these mutations are exon 20 insertions and the mutational status showed strong negative correlation with HPV DNA detection.[10] In addition, KRAS exon 2 mutations have been reported in a majority of oncocytic papillomas. The same EGFR and KRAS mutations are identified in the SCC associated with inverted and oncocytic papillomas, respectively.

CT appearance of inverted papillomas is nonspecific, with polypoid lesion originating from the lateral nasal wall. Occasionally it may originate from the nasal septum showing a lobulated mass. Focal bone remodeling and sclerosis can also be seen. Multiplanar CT is essential in assessing the extent of disease. MRI is rarely obtained for unsuspecting disease, but a characteristic columnar pattern may be seen reflecting layers of proliferating epithelium invaginating in the underlying stroma (see **Fig. 4**). The hyperplastic epithelium appears hypointense on T2-weighted images due to hypercellularity, and the underlying stroma shows hyperintensity on T1 postcontrast images due to hypervascularity (**Fig. 5**). The Krouse staging system for inverted papilloma is included in **Table 3**.[11]

Squamous Cell Carcinoma

SCC is the most frequent malignant tumor type, accounting for more than 60% of all sinonasal malignancies.[1] The maxillary sinus and nasal cavity are the most common sites of origin, with peak incidence in the sixth and seventh decades. There is also a male-to-female predominance at 2:1 ratio.[12] Multimodality therapy is the mainstay of treatment, depending on location and stage (**Table 4**). Imaging's main goal is to determine the extent of invasion, because SCC does not show specific CT or MRI findings (**Fig. 6**). Overall prognosis is poor (<50% 5-year survival rate), worsened with involvement of neighboring structures or multiple subsites.[13]

Histologically, a majority of sinonasal SCCs are characterized by the presence of irregular cohesive nests and cords of tumor cells with variable pleomorphism showing keratinization and intercellular bridges with an associated desmoplastic stromal reaction (**Fig. 7**). This keratinizing morphology, in addition to the classic immunoreactivity for high-molecular cytokeratin, p63 and p40, does not differ from SCC arising in other regions of the upper aerodigestive tract. In contrast to other head and neck sites, however, precursor lesions, like high-grade keratinizing intraepithelial dysplasia and carcinoma in situ, are rarely seen in isolation and are not well defined as in oral cavy and larynx.

Nonkeratinizing SCC is distinctive tumor type in the sinonasal tract that can be diagnostically problematic.[14] This variant has been referred in the literature as cylindrical cell carcinoma, Ringertz carcinoma, transitional cell carcinoma, and schneiderian carcinoma.[15,16] It is composed of nests and ribbons of pleomorphic, hyperchromatic cells

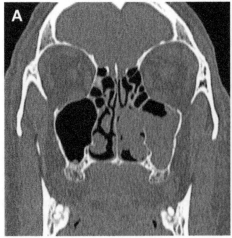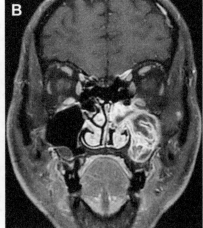

Fig. 5. (*A*) Biopsy-proven IP (Inverted Papilloma), CT without contrast. (*B*) MRI T1-weighted images, postcontrast. (*From* radiopaedia.org.)

Table 3
Krouse staging system for inverted papilloma
T1	Tumor totally confined to the nasal cavity, without extension into the sinuses. The tumor can be localized to 1 wall or region of the nasal cavity or can be bulky and extensive within the nasal cavity but must not extend into the sinuses or into any extranasal compartment. There must be no concurrent malignancy.
T2	Tumor involving the ostiomeatal complex, and ethmoid sinuses, and/or the medial portion of the maxillary sinus, with or without involvement of the nasal cavity. There must be no concurrent malignancy.
T3	Tumor involving the lateral, inferior, superior, anterior, or posterior walls of the maxillary sinus, the sphenoid sinus, and/or the frontal sinus, with or without involvement of the medial portion of the maxillary sinus, the ethmoid sinuses, or the nasal cavity. There must be no concurrent malignancy.
T4	All tumors with any extranasal/extrasinus extension to involve adjacent, contiguous structures, such as the orbit, the intracranial compartment, or the pterygomaxillary space. All tumors are associated with malignancy.

Data from Krouse JH. Development of a staging system for inverted papilloma. Laryngoscope 2000;110(6):965–8.

with increased nuclear to cytoplasmic ratio. Comedo-type necrosis is easily identified and the tumor shows brisk mitotic activity. Tumor cells are elongated to cylindrical and may show perpendicular arrangement to the underlying basement membrane. Non-keratinizing SCC exhibits a papillary architecture admixed endophytic growth with well-delineated pushing borders.[17] Transcriptionally active HPV is detected in approximately 40% of sinonasal nonkeratinizing SCC. In contrast to the oropharynx, however, a positive prognostic role of HPV has not been established in the sinonasal tract.[4,18,19]

Other morphological variants of SCC have been also described in the sinonasal tract, including basaloid, verrucous, spindle, and papillary. Verrucous SCC is a well-differentiated neoplasm with no metastatic potential that is characterized by an exophytic warty configuration with broad pushing borders. It is composed of a cellular proliferation with preserved maturation lacking cytological pleomorphism. The diagnosis of verrucous SCC is extremely challenging in biopsies and it can mimic benign epithelial proliferations. Its unequivocal diagnosis is better archived in resection specimens and after extensive sampling of the lesion.[20] Basaloid SCC is an aggressive neoplasm predominantly composed of high-grade basaloid cells arranged in solid nests with central comedo-type necrosis and peripheral palisading associated with hyalinized basement membrane material. Abrupt keratinization, associated surface dysplasia/carcinoma in situ, or focal areas of conventional SCC are seen.[21] Papillary SCC is a predominantly exophytic carcinoma characterized by papillary projections containing true fibrovascular cores and covered by a stratified squamous epithelium with overt features of malignancy. Even in the abscess of definite stromal invasion, this variant is considered invasive carcinoma by some authorities.[22] Spindle cell squamous carcinoma (also known as sarcomatoid carcinoma) is a poorly differentiated neoplasm predominantly composed of atypical spindle or pleomorphic cells showing variable positivity for cytokeratins and p63. Associated surface dysplasia/carcinoma in situ or focal admixed areas of conventional SCC can be seen in some cases. Morphologically, this variant can mimic mesenchymal neoplasms.[14]

Table 4
TNM classification for cancer of the nasal cavity and paranasal sinuses

Maxillary sinus

T1	Tumor limited to maxillary sinus mucosa with no erosion or destruction of bone
T2	Tumor causing bone erosion or destruction, including extension into the hard palate and/or middle nasal meatus, except extension to posterior wall of the maxillary sinus and pterygoid plates
T3	Tumor invades any of the following: bone of the posterior wall of the maxillary sinus, subcutaneous tissues, floor or medial wall of the orbit, pterygoid fossa, and ethmoid sinuses.
T4a	Moderately advanced local disease • Tumor invades the anterior orbital contents, skin of the cheek, pterygoid plates, infratemporal fossa, cribriform plate, sphenoid, or frontal sinuses.
T4b	Very advanced local disease • Tumor invades any of the following: orbital apex, dura, brain, middle cranial fossa, cranial nerves other than maxillary division of the trigeminal nerve (V2), nasopharynx, and clivus,

Nasal cavity and ethmoid sinus

T1	Tumor restricted to any 1 subsite, with or without bony invasion
T2	Tumor invading 2 subsites in a single region or extending to involve an adjacent region within the nasoethmoidal complex, with or without bony invasion
T3	Tumor extends to invade the medial wall or floor of the orbit, maxillary sinus, palate, or cribriform plate
T4a	Moderately advanced local disease—tumor invades any of the following: anterior orbital contents, skin of the nose or cheek, minimal extension to the anterior cranial fossa, pterygoid plates, sphenoid, and frontal sinuses
T4b	Very advanced local disease—tumor invades any of the following: orbital apex, dura brain, middle cranial fossa, cranial nerves other than maxillary division of trigeminal nerve (V2), nasopharynx, and clivus

Regional lymph nodes

N1	Metastasis in a single ipsilateral lymph node ≤3 cm in greatest dimension
N2a	Metastasis in a single ipsilateral lymph node >3 cm but not more than 6 cm in greatest dimension
N2b	Metastasis in multiple ipsilateral lymph nodes, none >6 cm in greatest dimension
N2c	Metastasis in bilateral or contralateral lymph nodes, none >6 cm in greatest dimension
N3	Metastasis in a lymph node >6 cm in greatest dimension

Distant metastasis

M0	No distant metastasis
M1	Distant metastasis

Histological grade

G1	Well differentiated
G2	Moderately differentiated
G3	Poorly differentiated
G4	Undifferentiated

Stage	T	N	M
I	T1	N0	M0
II	T2	N0	M0
III	T3	N0	M0
	T1	N1	M0
	T2	N1	M0
	T3	N1	M0
IVA	T4a	N0	M0
	T4a	N1	M0
	T1	N2	M0
	T2	N2	M0
	T3	N2	M0
	T4a	N2	M0
IVB	Any T	N3	M0
	T4b	Any N	M0
IVC	Any T	Any N	M1

The subsites within the nasal cavity include the septum; superior, middle, and inferior turbinates; and olfactory region of the cribriform plate.

Data from Deschler D, Moore M, Smith R. Quick reference guide to TNM staging of head and neck cancer and neck dissection classification. Alexandria (VA): American Academy of Otolaryngology- Head and Neck Surgery Foundation; 2014.

Sinonasal Undifferentiated Carcinoma

Sinonasal undifferentiated carcinoma (SNUC) is a highly aggressive tumor with only a brief history of symptoms with nasal obstruction and/or epistaxis, large tumor burden, and nodal disease at presentation (15%–20%). Similar to SCC, SNUC typically does not have distinctive imaging features (**Fig. 8**). Histologically, SNUC lacks definitive evidence of squamous or glandular differentiation.[23] It typically shows lobular and trabecular growth and is composed of medium to large polygonal cells with varying amount of cytoplasm and vesicular to hyperchromatic nuclei (**Fig. 9**). An increased degree of mitotic activity, individual cell necrosis, and large confluent areas of tumor necrosis are characteristic. Immunohistochemical studies consistently show diffuse and strong positivity for cytokeratin. Reactivity for p63 and neuroendocrine markers is variable and focal and does not show the typical staining pattern of a squamous cell or neuroendocrine carcinoma, respectively.[24] Multimodality treatment is advocated, but prognosis is poor with 5-year survival rate between 30% and 60%.

Sinonasal Neuroendocrine Carcinomas

Sinonasal neuroendocrine carcinomas (SNECs) are rare tumors that comprise a heterogenous group of malignant epithelial neoplasms characterized by the presence of neuroendocrine differentiation. Their prognosis is dependent on tumor type, and therefore different nomenclature schemas have been developed. The 2005 World Health Organization Classification of Head and Neck Tumors recognized different subtypes of SNECs: typical carcinoid, atypical carcinoid, small cell carcinoma, and "neuroendocrine carcinoma, not otherwise specified" (**Fig. 10**).[14] The last subtype was suggested for tumors that do not fit the aforementioned categories; however, many of those tumors are better classified today as large cell neuroendocrine carcinomas. Typical and atypical carcinoids are composed of small to medium-sized cells with moderate eosinophilic cytoplasm and uniform round to oval nuclei with stippled chromatin. A summary of the World Health Organization classification of neuroendocrine carcinomas of the head and neck is provided in **Table 5**.[25,26]

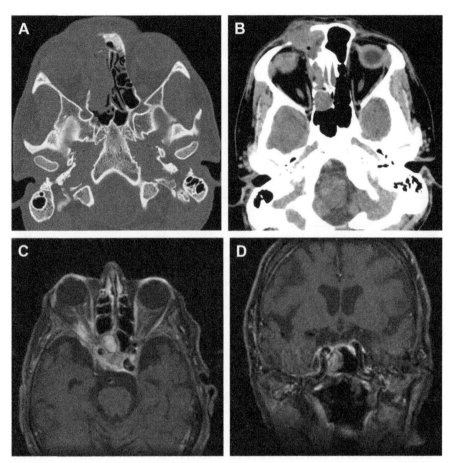

Fig. 6. (*A, B*) Biopsy-proven SCC. CT showed an infiltrating soft tissue mass with bony destruction of medial orbital wall, anterior wall of the frontal sinus and ethmoid cells. (*C, D*) MRI T1-weighted images postcontrast. Sphenoid SCC involving the orbital apex. (*From* radiopaedia.org.)

Adenocarcinoma and Adenoid Cystic Carcinoma

The histological spectrum of adenocarcinomas of the sinonasal tract includes salivary gland and nonsalivary gland adenocarcinomas. Among the former group, adenoid cystic carcinoma is the most common and its histological features are identical to that tumors arising in major and minor salivary glands.[14]

Adenoid cystic carcinoma is predominately composed of abluminal cells (modified myoepithelial cells) characterized by small to medium cell size, scant to moderate eosinophilic to clear cytoplasm and typical uniform, oval to sharply angulated nuclei with densely basophilic chromatin (**Fig. 11**). Scattered among the abluminal cells, there are ductal cells (luminal cells) with eosinophilic cytoplasm and round nuclei arranged in true glandular structures. Adenoid cystic carcinoma can exhibit 3 different architectural growth patterns and commonly displays perineural invasion. In the tubular pattern, ducts with true lumens separated by stroma are appreciated. The classic Swiss cheese configuration of the cribriform pattern is due to pseudocysts

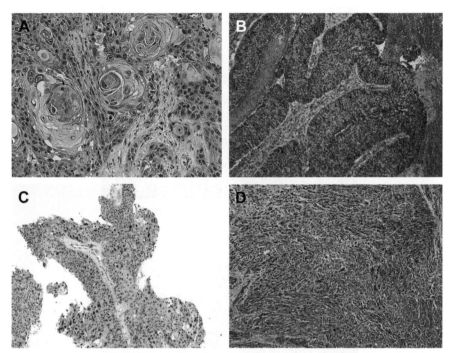

Fig. 7. (*A*) Hematoxylin-eosin slide of keratinizing SCC. (*B*) Nonkeratinizing SCC. (*C*) Papillary SCC. (*D*) Spindle cell squamous carcinoma.

containing amorphous basophilic extracellular material and/or hyalinized basement membrane material. In the solid pattern, tumor cells are arranged in sheets with few cyst spaces or tubules. The histological grading of adenoid cystic carcinoma mainly relies on the quantification of the 3 different patterns (**Table 6**). In addition, as the

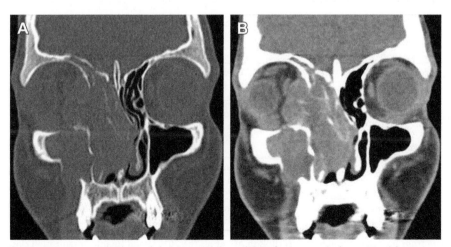

Fig. 8. Biopsy-proven SNUC. (*A*) Bone window. (*B*) Soft tissue window. CT with contrast showing a large sinonasal mass occupying the maxillary sinus and obliterating the ethmoids. Bony destruction is noted with erosion of the medial orbital wall and extraconal involvement. (*From* radiopaedia.org.)

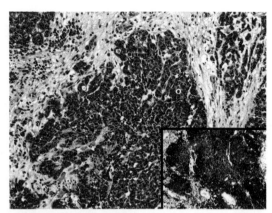

Fig. 9. Hematoxylin-eosin stain slide of SNUC. (*Inset*) Cytokeratin stain.

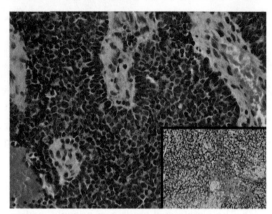

Fig. 10. SNECs. Small cell carcinoma. (*Inset*) Synaptophysin stain.

Table 5
2005 World Health Organization classification of neuroendocrine carcinomas of the head and neck

Classification	Criteria for Diagnosis
Carcinoid tumor	Tumor with neuroendocrine/carcinoid morphology Low mitotic rate (<2 mitoses per 10 HPF) Absence of necrosis
Atypical carcinoid tumor	Tumor with neuroendocrine/carcinoid morphology High mitotic rate (>2 mitoses per 10 HPF) Necrosis Non–small cell carcinoma
Small cell carcinoma	Tumor cells with small size High mitotic rate (>10 mitoses per 10 HPF) Necrosis
Neuroendocrine carcinoma, not otherwise specified	Neuroendocrine carcinoma that does not fit aforementioned categories

Data from Travis WD, Brambilla E, Nicholson AG, et al. The 2015 World Health Organization classification of lung tumors: impact of genetic, clinical and radiologic advances since the 2004 classification. J Thorac Oncol 2015;10(9):1243–60; and Kao HL, Chang WC, Li WY, et al. Head and neck large cell neuroendocrine carcinoma should be separated from atypical carcinoid on the basis of different clinical features, overall survival, and pathogenesis. Am J Surg Pathol 2012;36(2):185–92.

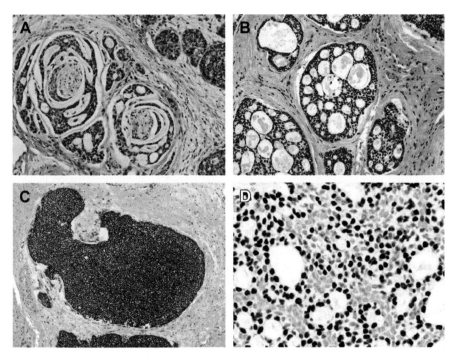

Fig. 11. Hematoxylin-eosin stain slide of adenoid cystic carcinoma. (*A*) Perineural invasion. (*B*) Classic cribriform pattern. (*C*) Solid pattern. (*D*) Tubular pattern.

grade increases, more nuclear polymorphism and mitotic activity are present. Rarely, adenoid cystic carcinoma undergoes high-grade transformation. Abluminal cells are variably positive for p63, p40, calponin, and smooth muscle actin, whereas epithelial membrane antigen, carcinoembryonic antigen, and c-kit (CD117) typically stain the luminal cells. Cytokeratin stains are positive in both cell types but tend to highlight the luminal cells.[27] Adenoid cystic carcinoma harbors a recurrent t(6;9) translocation involving the MYB gene and the NFIB gene. This molecular signature is detected by fluorescence in situ hybridization in approximately 30% to 40% of cases, but its detection improves to up to 86% by using more sensitive methods.[28,29]

Sinonasal nonsalivary gland adenocarcinomas can be classified as intestinal adenocarcinoma (ITAC) and non-ITAC types. There is a strong association with chronic exposure to wood dust and leather dust in ITAC, and the reported average

Table 6 Adenoid cystic carcinoma grading system by Perzin[30] and Szanto[31]	
Classification	
Grade I	Predominantly tubular, no solid
Grade II	Predominantly cribriform, <30% solid
Grade III	Solid component >30%

Data from Thompson LD, Penner C, Ho NJ, et al. Sinonasal tract and nasopharyngeal adenoid cystic carcinoma: a clinicopathologic and immunophenotypic study of 86 cases. Head Neck Pathol 2014;8(1):88–109.

exposure period is approximately 40 years. Ethmoid sinus is the most common location (40%), followed by nasal cavity (25%) and maxillary antrum (20%). Sporadic forms of ITAC are more frequent in women and show shorter survival times. Imaging produced by ITAC tumors shows mixed solid-fluid pattern (**Fig. 12**).

ITAC histologically and immunohistochemically resembles intestinal neoplasms (**Fig. 13**).[14] The classification scheme proposed by Barnes[32] further subdivided this category into 5 subtypes that correlate with clinical behavior: papillary, colonic, solid, mucinous, and mixed. The papillary type shows the less aggressive course and histologically looks like a tubulovillous adenoma. The most commonly encounter type is the colonic one, which is reminiscent of a conventional colorectal adenocarcinoma. The mucinous type is characterized by tumor cell lying in pools of mucin or by distended glands filled with mucin, whereas the solid type shows a diffuse proliferation lacking gland formation.[32] Regardless of the subtype, immunohistochemically, stains for CK20, CDX2, villin, and CK7 are positive in ITACs (**Table 7**).[14]

Non-ITACs lack histological or immunophenotypical features of ITACs or salivary-type adenocarcinomas. Typically, they are characterized by a back-to-back proliferation of glands without intervening stroma. The classic definition states that the glands are lined by a single layer of nonciliated cuboidal to columnar cells lacking myoepithelial or basal cells.[14] Few cases have been described, however, in which a myoepithelial component is identified. Based on the degree of cytomorphological characteristics, including pleomorphism, mitotic activity, and necrosis, non-ITACs can be further divided into low-grade and high-grade tumors.[33,34]

Chordoma

Chordomas represent rare, malignant nonepithelial tumors derived from notochordal tissue. These lesions are low grade because they present with aggressive local invasion but low risk for distant metastasis.[35] The skull base is the second most common location, with the sacrum the most common site. There are 2 variants: chondroid and myxoid, with chondroid variants containing cartilage.

A majority of skull base chordomas originate from the spheno-occipital synchondrosis, with patients complaining of headaches and diplopia on lateral gaze of the affected side. Cranial nerve VI palsy is related to the mass effect because the path

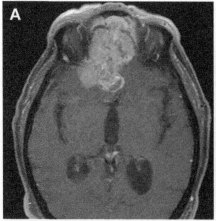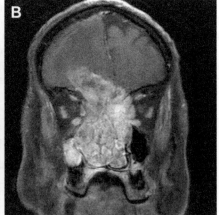

Fig. 12. (*A*) Axial view. (*B*) Coronal view. Biopsy-proven sinonasal ITAC, colonic type. MRI T1-weighted images postcontrast, mass extends through cribriform plate into the frontal lobes. (*From* radiopaedia.org.)

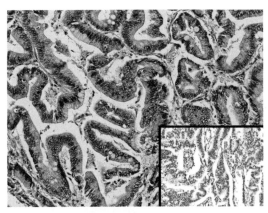

Fig. 13. ITAC, papillary type. (*Inset*) CDX2 staining.

of the cranial nerve is close in proximity to the spheno-occipital fissure. Radiographically, chordomas present with lytic bone lesions arising from the clivus with intratumoral calcifications (**Fig. 14**). CT is usually adequate for generating a diagnosis, but MRI is used extensively for treatment planning. Total to subtotal resection is the optimal treatment, with adjuvant radiotherapy for residual disease. Overall 5-year survival rate approaches 50%. Histologically, the tumor consists of physaliphorous cells with multiple cytoplasmic vacuoles within myxoid stroma. Cells stain strongly with epithelial markers (pan cytokeratin, epithelial membrane antigen, and S100).

TUMOR TYPES: NONEPITHELIAL TUMORS
Esthesioneuroblastoma

Also referred as olfactory neuroblastoma, esthesioneuroblastoma is a rare, malignant neuroectodermal tumor arising from the olfactory epithelium, which extends from the cribriform plate and extends to the ethmoid roof, upper nasal septum, and superior turbinates. There is a bimodal incidence (second and fifth decades) and slight male predominance.

Esthesioneuroblastoma is clinically staged by the Kadish classification and histologically graded by the Hyams system (**Table 8**).[36,37] Most tumors are diagnosed in an advanced stage, with cross-section imaging showing the lesion spanning across the cribriform plate (**Fig. 15**). Treatment consists of surgical resection with negative margins, followed by chemoradiotherapy.

Table 7 Adenocarcinoma subtypes by Barnes	
Intestinal-type Adenocarcinoma	**Non–intestinal-type Adenocarcinoma**
Papillary	Low grade
Colonic	High grade
Solid	
Mucinous	
Mixed	

Data from Barnes L. Intestinal-type adenocarcinoma of the nasal cavity and paranasal sinuses. Am J Surg Pathol 1986;10(3):192–202.

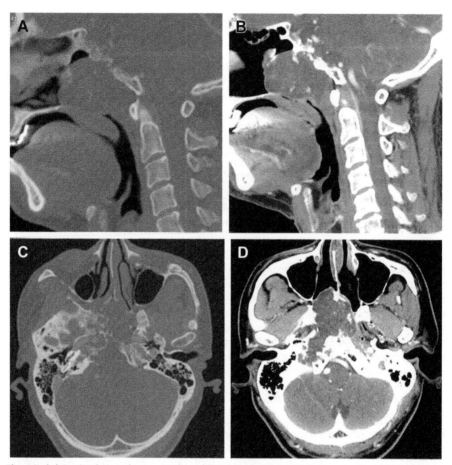

Fig. 14. (*A*) Sagittal view, bone window. (*B*) Sagittal view, soft tissue window. (*C*) Axial view, bone window. (*D*) Sagittal view, soft tissue window. Biopsy-proven chordoma. CT without and with contrast showing clival destruction. (*From* radiopaedia.org.)

Table 8
Kadish and Hyams grading for esthesioneuroblastoma

Kadish Classification		Hyams Histological Grading				
A	Tumor limited to nasal cavity	Microscopic features	1	2	3	4
B	Tumor limited to nasal cavity and paranasal sinuses	Pleomorphism	–	+	++	+++
C	Tumor extends into skull base, intracranial compartment, orbit, distant metastatic disease	Lobular architecture	+	+	+/–	+/–
		Neurofibrillary matrix	+++	+	+/–	–
		Rosettes	+	+	+/–	+/–
		Mitoses	–	–	+	+++
		Necrosis	–	–	+	+++

Data from Kadish S, Goodman M, Wang CC. Olfactory neuroblastoma. A clinical analysis of 17 cases. Cancer 1976;37(3):1571–6; and Van Gompel JJ, Giannini C, Olsen KD, et al. Long-term outcome of esthesioneuroblastoma: hyams grade predicts patient survival. J Neurol Surg B Skull Base 2012;73(5):331–6.

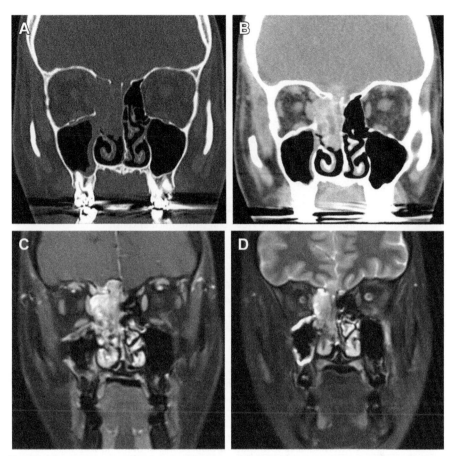

Fig. 15. Biopsy-proven esthesioneuroblastoma. (*A*) CT without contrast showing soft tissue extending intracranially through the cribriform plate and laterally through the lamina papyracea into the orbit. (*B* [*top*]) CT with contrast showing heterogenous enhancement. (*C*) MRI T1-weighted image postcontrast. (*D*) MRI T2-weighted image. (*From* radiopaedia.org.)

Histologically, esthesioneuroblastoma often shows prominent fibrillary or reticular background, with sheets of small cells with scant cytoplasm. Some show nuclear pleomorphism, with variable mitotic figures and Homer-Wright rosettes (**Fig. 16**). Necrosis is a poor prognostic factor, and the Hyams histological grading system is detailed in **Table 8**. Low-grade tumors (Hyams 1–2) show absence of low mitotic activity (<5 mitoses per 10 high-power fields [HPFs]) whereas high-grade tumors (Hyams 3–4) show high mitotic index. Grade 4 tumors often show severe necrosis and anaplasia.

Malignant Melanoma

Sinonasal mucosal melanoma arises from melanocytes that migrated from the neural crest to the nasal cavity mucosa. It comprises 1% of all melanomas, with the nasal septum and lateral nasal wall the most common sites of origin. Established risk factors for cutaneous melanoma, such as sun damage, family history, and atypical nevi, do not apply to mucosal melanoma. Peak incidence is observed in the sixth decade,

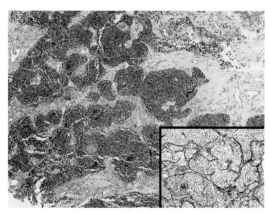

Fig. 16. Esthesioneuroblastoma. (*Inset*) S100 stain (sustentacular cells).

with no gender preference. TNM classification of mucosal melanoma is summarized in **Table 9**.

On MRI, mucosal melanoma appears as a solid soft tissue with local invasion frequent on presentation. A peculiar T1-weighted hyperintensity can be noted due to the paramagnetic properties of melanin and hemorrhage. The lesion also returns hyperintensity after contrast on T1-weighted images and moderate enhancement on

Table 9			
TNM classification for mucosal melanoma of the head and neck			
Primary tumor			
T3	Mucosal disease		
T4a	Moderately advanced disease • Involving deep soft tissue, cartilage, bone, or overlying skin		
T4b	Very advanced disease • Tumor involving brain, dura, skull base, lower cranial nerves (IX, X, XI, and XII), masticator space, carotid artery, prevertebral space, or mediastinal structures		
Reginal lymph nodes			
N1			Regional lymph node metastases present
Distant metastasis			
M0			No distant metastasis
M1			Distant Metastasis
Stage	*T*	*N*	*M*
III	T3	N0	M0
IVA	T4a	N0	M0
	T3	N1	M0
	T4a	N1	M0
IVB	T4b	Any N	M0
IVC	Any T	Any N	M1

Data from Deschler D, Moore M, Smith R. Quick reference guide to TNM staging of head and neck cancer and neck dissection classification. 2014.

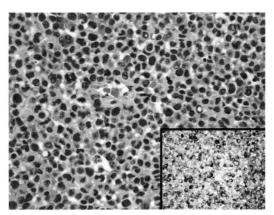

Fig. 17. Epithelioid melanoma. (*Inset*) HMB45 stain.

T2-weighted images. Wide local excision with negative margins is the mainstay of treatment, but overall prognosis is poor, with distant metastasis occurring in more than 50% of cases.

Histologically, mucosal melanoma is often ulcerated and necrotic, with small uniform cells. A nesting growth pattern can be observed, and 70% of the cells have pigment. There is frequent vascular and deep tissue invasion, and other patterns are small blue cell, spindle cell, and pleomorphic cell types (**Fig. 17**).

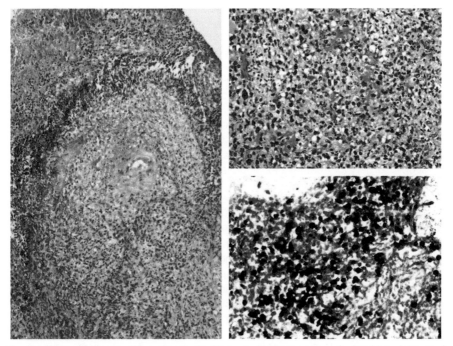

Fig. 18. Natural killer/T-cell lymphoma. (*Left*) Angiodestructive growth. (*Right top*) Atypical polymoprhic proliferation. (*Right bottom*) EBV-encoded RNA (*EBER*).

Lymphoma

In the sinonasal region, 2 main extranodal, extralymphatic non-Hodgkin lymphomas can be observed. Diffuse B-cell lymphoma appears as a soft tissue mass with surrounding bone erosion, possibly originating from Waldeyer ring. It most commonly affects the maxillary sinus and without necrosis. Natural killer/T-cell lymphoma involves the nasal cavity, presenting as a midline lesion with erosion of the nasal septum, inferior turbinates, and palate. The tumor is destructive, often with areas of necrosis (**Fig. 18**) leading to variable enhancement on CT.

SUMMARY

Most sinonasal and ventral skull base malignancies present with nonspecific symptoms. Diagnosis of initial tumor growth requires thorough history taking with a high index of suspicion on physical examination. Modern imaging techniques often help define tumor extension and treatment planning, but diagnosis can only be confirmed histologically, because they are radiographically indistinct. The wide variety of pathology reflects the tissue types in the sinonasal area, leading to a broad differential diagnosis preoperatively.

REFERENCES

1. Maroldi R, Nicolai P, Battaglia G. Imaging in treatment planning for sinonasal diseases. Berlin: Springer; 2005.
2. Gras Cabrerizo JR, Sarandeses Garcia A, Montserrat IGJR, et al. Revision of carcinomas in paranasal sinuses. Acta Otorrinolaringol Esp 2007;58(6):266–75 [in Spanish].
3. Thompson LD. Schneiderian papilloma of the sinonasal tract. Ear Nose Throat J 2015;94(4–5):146–8.
4. Lewis JS Jr, Westra WH, Thompson LD, et al. The sinonasal tract: another potential "hot spot" for carcinomas with transcriptionally-active human papillomavirus. Head Neck Pathol 2014;8(3):241–9.
5. Kaufman MR, Brandwein MS, Lawson W. Sinonasal papillomas: clinicopathologic review of 40 patients with inverted and oncocytic schneiderian papillomas. Laryngoscope 2002;112(8 Pt 1):1372–7.
6. Barnes L, Bedetti C. Oncocytic Schneiderian papilloma: a reappraisal of cylindrical cell papilloma of the sinonasal tract. Hum Pathol 1984;15(4):344–51.
7. Lombardi D, Tomenzoli D, Butta L, et al. Limitations and complications of endoscopic surgery for treatment for sinonasal inverted papilloma: a reassessment after 212 cases. Head Neck 2011;33(8):1154–61.
8. Barnes L. Schneiderian papillomas and nonsalivary glandular neoplasms of the head and neck. Mod Pathol 2002;15(3):279–97.
9. Lawson W, Schlecht NF, Brandwein-Gensler M. The role of the human papillomavirus in the pathogenesis of Schneiderian inverted papillomas: an analytic overview of the evidence. Head Neck Pathol 2008;2(2):49–59.
10. Udager AM, Rolland DC, McHugh JB, et al. High-frequency targetable EGFR mutations in sinonasal squamous cell carcinomas arising from inverted sinonasal papilloma. Cancer Res 2015;75(13):2600–6.
11. Krouse JH. Development of a staging system for inverted papilloma. Laryngoscope 2000;110(6):965–8.
12. Samant S, Kruger E. Cancer of the paranasal sinuses. Curr Oncol Rep 2007;9(2): 147–51.

13. Suarez C, Llorente JL, Fernandez De Leon R, et al. Prognostic factors in sinonasal tumors involving the anterior skull base. Head Neck 2004;26(2):136–44.
14. Thompson L. World Health Organization classification of tumours: pathology and genetics of head and neck tumours. Ear Nose Throat J Feb 2006;85(2):74.
15. Kumar M, Bahl A, Sharma DN, et al. Cylindric cell carcinoma of the base of the tongue: a rare variant of squamous cell carcinoma. J Cancer Res Ther 2009; 5(2):124–6.
16. McKenzie J. Ringertz tumour with an unusual presentation. J Laryngol Otol 1962; 76:1002–4.
17. Thompson LDR. Sinonasal carcinomas. Curr Diagn Pathol 2006;12(1):40–53.
18. Bishop JA, Guo TW, Smith DF, et al. Human papillomavirus-related carcinomas of the sinonasal tract. Am J Surg Pathol 2013;37(2):185–92.
19. Larque AB, Hakim S, Ordi J, et al. High-risk human papillomavirus is transcriptionally active in a subset of sinonasal squamous cell carcinomas. Mod Pathol 2014;27(3):343–51.
20. Durden FL Jr, Moore CE, Muller S. Verrucous carcinoma of the paranasal sinuses: a case report. Ear Nose Throat J 2010;89(7):E21–3.
21. Wieneke JA, Thompson LD, Wenig BM. Basaloid squamous cell carcinoma of the sinonasal tract. Cancer 1999;85(4):841–54.
22. Suarez PA, Adler-Storthz K, Luna MA, et al. Papillary squamous cell carcinomas of the upper aerodigestive tract: a clinicopathologic and molecular study. Head Neck 2000;22(4):360–8.
23. Frierson HF Jr, Mills SE, Fechner RE, et al. Sinonasal undifferentiated carcinoma. An aggressive neoplasm derived from schneiderian epithelium and distinct from olfactory neuroblastoma. Am J Surg Pathol 1986;10(11):771–9.
24. Ejaz A, Wenig BM. Sinonasal undifferentiated carcinoma: clinical and pathologic features and a discussion on classification, cellular differentiation, and differential diagnosis. Adv Anat Pathol 2005;12(3):134–43.
25. Travis WD, Brambilla E, Nicholson AG, et al. The 2015 World Health Organization classification of lung tumors: impact of genetic, clinical and radiologic advances since the 2004 classification. J Thorac Oncol 2015;10(9):1243–60.
26. Kao HL, Chang WC, Li WY, et al. Head and neck large cell neuroendocrine carcinoma should be separated from atypical carcinoid on the basis of different clinical features, overall survival, and pathogenesis. Am J Surg Pathol 2012;36(2): 185–92.
27. Thompson LD, Penner C, Ho NJ, et al. Sinonasal tract and nasopharyngeal adenoid cystic carcinoma: a clinicopathologic and immunophenotypic study of 86 cases. Head Neck Pathol 2014;8(1):88–109.
28. Rettig EM, Tan M, Ling S, et al. MYB rearrangement and clinicopathologic characteristics in head and neck adenoid cystic carcinoma. Laryngoscope 2015; 125(9):E292–9.
29. Brill LB 2nd, Kanner WA, Fehr A, et al. Analysis of MYB expression and MYB-NFIB gene fusions in adenoid cystic carcinoma and other salivary neoplasms. Mod Pathol 2011;24(9):1169–76.
30. Perzin KH, Gullane P, Clairmont AC. Adenoid cystic carcinomas arising in salivary glands; a correlation of histologic features and clinical course. Cancer 1978;42: 265–82.
31. Szanto PA, Luna MA, Tortoledo ME, et al. Histologic grading of adenoid cystic carcinoma of the salivary glands. Cancer 1984;54(6):1062–9.
32. Barnes L. Intestinal-type adenocarcinoma of the nasal cavity and paranasal sinuses. Am J Surg Pathol 1986;10(3):192–202.

33. Heffner DK, Hyams VJ, Hauck KW, et al. Low-grade adenocarcinoma of the nasal cavity and paranasal sinuses. Cancer 1982;50(2):312–22.
34. Stelow EB, Jo VY, Mills SE, et al. A histologic and immunohistochemical study describing the diversity of tumors classified as sinonasal high-grade nonintestinal adenocarcinomas. Am J Surg Pathol 2011;35(7):971–80.
35. Erdem E, Angtuaco EC, Van Hemert R, et al. Comprehensive review of intracranial chordoma. Radiographics 2003;23(4):995–1009.
36. Kadish S, Goodman M, Wang CC. Olfactory neuroblastoma. A clinical analysis of 17 cases. Cancer 1976;37(3):1571–6.
37. Van Gompel JJ, Giannini C, Olsen KD, et al. Long-term outcome of esthesioneuroblastoma: hyams grade predicts patient survival. J Neurol Surg B Skull Base 2012;73(5):331–6.

Anatomic Considerations for Sinonasal and Ventral Skull Base Malignancy

 CrossMark

Thomas J. Willson, MD[a], Juan C. Fernandez-Miranda, MD[b],*,
Cristian Ferrareze Nunes, MD[b], Stefan Lieber, MD[b],
Eric W. Wang, MD[a]

KEYWORDS

- Anatomy • Skullbase • Endoscopic • Endonasal

KEY POINTS

- Sinonasal malignancy is rare in general but with an understanding of anatomy from an endonasal perspective many of these lesions may be dealt with using a totally endoscopic approach.
- Preservation of normal nasal structures should be given consideration when possible to restore function to the nose following surgery.
- The sphenoid bone is central in the nasal cavity and contains several landmarks of great importance. An understanding of this anatomy is crucial to endonasal surgery.
- The clivus may be subdivided into thirds, which extend from the dorsum sella superiorly to the region just deep to the nasopharynx inferiorly.
- Knowledge of the anatomic structures surrounding the pterygopalatine space and pterygoid region allows lateral dissection when lesions dictate this approach.

INTRODUCTION

Malignancies of the sinonasal region and ventral skull base include a varied group of uncommon tumors that are a challenge to treat. These malignancies, with few exceptions, often present late because of their insidious growth and bland symptomatology. Common symptoms include sinusitis, nasal obstruction, facial pain, epistaxis, and headache. Patients often suffer a protracted course to diagnosis given these inconspicuous symptoms and tend to present with advanced lesions. As with malignancies of other sites, the primary goal in surgical management is complete resection with

[a] Department of Otolaryngology—Head & Neck Surgery, UPMC Eye & Ear Institute, University of Pittsburgh Medical Center, Suite 500, 203 Lothrop Street, Pittsburgh, PA 15213, USA;
[b] Department of Neurological Surgery, UPMC Presbyterian, University of Pittsburgh Medical Center, Suite B-400, 200 Lothrop Street, Pittsburgh, PA 15213, USA
* Corresponding author.
E-mail address: fernandezmirandajc@upmc.edu

Otolaryngol Clin N Am 50 (2017) 245–255
http://dx.doi.org/10.1016/j.otc.2016.12.003
0030-6665/17/© 2016 Elsevier Inc. All rights reserved.

oto.theclinics.com

negative margins. This presents a unique surgical challenge in that these lesions lie within a region of densely populated anatomic real estate where extension of tumors beyond the confines of their site of origin may put highly important structures at great risk. This fact reinforces the importance of complete preoperative work-up and a sound anatomic understanding.

ANTERIOR VENTRAL SKULL BASE
Nasal Cavity

The nasal cavity forms the corridor though which sinonasal and ventral skull base malignancies may be approached. This corridor serves many physiologic functions that can be compromised during endonasal surgery of these lesions. The nasal cavity is lined with ciliated respiratory epithelium, which aids in transport of a bilayer mucus blanket designed as a first line of defense against pathogens and irritants. Dysfunction of this mucosal lining may lead to stagnation of mucus, crusting, infection, and secondary osteitis. This mucosa may be used to reconstruct defects created by surgery in the form of local axial flaps. The nasoseptal flap and the inferior turbinate or lateral wall flap are two examples. In the midline the nasal septum is formed as a coalescence of the quadrangular cartilage anteriorly, the vomer inferior and posteriorly, and the perpendicular plate of the ethmoid bone superior and posteriorly. The mucosa covering the septum receives its blood supply from multiple sources, chiefly the labial artery anteriorly, the anterior and posterior ethmoidal arteries, and the posterior septal branch of the sphenopalatine artery at the posterior aspect. The posterior septal branch is preserved and used to form the pedicle for the nasoseptal flap. The high septal mucosa is termed olfactory epithelium because it harbors the olfactory fila transmitted via the cribriform plate. These are preserved if the dissection does not travel high into the nasal vault until the head of the middle turbinate, a rough landmark for the anterior limit of the cribriform, is reached. Along the lateral wall of the nasal cavity lie the turbinates. The inferior turbinate is a process of the maxillary bone and posteriorly the palatine bone. Its role in the nasal cavity seems to be related to aid in the dispersion of airflow throughout the nasal cavity allowing for efficient warming and humidification of air before passing to the lungs. These structures can become enlarged affecting transnasal surgical access; however, caution should be taken when considering removal unless tumor dictates. Complete removal of the inferior turbinate is a risk factor for development of paradoxic congestion despite adequate airway space, often with associated crusting and nasal dryness.[1] "Outfracture" or lateralization of these structures is often sufficient to provide additional space after topical decongestion has been performed. The middle turbinate is a product of the ethmoid bone and is situated in the mid nasal cavity forming the medial aspect of the middle meatus. It has multiple attachment sites, one oriented vertically attaching to the skull base and the other, termed the basal lamella, to the lateral wall. The basal lamella anatomically separates the anterior and posterior ethmoid air cells, and it is just anterior to this structure that the sphenopalatine artery emerges from the pterygopalatine space. The middle turbinate increases the overall surface area of the nasal mucosa and when pneumatized has been postulated to have a protective effect against allergens.[2] When using the nasal cavity as a corridor for tumor extirpation, this structure presents a challenge in terms of access and management. Some argue for preservation of these structures when possible, whereas others advocate removal. For tumors of the anterior ventral skull base the middle turbinate is generally removed early. Studies looking at the effects of turbinate removal have not brought consensus as to the effect of this removal.[3] When approaching the posterior skull base, the middle turbinate may be preserved by lateralization with firm but gentle pressure so as to minimize mucosal trauma and subsequent bleeding. This significantly narrows the middle meatus and the turbinate does not typically recover its normal position. Lateralization has been studied after sinus surgery and it does not seem to correlate with increase in patient symptoms.[4] The group did elucidate that the frontal sinus may be affected by this phenomenon; however, this is likely secondary to scarring after the frontal recess has been dissected for sinus disease.

The Skull Base

The anterior ventral skull base is comprised chiefly of the ethmoid and frontal bones, with the posterior third being formed by the planum sphenoidale. The components of the ethmoid bone are the cribriform plate and crista gali centrally; the roof or fovea ethmoidalis superiorly; the lamina papyracea laterally; and the perpendicular plate, which joins with the vomer inferiorly. The ethmoidal air cells lie within the bounds of the frontal recess anteriorly to the face of the sphenoid sinus posteriorly. The most anterior ethmoid air cell is termed the agger nasi cell and endoscopically appears as a bulge of the lateral wall at the axilla of the middle turbinate. The agger nasi cell is consistently present in more than 90% of cases.[5] Removal of this cell and its roof or "cap" is a key in the operative unveiling of the frontal sinus outflow pathway. Beyond the frontal outflow, moving posteriorly, lies the supraorbital ethmoid cell. This cell is present in just over 50% of cases and helps one to identify the position of the anterior ethmoidal artery.[6] The anterior ethmoidal artery may persist within a mesentery below the skull base within the posterior wall of this cell, or be found at the anterior ventral skull base just beneath a thin layer of bone. In any case it is reliably found within, or in continuity with, the posterior wall of the supraorbital ethmoid cell.[6] Its trajectory is oblique, moving anteriorly as is courses from the medial orbit across the skull base medially (**Fig. 1**A). This subtle finding is helpful in cases where the artery is not obvious. Proceeding more posterior, the posterior ethmoidal artery is encountered after a distance of 10 to 12 mm from the anterior ethmoidal artery as it exits the orbit. This artery is typically found within the bone of the anterior ventral skull base, taking a more direct course medially as it traverses the skull base. After the ethmoid air cells have been cleared from the skull base and the ethmoidal arteries controlled, completion of a

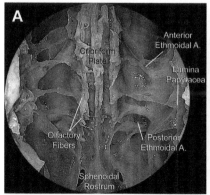 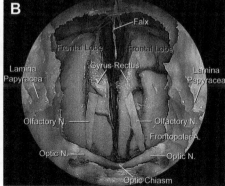

Fig. 1. (A) Endoscopic view of the anterior cranial base following complete ethmoidectomy and resection of the middle turbinates. Mucosa is removed. Note the anterior ethmoid artery running in the posterior wall of the suprabullar cell at *left*. (B) Endoscopic view of the anterior cranial fossa after osteotomy and dural resection are completed.

Draf III frontal sinusotomy may be performed. This procedure removes a portion of the high anterior septum just in front of the middle turbinate and unifies the frontal sinuses into a common cavity (horseshoe shaped) allowing access to the anterior portion of the cribriform. Traditionally, the first olfactory fila was identified along the lateral lamella of the cribriform heralding the posterior limit of the dissection at the outside. In recent years this practice has fallen out of vogue with some citing a risk of creating a cerebrospinal fluid leak. In any case these fibers are often seen at some point in the course of the dissection. After completing the Draf III, osteotomies along the fovea ethmoidalis bilaterally are made. The anterior osteotomy should only be made after dissecting the crista gali free from the falx cerebri. After bony removal is completed only the dura separates the surgeon from the fronto-orbital branches of the anterior cerebral artery (**Fig. 1**B). These vessels supply the olfactory bulbs and the cortical surface. Medially the frontopolar vessels run within the interhemispheric fissure. When tumor is present care must be taken as dissection is carried to the superior aspect of the tumor because the fronto-orbital vessels often lie draped over the top. These vessels are intimately associated with the gyrus rectus and olfactory bulbs on each side of the falx.

Olfaction is an important sensory function unique to the nasal cavity and an important part of the human experience. The olfactory bulbs lie within the ventral skull base on the intracranial side of the cribriform plate transmitting sensory fila via tiny perforations in the bone. Overlying these fila is the olfactory epithelium, which exists in specific distributions within the nasal cavity. This lining may be preserved in some cases of malignancy to maximize the chance of olfaction postsurgically. However, this should not influence the decision to obtain negative surgical margins intraoperatively. The anterior ventral skull base is a region often involved in sinonasal malignancy. Intricate knowledge of the vascular anatomy is important because these vessels are often involved as "feeder" vessels to tumors. Appropriate patient counseling regarding expected functional outcomes after surgery with regard to sense of smell is also important because this is often impacted during surgery in this region.

SPHENOID SINUS AND POSTERIOR VENTRAL SKULL BASE
Sphenoid Sinus

The sphenoid sinus lies at the far posterior aspect of the nasal cavity. The sphenoid ostium lies at the inferomedial aspect of the sphenoethmoidal recess, usually veiled behind the superior turbinate. The superior turbinate also arises from the ethmoid bone, and contains a small fraction of olfactory epithelium. It is a reliable landmark for the sphenoid ostium, which lies inferomedially to it. The superior turbinate is sometimes resected during sphenoid sinus exposure. After removal of the inferior half of the superior turbinate, the ostium usually comes into view. The sinus should be entered in a safe fashion, low and medial, to avoid injury to critical structures that lie beyond. Whether a transethmoidal approach or transnasal approach is taken, the point of entry is the same. In the case of an Onodi cell, the posterior-most ethmoid cell may extend beyond the face of the sphenoid pushing it inferiorly. This is significant because the optic canal often has bony dehiscences, and if the surgeon presumes to be in the sphenoid when actually in an Onodi cell, there is potential for injury to the optic nerve. This finding is easily noted preoperatively by careful examination of the preoperative imaging. Within the sphenoid sinus are several important anatomic landmarks that are easily seen in a well-pneumatized sinus (**Fig. 2**). These landmarks serve as a roadmap for surgical dissection, but also demonstrate the proximity of the sinus to crucial structures. The sphenoid pneumatization is generally categorized into one of three

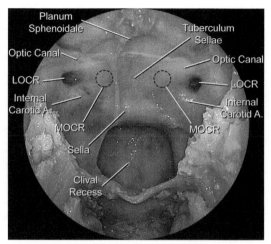

Fig. 2. Close-up image of the sellar anatomy from endoscopic transphenoidal approach. LOCR, lateral opticocarotid recess; MOCR, medial opticocarotid recess.

distinct classifications: (1) conchal, (2) presellar, or (3) sellar (although a postsellar configuration has been described). Identification of landmarks is typically the most challenging in the conchal pattern because of masking by thick bone. Pneumatization of the lateral recess of the sphenoid sinus expands the cavity further in some cases. The sella turcica lies centrally and is situated above the clival recess in a pneumatized sinus. The lateral aspects of the clival recess may at times look like pillars because of the bony covering of the paraclival carotid artery segments. Adjacent to the sella, the carotid prominences may be seen often given away by a telltale pinkish hue appreciated by the keen observer. The carotid prominence, or paraclinoidal carotid segment, is the anterior-most projection of the carotid because it loops back on itself wrapping about a small bony depression. This depression is the middle clinoid, which may be removed in cases where a complete bony ring connecting the anterior and middle is not present. Superolateral to the prominence lies a depression in the bone indicating the lateral opticocarotid recess, and the optic nerve immediately superior. The medial opticocarotid recess lies approximately 5 mm medial to the lateral opticocarotid recess and is also a consistent landmark (see **Fig. 2**).[7] The ophthalmic artery approaches the orbit along a path in the roof of the lateral opticocarotid recess nestled beneath the optic nerve. This becomes crucial during optic decompression because the dura around the optic nerve is always incised superiorly so as not to inadvertently injure this artery.

The Clivus

The clivus (latin for slope) extends from the dorsum sella and posterior clinoids to the foramen magnum, and is formed as a union of the sphenoid and occipital bones. It may be divided into thirds with the upper third discussed as the "sellar" clivus, which extends from the superior-most aspect down to sellar floor. Just below the level of the sellar floor, Dorello canal exists as a dural fold and carries the abducens nerve (cranial nerve [CN] VI). To gain surgical access in this region the exposure required is analogous to that of a transphenoidal pituitary approach. The lateral extent of the exposure proceeds to the cavernous sinus on both sides of the sella (**Fig. 3**A). The pituitary gland may be transposed to provide access to the posterior clinoids, and this may be

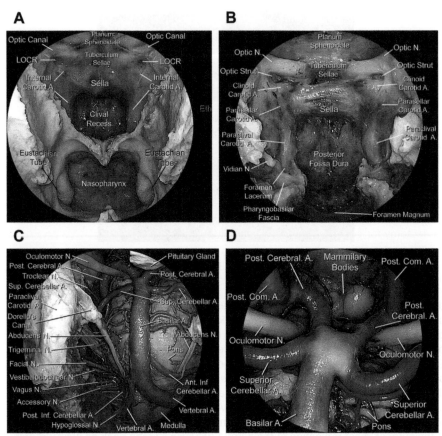

Fig. 3. (*A*) Bony anatomy of posterior nasal cavity following septectomy and dissection of the sphenoid sinus. (*B*) Bone removed over the tuberculum and extending inferiorly to the foramen magnum. (*C*) Endoscopic view following dural resection and posterior clinoidectomy to view posterior fossa contents. (*D*) Endoscopic view following dural resection and posterior clinoidectomy to view superior posterior fossa contents. LOCR, lateral optico-carotid recess.

performed in one of three fashions: (1) interdural, (2) intradural, or (3) extradural. Extradural dissection offers the least amount of manipulation to the gland and portends a lesser risk of postprocedural hypopituitarism. However, if further access is needed interdural dissection provides wider exposure to the posterior clinoid. When this is undertaken the anterior wall of the cavernous sinus is entered and the sinus bleeding must be packed off. The inferior hypophyseal artery, which provides nondominant supply to the gland, crosses the field and is transposed or sacrificed. Once the posterior clinoidectomy is performed and dura entered, the mammillary bodies are exposed along with the floor of the third ventricle, basilar artery, posterior and superior cerebellar arteries, and oculomotor (**Fig. 3**B).

The middle third of the clivus then begins and extends from the floor of the sella inferiorly to the level of the outer floor of the sphenoid sinus and foramen lacerum, where the carotid becomes horizontal and turns laterally. The foramen lacerum lies at the level of the superior aspect of the torus tubaris in close relationship to the cartilaginous eustachian tube.[8,9] Exposure through the mid clivus posteriorly opens into the prepontine cistern and reveals several crucial anatomic structures. Beyond the dura lie the basilar trunk, anterior inferior cerebellar artery, CN VI, and the ventral pons with perforators arising from the basilar trunk. If the paraclival carotid artery is freed of bony obstruction and is lateralized, access to the petrous apex, tentorium, trochlear nerve, and posterior root of the trigeminal nerve (CN V) may be obtained.

Inferiorly, the lower clivus is covered by pharyngobasilar fascia, and the longus capitus and rectus capitus muscles. Access to the anterior surface of foramen magnum, C1, occipital condyles, apical ligament, and atlanto-occipital joint is gained following detachment of the previously mentioned musculature (**Fig. 3**C). Beyond this lies the premedullary cistern, which houses the vertebral arteries at their junction with the basilar artery, the posterior inferior cerebellar artery, anterior spinal arteries, hypoglossal canal and nerves, the lower CNs, and the ventral medulla (**Fig. 3**D).

The middle and lower clivus may serve as a surgical corridor for pathologies, such as chondrosarcoma, chordoma, and any tumor with an origin in the clivus. Again, access in this region begins with a large sphenoidotomy, and in this case posterior low septectomy for access. The paraclival carotid arteries are identified but not necessarily exposed unless surgery dictates. Fascia is elevated from the inferior margin of the sphenoidotomy and a nasopharyngectomy is performed typically using needle-tipped cautery and suction or microdebrider. Here, thought may be given to preserving a portion of the nasopharyngeal mucosa and musculature to aid in reconstruction where dural disruption or resection is anticipated. At the lateral aspect of the dissection the supracondylar groove is identified, which aids in locating the hypoglossal canal. This structure is a ridge of bone onto which the rectus capitus muscle attaches. After clearing the fascia from the superior aspect at the sphenoid floor, to the inferior aspect at the foramen magnum, drilling may proceed. Beginning superiorly, the floor of the sphenoid is taken posteriorly to the limit of the clival recess in a pneumatized sinus. If underpneumatization is present a recess must be created and in either case the lateral limit is the paraclival carotid artery. When pneumatization is suboptimal, Doppler sonography and image guidance aid to identify the carotid arteries. After the superior drilling is complete, the remaining inferior clivus is drilled to the level of the inner cortex, thinned, and removed with a Kerrison rongeur. Proceeding through the dura, one should be aware of the presence of the venous plexus, which lies sandwiched between the periosteal and meningeal layers of the dura. This plexus may be packed off with flowable gelfoam. The basilar artery is identified with Doppler before entering the meningeal layer, and care should be taken also to identify and avoid the abducens nerves.

PTERYGOPALATINE FOSSA AND BEYOND
The Maxillary Sinus

The maxillary sinus lies lateral to the nasal cavity and inferior to the orbit, and may serve as a potential site of growth for malignant lesions. The orbital floor bounds the cavity superiorly, and carries within it the second branch of the CN V, or V2. Larger lesions may extend their reach beyond the sinus and into the orbit through this very thin bone. Furthermore, the presence of V2 provides a potential route of spread intracranially via the foramen rotundum.

Posteriorly, the sinus is bounded by the pterygopalatine fossa (PPF). Within this small space there are contained several important neurovascular structures. The internal maxillary artery (IMAX) gives rise to several branches that supply the nasal cavity and lies within the PPF exiting medially via a foramen hidden just posterior to the bony structure, the crista ethmoidalis (**Fig. 4**A). If not needed for reconstructive purposes

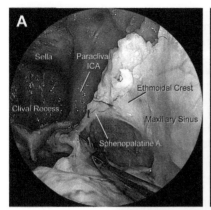
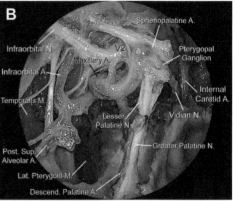
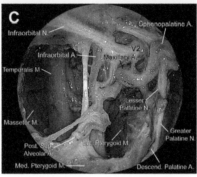

Fig. 4. (A) Endoscopic view of lateral nasal wall (*left*) with mucosa reflected and middle turbinate removed. (B) Endoscopic view of the pterygopalatine space with bone and fat removed. (C) Endoscopic view of the pterygopalatine space and infratemporal fossa contents, looking slightly more lateral than in B. ICA, internal carotid artery.

the artery should be dealt with definitively to prevent blood loss. The vidian nerve, made of contributions from the greater superficial petrosal nerve and the deep petrosal nerve, carries preganglionic parasympathetics to the pterygopalatine ganglion via the greater superficial petrosal nerve, whereas the deep petrosal nerve contributes sympathetics (which do not synapse at the ganglion). The pterygopalatine ganglion lies within the PPF space, and gives rise to postganglionic parasympathetic fibers (**Fig. 4**B). The parasympathetic and sympathetic branches supply the mucosa of the nose, soft palate, tonsils, uvula, hard palate, upper lip, gums, and upper pharynx. There is additional parasympathetic contribution to the lacrimal gland carried via the zygomatic branches of the ophthalmic nerve (V1) entering the orbit via the inferior orbital fissure. Disruption of these fibers may lead to dry eye and thus should be kept in mind when extirpation of tumors from this region requires their sacrifice. The descending palatine artery and nerves are transmitted inferiorly to supply the hard palate via the greater palatine foramen.

The medial wall of the sinus is made up of contributions from the palatine bone. At its anterior-most aspect lies the natural ostium of the sinus and just beyond this the lacrimal sac, which lies within the frontal process of the maxilla. The mucocilliary flow within the sinus directs all sinus output via this singular ostium, therefore it is optimal for this to remain as undisturbed as possible. The inferior turbinate originates from this medial wall and overrides the valve of Hasner (nasolacrimal duct opening).

Tumor invasion of the sac or postsurgical scarring of the valve may lead to epiphora. Attention to this preoperatively may indicate intraoperative dacrocystorhinostomy to avoid this complication. If the valve or sac must be taken for margins or involvement, it is best to use cold steel as opposed to cautery because the latter method may encourage scar more than the former. The anterior and lateral boundaries are the malar region anteriorly with maxillary bone and the lateral portion of the maxilla, which opens toward the masticator space. Inferiorly, the floor is made up of the maxilla. Opening of the maxillary sinus is an integral step in several approaches to sinonasal and ventral skull base tumors and should be done in a manner that preserves function when possible and yet allows visualization of important landmarks.

Transpterygoid Approach

As tumors transgress into the lateral recess of the sphenoid, middle fossa, infrapetrous skull base, medial infratemporal fossa (ITF), and Meckel cave, the PPF and pterygoid serve as an anatomic corridor for endonasal access.[10,11] Discussed previously are a great number of important structures one must consider when embarking though this corridor. The transpterygoid approach uses knowledge of boundaries and structures to allow the resection to proceed more laterally. Importantly, preservation of some of these structures along this corridor may be achieved. To proceed through this corridor, a maxillary antrostomy is usually made to expose the posterior wall of the sinus. The crista ethmoidalis is used as a bony landmark to identify the position of the Sphenopalatine Artery branch emerging into the nasal cavity. This opening is then used to begin removing the posterior wall of the sinus, exposing the PPF contents still encased in their periosteal lining. Inferomedially lies the greater palatine canal and its contents. This canal forms a groove at the intersection the maxillary bone and the perpendicular plate of the palatine bone. The vidian nerve is typically identified as it tracks posteriorly eventually passing lateral to the petrous carotid artery. Subperiosteal dissection of the PPF contents proceeds to expose the foramen rotundum, maxillary strut, and inferior orbital fissure. Once anterior exposure has been achieved, the medial dissection can begin. The orbital, sphenoid, and perpendicular processes of the palatine bone may be removed. As the sphenoid process is dissected, the palatovaginal canal and its pharyngeal artery are identified. This artery is generally transected to remove the sphenoid sinus floor. If preservation of the vidian nerve is desired, the vidian canal can be exposed along its length and the bone flaked off with a dissector. This maneuver allows the pterygoid plates to be exposed and drilled away.

Transmaxillary Approach

The contralateral transmaxillary approach expends the lateral extent of the surgical field and may be combined with a transpterygoid approach on the ipsilateral side if necessary. The concept is much the same as striking the ideal billiard shot aiming across the table toward the corner as opposed to aiming down the length of the table. To make this approach work a "mega antrostomy" or medial maxillectomy and a posterior septectomy must be performed to accommodate the instruments and scope reaching across the nasal cavity.[12,13] Once completed, a gingivobuccal sulcus incision is made, taking care to preserve a cuff of mucosa along the gingiva as is performed when approaching the maxilla for trauma. Periosteal elevators of choice are used to expose the face of the maxilla and the infraorbital nerve preserved when possible. The key landmark is a depression in the face just superior to the canine tooth root appropriately named the canine fossa. The location is a reliable landmark; however, confirming with imaging guidance aids in the avoidance of tooth roots, a potential complication of this approach. The canine fossa is an area of thin bone and is entered with a small 3- to 5-mm drill. Often, the aperture is widened with Kerrison rongeurs to the desired size. Logically, expansion of the opening laterally extends the angle of approach to the contralateral side. This "third" aperture shifts the port of entry to the contralateral side of the surgical field by delivering the scope and a suction or dissector through the maxillary sinus and the second suction or dissector via the adjacent nostril. This approach alters the angle of approach in the coronal plane substantially allowing far lateral dissection to proceed in a safe fashion.

Infratemporal Fossa

The ITF is a space located beneath the floor of the middle cranial fossa and posterior to the maxilla that contains the parapharyngeal and masticator spaces. Tumors in this region have traditionally been approached via open surgical approaches, but may be accessed endoscopically. This space is in continuity with the PPF via the pterygomaxillary fissure. The parapharyngeal space is divided into a prestyloid and poststyloid compartment by the styloid and the stylopharyngeal aponeurosis. The prestyloid space is fat containing and situated between the medial pterygoid and the tensor veli palatini muscles. The poststyloid compartment houses the internal carotid artery, internal jugular vein, and lower CNs (IX–XII). The masticator space contains the medial and lateral pterygoid muscles, the temporalis tendon insertion onto the coronoid process, the IMAX, the mandibular branch of CN V (V3), the tensor and levator veli palatini muscles, the styloid diaphragm, and the eustachian tube. To access this space and the contents within, the steps to a transpterygoid approach are followed. The descending palatine bundle is typically sacrificed to access deeper and more lateral structures in this case. The orbital process of the palatine bone is removed and the PPF contents are mobilized laterally. The vidian nerve is identified but may require sacrifice to mobilize tissues to access the ITF. The medial pterygoid plate must be completely removed to expose the underlying musculature attaching to the medial aspect of the lateral pterygoid plate (**Fig. 4**C). The anterior genu and horizontal carotid segments of the carotid are identified and IMAX branches ligated as appropriate. This approach is typically sufficient to allow resection of tumors near the cartilaginous segment of the eustachian tube.[14] If further access is needed the lateral pterygoid must be addressed. First the attaching muscles (medially the medial pterygoid muscle, and laterally the lateral pterygoid muscle) must be dissected away from the plate itself. Muscle bleeding is controlled via bipolar cautery, hemostatic agents, or pressure. In these cases, postoperative outcome is sacrificed for tumor control in that the resection/dissection of the pterygoid musculature generally leads to trismus secondary to scarring.

SUMMARY

Endoscopic technology has greatly changed the way in which sinonasal and ventral skull base malignancy is approached surgically. The anatomy of this region is dense and complex, with many structures lying encased in bone. In light of this, a detailed understanding of the important anatomy must be obtained and understood. The "inside out" approach coming from an endonasal perspective presents unique surgical challenges while offering the possibility of decreased morbidity and increased patient safety. Continued education and research to this end adds to the collective knowledge and experience, effectively pushing the frontiers and challenging surgical dogma.

REFERENCES

1. Scheithauer MO. Surgery of the turbinates and "empty nose" syndrome. GMS Curr Top Otorhinolaryngol Head Neck Surg 2010;9:Doc03.

2. Worrall DM, Campbell RG, Palmer JN, et al. Concha bullosa: a shield against allergens? ORL J Otorhinolaryngol Relat Spec 2015;77:281–6.
3. Choby GW, Hobson CE, Lee S, et al. Clinical effects of middle turbinate resection after endoscopic sinus surgery: a systematic review. Am J Rhinol Allergy 2014; 28:502–7.
4. Bassiouni A, Chen PG, Naidoo Y, et al. Clinical significance of middle turbinate lateralization after endoscopic sinus surgery. Laryngoscope 2015;125:36–41.
5. Bolger WE, Butzin CA, Parsons DS. Paranasal sinus bony anatomic variations and mucosal abnormalities: CT analysis for endoscopic sinus surgery. Laryngoscope 1991;101:56–64.
6. Jang DW, Lachanas VA, White LC, et al. Supraorbital ethmoid cell: a consistent landmark for endoscopic identification of the anterior ethmoidal artery. Otolaryngol Head Neck Surg 2014;151:1073–7.
7. Nunes CF, Prevedello DM, Carrau RL, et al. Morphometric analysis of the medial opticocarotid recess and its anatomical relations relevant to the transsphenoidal endoscopic endonasal approaches. Acta Neurochir (Wien) 2016;158:319–24.
8. Liu J, Pinheiro-Neto CD, Fernandez-Miranda JC, et al. Eustachian tube and internal carotid artery in skull base surgery: an anatomical study. Laryngoscope 2014; 124:2655–64.
9. Sreenath SB, Recinos PF, McClurg SW, et al. The endoscopic endonasal approach to the hypoglossal canal: the role of the eustachian tube as a landmark for dissection. JAMA Otolaryngol Head Neck Surg 2015;141:927–33.
10. Pinheiro-Neto CD, Fernandez-Miranda JC, Prevedello DM, et al. Transposition of the pterygopalatine fossa during endoscopic endonasal transpterygoid approaches. J Neurol Surg B Skull Base 2013;74:266–70.
11. Patel CR, Fernandez-Miranda JC, Wang WH, et al. Skull base anatomy. Otolaryngol Clin North Am 2016;49:9–20.
12. Harvey RJ, Sheehan PO, Debnath NI, et al. Transseptal approach for extended endoscopic resections of the maxilla and infratemporal fossa. Am J Rhinol Allergy 2009;23:426–32.
13. Wang EW, Gullung JL, Schlosser RJ. Modified endoscopic medial maxillectomy for recalcitrant chronic maxillary sinusitis. Int Forum Allergy Rhinol 2011;1:493–7.
14. Taylor RJ, Patel MR, Wheless SA, et al. Endoscopic endonasal approaches to infratemporal fossa tumors: a classification system and case series. Laryngoscope 2014;124:2443–50.

Staging of Sinonasal and Ventral Skull Base Malignancies

Dipan D. Desai, BS[a], Bryan M. Brandon, MD[a],
Elizabeth L. Perkins, MD[a], Charles S. Ebert, MD, MPH[a],
Adam M. Zanation, MD[a,b], Brian D. Thorp, MD[a,*]

KEYWORDS

- Paranasal sinus malignancy • Cancer staging • Skull base • Head and neck cancer

KEY POINTS

- Sinonasal and skull base malignancies typically present at a late stage and have poor overall prognosis.
- This understudied group of tumors includes an incredibly diverse set of pathologies with varying characteristics and etiologies.
- The American Joint Committee on Cancer has established a common staging system for all sinonasal malignancies.
- Many staging systems exist for a specific pathology and often have established prognostic value.
- Thorough evaluation and imaging, and an awareness of certain characteristic tumor patterns of spread, are keys to accurate staging and guide optimal treatment.

INTRODUCTION

Paranasal sinus and skull base malignancies include a heterogeneous group of tumors with widely varying histology and prognosis. Because of typically late presentation and the frequent involvement of critical structures, including the orbit and brain, these tumors represent a great challenge for head and neck surgeons and oncologists.

Perhaps adding to this complexity is that paranasal sinus malignancies remain an uncommon and rare entity in Western countries. The incidence of these cancers is estimated to be less than 1 per 100,000 individuals per year, and they represent

Conflict of Interest Statement: There are no conflicts of interest in the production of this article.
[a] Department of Otolaryngology/Head and Neck Surgery, 170 Manning Drive, CB 7070, Chapel Hill, NC 27599, USA; [b] Department of Neurosurgery, 170 Manning Drive, CB 7060, Chapel Hill, NC 27599, USA
* Corresponding author.
E-mail address: brian_thorp@med.unc.edu

Otolaryngol Clin N Am 50 (2017) 257–271
http://dx.doi.org/10.1016/j.otc.2016.12.004
oto.theclinics.com

only a small fraction of the total number of head and neck cancers.[1,2] Most of these cancers are located in either the maxillary sinus or nasal cavity, with cancers of other sinuses occurring more infrequently. Although varied based on specific tumor histology, these cancers are most frequently diagnosed during or after the sixth decade of life.[2] These neoplasms also have unique risk factors. Contributing factors for other head and neck cancers, such as tobacco use, alcohol abuse, and human papillomavirus, do not seem to be strongly correlated with these tumors. Instead, occupational hazards and long-term inhalation of industrial toxins have historically been linked to the development of paranasal sinus malignancies, possibly by promoting chronic inflammation.[3] Specifically, workers in the furniture, textile, and leather industries have been shown to be at increased risk.[4–6]

Although often discussed as a group because of their rarity, paranasal sinus and ventral skull base malignancies include more than 40 unique histologies (**Box 1**), as classified by the World Health Organization.[7] These etiologies are broadly subclassified into epithelial or nonepithelial malignancies. Squamous cell carcinoma (SCC), adenocarcinoma, and sinonasal undifferentiated carcinoma (SNUC) are common epithelial pathologies, whereas rhabdomyosarcoma and lymphomas are well-known nonepithelial tumors that occur in this region. Overall, SCC has been reported to be the most common of these histologies and comprises between 36% and 58% of all paranasal sinus cancers, followed in frequency by adenocarcinoma, mucosal melanoma, esthesioneuroblastoma (ENB), and adenoid cystic carcinoma.[1,2,8]

STAGING

Because of this remarkably wide variety of histologies, the development of a comprehensive staging system with prognostic relevance for each tumor subtype and anatomic location has historically presented a unique challenge. The first major effort to elucidate prognostic variables was made by Ohngren in 1936.[9] He proposed an imaginary line, now referred to as the Ohngren line, running from the angle of the mandible to the medial canthus. He described that lesions located anterior and/or inferior to this line seemed to have an improved prognosis and higher likelihood of complete resection. In contrast, tumors located posterior and/or superior to this line, including those of the frontal, ethmoid, and sphenoid sinus, were more difficult to resect and frequently involved high-value structures of the head and neck, thus portending an overall poorer prognosis.

Today, the paranasal sinuses and nasal cavity are incorporated into conventional TNM classifications by the American Joint Committee on Cancer (AJCC).[10] This system is primarily structured by the extent of tumor invasion (**Table 1**). Because of this focus on the involvement of specific structures rather than the total lesion size, the system features separate "T" classifications for maxillary tumors and nasal cavity/ethmoid tumors. Of note, this AJCC staging system does not include "T" staging for either sphenoid or frontal tumors. This TNM system is also used to further categorize these malignancies into stages I to IV for prognostic purposes. Using data from the National Cancer Data Base for patients diagnosed with any nasal or sinus malignancy in 1998 to 1999, the AJCC reported a relative 5-year survival rate of 63% for stage I tumors, 61% for stage II tumors, 50% for stage III, and only 35% for stage IV.[10]

Unfortunately, because specific cancer pathology is a major determinant of survival and neck metastases are relatively uncommon for paranasal sinus and ventral skull base malignancies, this TNM classification system may not be as clinically useful for

Box 1
Histologic classification of paranasal sinus malignancies

Epithelial Malignancies

Squamous cell carcinoma
  Verrucous carcinoma
  Papillary squamous cell carcinoma
  Basaloid squamous cell carcinoma
  Spindle cell carcinoma
  Adenosquamous carcinoma
  Acantholytic squamous cell carcinoma

Lymphoepithelial carcinoma

Sinonasal undifferentiated carcinoma

Adenocarcinoma
  Intestinal-type adenocarcinoma
  Nonintestinal-type adenocarcinoma

Salivary gland-type carcinomas
  Adenoid cystic carcinoma
  Acinic cell carcinoma
  Mucoepidermoid carcinoma
  Epithelial-myoepithelial carcinoma
  Clear cell carcinoma not otherwise specified
  Myoepithelial carcinoma
  Carcinoma ex pleomorphic adenoma
  Polymorphous low-grade adenocarcinoma

Neuroendocrine tumors
  Typical carcinoid
  Atypical carcinoid

Small cell carcinoma, neuroendocrine type

Nonepithelial Malignancies

Soft tissue malignancies
  Fibrosarcoma
  Malignant fibrous histiocytoma
  Leiocyosarcome
  Rhabdomyosarcoma
  Angiosarcoma
  Malignant peripheral nerve sheath tumor

Bone and cartilage malignancies
  Chondrosarcoma
  Mesenchymal chondrosarcoma
  Osteosarcoma
  Chordoma

Hematolymphoid malignancies
  Extranodal natural killer/T-cell lymphoma
  Diffuse large B-cell lymphoma
  Extramedullary plasmacytoma
  Extramedullary myeloid sarcoma
  Histiocytic sarcoma
  Langerhans cell histiocytosis

Neuroectodermal malignancies
  Ewing sarcoma
  Primitive neuroectodermal tumor
  Olfactory neuroblastoma

Melanotic neuroectodermal tumor of infancy
Mucosal malignant melanoma

Germ cell malignancies
Teratoma with malignant tranformation
Sinonasal teratocarcinosarcoma

Adapted from Ho AS, Zanation A, Ganly I. Malignancies of the paranasal sinus. Cummings otolaryngology. 6th edition. Philadelphia: Elsevier; 2015. p. 1176–201; with permission.

determining prognosis as comparable systems for other head and neck cancers.[11] Because of this complexity, a variety of alternative or modified staging systems have been developed for specific tumor subtypes. This article reviews specific systems of staging for common sinonasal/ventral skull base pathologies and their utility in determining prognosis.

EVALUATION

The presenting symptoms of sinonasal and ventral skull base malignancies are typically nonspecific and, therefore, can make early diagnosis difficult. This is in part because many of the most frequently seen symptoms of these tumors, namely nasal obstruction, pain, swelling, and nasal discharge, are also seen with benign inflammatory or allergic disease processes.[12] However, certain features at the time of presentation may provide specific value. New-onset of unilateral sinonasal symptoms or obstruction in a previously healthy patient should raise the index of suspicion for a potential malignancy.[13] Additionally, if a malignancy is suspected, evidence of local tumor invasion may be present. Signs of tumor invasion vary based on the involved anatomic structure and can include diplopia (orbital involvement), trismus (pterygoid musculature invasion), hearing loss (Eustachian tube or prevertebral musculature involvement), epiphora (lacrimal duct invasion), and/or cranial nerve palsy or paralysis.[14] Additionally, cervical lymphadenopathy, when present, may narrow the differential diagnosis to certain pathologies and typically indicates a worse prognosis.[15] Overall, the presence of these symptoms offers valuable clinical risk stratification and a preliminary understanding of disease progression and prognosis.

IMAGING AND TESTING

Thorough imaging is a prerequisite of sinonasal cancer staging and plays a crucial role in determining appropriate treatment plans. To fully evaluate the lesion, a fine-cut computed tomography (CT) in all three planes and MRI are needed. These technologies each provide complementary information and together allow for near-ideal determination of tumor extension.[16] The CT is a convenient and easily tolerated imaging modality that highlights bony involvement and allows the surgeon to determine whether the tumor has extended beyond the bony borders of the originating sinus or into adjacent structures, such as the lamina papyracea and/or ventral skull base. Additionally, because CT imaging also highlights calcified deposits and cartilage, it may provide evidence of a particular tumor etiology, such as certain sarcomas or ENB.[14] In contrast, MRI offers a superior view of soft tissues because of its variety of sequences. Thus, it provides a more precise delineation of dural, vascular, and/ or muscular involvement.[17] Because involvement of many of these anatomic structures is a major component of the paranasal sinus cancer TNM staging criteria, evaluation of CT and MRI is of the utmost importance.

Table 1	
AJCC staging system for cancer of paranasal sinuses	
Primary Tumor (T)	
Maxillary sinus	
TX	Primary tumor cannot be assessed
T0	No evidence of primary tumor
Tis	Carcinoma in situ
T1	Tumor only in maxillary sinus mucosa, does not invade into bone
T2	Tumor invades bone, including extension into the hard palate and/or middle nasal meatus. Excludes extension into posterior wall of the maxillary sinus and pterygoid plates
T3	Tumor invasion into any of the following: posterior wall of the maxillary sinus, subcutaneous issues, floor or medial wall of the orbit, pterygoid fossa, ethmoid sinuses
T4a	Moderately advanced local disease: tumor invades the anterior orbital contents, skin of the cheek, pterygoid plates, infratemporal fossa, cribriform plate, sphenoid or frontal sinuses
T4b	Very advanced local disease: tumor invades any of the following: orbital apex, dura, brain, middle cranial fossa, cranial nerves other than maxillary division of trigeminal nerve (V2), nasopharynx, or clivus
Nasal cavity and ethmoid sinus	
TX	Primary tumor cannot be assessed
T0	No evidence of primary tumor
Tis	Carcinoma in situ
T1	Tumor only in the nasal cavity or one ethmoid sinus, with or without bony invasion
T2	Tumor invading multiple subsites in a single region or extending to involve an adjacent region within the nasoethmoidal complex, with or without bony invasion
T3	Tumor extends to invade the medial wall or floor of the orbit, maxillary sinus, palate, or cribriform plate
T4a	Moderately advanced local disease: tumor invades any of the following: anterior orbital contents, skin of the nose or cheek, minimal extension to the anterior cranial fossa, pterygoid plates, sphenoid or frontal sinuses
T4b	Tumor invades any of the following: orbital apex, dura, brain, middle cranial fossa, cranial nerves other than maxillary division of trigeminal nerve (V2), nasopharynx, or clivus
Regional Lymph Nodes (N)	
NX	Regional nodes cannot be assessed
N0	No regional lymph node metastasis
N1	Metastasis in a single ipsilateral lymph node ≤3 cm in greatest dimension
N2	Any of the following three conditions:
N2a	Metastasis in single ipsilateral lymph node >3 cm but not more than 6 cm in greatest dimension
N2b	Metastasis in multiple ipsilateral lymph nodes, none >6 m in greatest dimension

(continued on next page)

Table 1 (continued)			
Regional Lymph Nodes (N)			
N2c	Metastasis in bilateral or contralateral lymph nodes, none >6 cm in greatest dimension		
N3	Metastasis in a lymph node >6 cm in greatest dimension		
Distant Metastasis (M)			
M0			No distant metastasis
M1			Distant metastasis
Stage	**T**	**N**	**M**
0	Tis	N0	M0
I	T1	N0	M0
II	T2	N0	M0
III	T3	N0	M0
	T1	N1	
	T2	N1	
	T3	N1	
IVA	T4a	N0	M0
	T4a	N1	
	T1	N2	
	T2	N2	
	T3	N2	
	T4a	N2	
IVB	T any	N3	M0
	T4b	N any	
IVC	T any	N any	M1

Adapted from Edge S, Byrd DR, Compton CC, et al, editors. AJCC cancer staging manual. 7th edition. New York: Springer; 2011; with permission.

After obtaining comprehensive imaging, biopsy is necessary to establish a definitive tissue diagnosis. Although the nasal passages sometimes allow for direct access to sinonasal tumors, care must be taken not to violate normal tissue planes and complicate later resection. Difficult biopsies can instead be performed under general anesthesia.[13] Because of the histologic complexity of these cancers and potential for misdiagnosis, tissue diagnosis should ideally be made by an experienced head and neck pathologist.

Additional testing may become necessary in special circumstances, often based on the tumor histology. PET/CT is used to detect regional and distant metastases for advanced disease. Additionally, certain tumors have characteristic patterns of spread and may require pretreatment imaging of the chest/abdomen or a radionucleotide bone scan. Along with CT, MRI, and tissue biopsy, these tests ensure accurate staging and optimal treatment.

PATHOLOGIES
Sinonasal Esthesioneuroblastoma

Also known as olfactory neuroblastoma, ENB is a rare, sinonasal/ventral skull base malignancy that represents an estimated 3% to 6% of sinonasal/skull base cancers and has a peak incidence in the sixth decade of life.[2,18,19] Proper histologic diagnosis is difficult, and these tumors have frequently been mistaken for SNUC.[20,21] Because these cancers are believed to arise from neuroepithelial olfactory cells of the superior nasal cavity, they have a propensity to invade intracranially through the cribriform plate and anterior ventral skull base.[22] Additionally, ENB is notorious for producing local recurrence and distant metastasis, often up to 10 years after original treatment.[23–25] A meta-analysis by Gore and Zanation in 2009 evaluated a total of 678 patients and found a 20.2% rate of cervical metastasis. Among this subgroup, 61.7% had cervical metastasis that presented more than 6 months after time of diagnosis.[24] Furthermore, a recently published, multicenter study by Nalavenkata and colleagues[26] reported similar findings. In this study, 18 of 113 (15.9%) patients with ENB had cervical metastasis, and 55.5% of those were delayed.

Because of these unique patterns of spread and risk of metastasis, several specific staging systems have been developed.[27] Kadish and colleagues[28] first proposed an ENB staging system in 1976 that classified tumors into three categories (A–C) by location and extension but did not include either cervical or distant metastasis as staging variables. Recognizing that metastasis is a strong predictor of poor survival, Morita and colleagues[19] later updated the original Kadish system to include this information by a redefined stage C and introducing a new stage D (**Table 2**). This modified Kadish system typically allows for accurate staging using only standard CT and MRI imaging. Thus, it remains the most widely used clinical staging system today and has been shown to successfully predict outcomes and prognosis.[29,30] Additionally, the Hyams grading system assigns ENB tumors a grade of I to IV based on a variety of histopathologic findings, including nuclear polymorphism, mitotic activity, necrosis, architecture, and rosette formation (**Table 3**).[31] Recent studies by Kaur and colleagues[32] and Malouf and colleagues[33] have suggested that the Hyams grading system independently predicts prognosis for ENB and is complementary to staging, especially in advanced disease.

The rarity of this disease and its previous confusion with SNUC has made large-scale comparisons of the Kadish staging and Hyams grading systems difficult. The largest, single-institution series to date was conducted by Bell and colleagues[34] at MD Anderson. In this series, the 5- and 10-year overall survival was 75% and 55%, respectively. Of the 124 cases identified, 61% were low-grade, Hyams I/II tumors. Of note, these low-grade cases were less likely to recur and high-grade histology was significantly associated with reduced disease-specific survival. When using the Kadish staging system for the same cases, no significant differences in recurrence or survival were seen when comparing T, N, M, or overall stage. A large meta-analysis conducted by Dulguerov and coworkers[35] with a total of 390 patients from 26 studies revealed that for studies that included Hyams grading, patients with grade I and II tumors had a mean survival of 56%, as compared with 25% for those with grades III and IV. Meanwhile, 21 included studies that reported Kadish staging information revealed a mean survival of 72%, 59%, and 47% for stage A, B, and C tumors,

Table 2
Modified Kadish esthesioneuroblastoma staging system

Stage	Tumor Boundaries
A	Limited to nasal cavity
B	Confined to nasal and paranasal sinuses
C	Extending to cribriform plate, skull base, orbit, or intracranial cavity
D	Cervical or distant metastasis

Adapted from Morita A, Ebersold MJ, Olsen KD, et al. Esthesioneuroblastoma. Neurosurgery 1993;32(5):706–15.

Table 3
Hyams grading system for esthesioneuroblastoma

	Histologic Features				
Grade	Architecture	Mitotic Activity	Nuclear Pleomorphism	Rosettes	Necrosis
1	Lobular	Absent	Absent	HW ±	Absent
2	Lobular	Present	Moderate	HW ±	Absent
3	Variable	Prominent	Prominent	FW ±	± Present
4	Variable	Marked	Marked	Absent	Common

Abbreviations: FW, Flexner-Wintersteiner rosette; HW, Homer Wright pseudorosette.
Adapted from Hyams V. Tumors of the upper respiratory tract and ear. In: Hyams V, Batsakis L, Michaels L, editors. Atlas of tumor pathology. Washington, DC: Armed Forces Institute of Pathology; 1988. p. 240–8.

respectively.[35] Additional research is needed to fully elucidate the ideal use and prognostic relationship between the grading and clinical staging systems.

Sinonasal Undifferentiated Carcinoma

SNUC was originally described by Frierson and colleagues in 1986.[36] Since that time, it has become recognized as a rapidly progressive neuroendocrine malignancy with an age-adjusted incidence of about 0.02 per 100,000 individuals and a median age of diagnosis in the sixth decade of life.[37] These high-grade neoplasms lack squamous or glandular differentiation and frequently arise from the ethmoid sinuses. Immunohistochemistry analysis is often required to distinguish between SNUC and ENB pathology.[27] Most patients with SNUC are typically diagnosed with advanced disease extending beyond the paranasal sinuses. The most common sites of regional invasion in these patients are the orbit (53%) and ventral skull base (41%), and involvement of these sites is an indicator of poor prognosis.[38,39] In addition, cervical spread and distant metastasis to organs, such as the lungs and liver, are commonly present and further complicate treatment of these malignancies.[39] Each of these factors must be carefully evaluated when initially staging a patient with SNUC. SNUC is typically staged using the Kadish system, as described for ENB tumors or the AJCC TNM staging system for paranasal sinus malignancies (see **Table 1**).

Although outcomes have improved substantially from the median survival of 4 months originally reported by Frierson and colleagues, the prognosis for SNUC remains poor. A recent study by Chambers and colleagues[37] found a median survival of 22.1 months, and the 5-year overall survival has been reported to be between 22% and 35%.[2,39] A 2012 meta-analysis by Reiersen and colleagues[38] analyzed a total of 167 patients and found that nearly 50% of patients initially present with Kadish stage C disease. The prognostic impact of the Kadish staging system was relatively unclear because overall survival was 57.44% for Kadish stage A tumors, 34.21% for stage B tumors, and 47.56% for stage C tumors, albeit with shorter mean follow-up time for the stage C group. A recent study conducted by Kuan and colleagues[40] stratified survival by modified Kadish staging. Interestingly, in contrast to the previous meta-analysis, these authors found that increasing modified Kadish staging score was associated with significant decreases in overall and disease-specific survival. This finding was seen on univariate and multivariate analysis. The relative prognostic significance of commonly used staging systems for SNUC has yet to be fully evaluated and will likely be the topic of future research efforts.

Sinonasal Mucosal Melanoma

Mucosal melanoma is a rare malignancy, representing approximately 1% of total melanoma cases.[41] However, among these mucosal melanomas, more than half occur within the head and neck, often in the nasal cavity and paranasal sinuses.[42] As with many other sinonasal malignancies, these tumors occur most frequently in elderly patients. Of note, sinonasal mucosal melanoma may have unique characteristics that differ from its cutaneous counterparts, and classically important factors, such as depth of invasion and lactate dehydrogenase, are of less utility.[14] Furthermore, these neoplasms are remarkably aggressive and can often feature a rapid progression from initially asymptomatic disease to distant metastasis and mortality.[43]

Because of these characteristics and aggressive course, staging systems specifically adapted for sinonasal mucosal melanomas are of great importance and several have been proposed. Ballantyne[44] initially developed a simple staging system with three stages: confined to primary site (stage I), regional lymph node metastasis (stage II), and distant metastasis (stage III). Later, Prasad and colleagues[45] updated this system and incorporated depth of invasion to subcategorize Ballantyne stage I lesions into three levels. Notably, Thompson and colleagues[46] proposed a staging system based on a comprehensive survival analysis of 115 patients with mucosal melanoma. This system is similar to TNM staging and incorporates the classic primary determinants of prognosis: size, anatomic location, and presence of distant spread (**Table 4**). Classification of T1 versus T2 disease is based on the number of anatomic sites involved. Here, anatomic site refers to the nasal cavity, each of the major paranasal sinuses, and the nasopharynx. This staging system was found to significantly predict the likelihood of patient mortality in their group.[46]

Currently, the AJCC staging system for mucosal melanoma of the head and neck is the most commonly used and is in a classic TNM format (**Table 5**). Because of the aggressive nature and poor prognosis of these malignancies, mucosal melanomas are classified as T3 and therefore stage III at a minimum. Shuman and colleagues[47]

Table 4
Thompson staging system for sinonasal tract and nasopharynx mucosal malignant melanoma

Primary tumor (T)	
T1	Single anatomic site[a]
T2	Multiple anatomic sites[a]
Regional lymph nodes (N)	
N1	Any lymph node metastasis
Distant metastasis (M)	
M1	Distant metastasis
Stage grouping	
Stage I	T1 N0 M0
Stage II	T2 N0 M0
Stage III	Any T any N M1
Stage IV	Any T any N M1

[a] Anatomic sites: maxillary sinus, frontal sinus, sphenoid sinus, ethmoid sinus, nasopharynx, and nasal cavity.

Adapted from Thompson LDR, Wieneke JA, Miettinen M. Sinonasal tract and nasopharyngeal melanomas: a clinicopathologic study of 115 cases with a proposed staging system. Am J Surg Pathol 2003;27(5):594–611.

Table 5
AJCC staging of mucosal melanoma of the head and neck

Primary tumor (T)	
T3	Mucosal disease
T4a	Involvement of deep soft tissue, cartilage, bone, or overlying skin
T4b	Involvement of the brain, dura, skull base, lower cranial nerves, carotid artery, masticator space, or prevertebral space
Regional lymph nodes (N)	
NX	Regional lymph nodes cannot be assessed
N0	No regional lymph node metastases
N1	Regional lymph node metastases exists
Distant metastasis (M)	
M0	No distant metastasis
M1	Distant metastasis exists
Stage grouping	
Stage III	T3, N0, M0
Stage IVA	T4a, N0, M0 T3-T4a, N1, M0
Stage IVB	T4B, any N, M0
Stage IVC	Any T or N, M1

Adapted from Edge S, Byrd DR, Compton CC, et al, editors. AJCC cancer staging manual. 7th edition. New York: Springer; 2011; with permission.

conducted a study evaluating this system's prognostic value and found that individual T, N, and M stage, and overall AJCC stage, were each highly predictive of decreased overall and disease-free survival. Koivunen and colleagues[48] also studied this topic in a group of 50 patients with sinonasal mucosal melanoma. In this study, the overall 5-year survival was 27%, and T stage and AJCC stage were again found to be significantly associated with worse prognosis. These authors also evaluated the impact of tumor extension into local sites that are not currently included in the AJCC system. Of these, only sphenoid sinus involvement was significantly associated with differing prognosis.

Sinonasal Rhabdomyosarcoma

Rhabdomyosarcoma originates from primitive myogenic cells and is the most common sinonasal malignancy among children. These tumors appear as small round blue cells and are further classified into four distinct histologic groups with varying prognosis.[49] These subtypes (embryonic, alveolar, anaplastic, and undifferentiated), TNM staging, and postsurgical status have all been integrated into a single rhabdomyosarcoma staging system (**Table 6**). Of note, TNM staging for these neoplasms specifically includes a site of disease component, in addition to the typical tumor size, nodal involvement, and metastasis variables. Under this TNM system, rhabdomyosarcomas of the head and neck or orbit are classified as TNM stage I and have a relatively good prognosis, whereas parameningeal sites typically are classified as stage II or III with a worse prognosis. The postsurgical component of the staging system classifies surgical end results into four stages based on feasibility and completeness of resection.[50] Additionally, an embryonal histology decreases the overall risk category because it has a favorable prognosis and 5-year survival

Table 6				
Rhabdomyosarcoma staging				
TNM Stage	**Site**	**Tumor Size**	**Nodal Involvement**	**Metastasis**
I	Orbit Head and neck Genitourinary (nonbladder/ nonprostate)	<5 cm or >5 cm	Any N	M0
II	Bladder/prostate Extremity/trunk Parameningeal Other	<5 cm	N0	M0
III	Bladder/prostate Extremity/trunk Parameningeal Other	>5 cm <5 cm	Any N N1	M0
IV	All	—	—	M1

Clinical Group	**Definition**
I	Localized disease and completely removed Ia. Confined to original muscle/organ Ib. Invasion of outside muscle/organ and no regional nodes involved
II	Total gross resection with evidence of regional spread IIa. Grossly resected tumor with microscopic residual disease IIb. Regional disease with involved nodes, completely resected with no microscopic residual disease IIc. Regional disease with involved nodes. Grossly resected, but with evidence of microscopic residual and/or histologic involvement of the most distal regional node in the dissection
III	Incomplete resection
IV	Distant metastasis

Risk Group	**Definition**
Low	Stage I; embryonal histology; and clinical groups 1, 2, or 3 Stage II or III, embryonal histology, and clinical groups 1 or 2
Intermediate	Stage II or III, embryonal histology, and clinical group 3 Stage I, II, or III; alveolar histology
High	Stage IV

Adapted from Radzikowska J, Kukwa W, Kukwa A, et al. Rhabdomyosarcoma of the head and neck in children. Contemp Oncol (Pozn) 2015;19(2):98–107; with permission.

rate of 80%, compared with a corresponding rate of only 52% for alveolar subtypes.[51]

Sinonasal Squamous Cell Carcinoma

Among the many histologic subtypes of sinonasal and ventral skull base malignancies, SCC is the most common. SCC represents about 41% to 51% of these cancers and occurs most often in the nasal cavity and maxillary sinus.[2,52] Similar to other malignancies of this region, SCC typically has an insidious onset, and most patients present with advanced disease, often involving critical local structures or lymphatic metastasis.[53] Particularly high-risk subsites for neck metastasis include the nasal septum or columella.[13] SCC has also been shown to recur relatively rapidly, often within a

period of 3 years.[54] In addition to the previously mentioned industrial risk factors, human papillomavirus, specifically subtypes 6 and 11, also seems to play a role in development of SCC by promoting malignant transformation of sinonasal inverted papillomas.[55]

The current clinical consensus is that AJCC staging is appropriate for SCC and is predictive of survival. The relative 5-year survival for sinonasal SCC has been reported at about 53%.[2,52] Ansa and colleagues[56] conducted a study of sinonasal SCC using the Surveillance, Epidemiology and End Results program. These authors reported that increasing AJCC T stage was significantly associated with worse survival, even after controlling for other patient and tumor variables. The reported hazard ratios were 1.77 for T2 disease, 2.49 for T3, and 3.64 for T4 disease. Additionally, regional and distant disease stage, which correspond to modern N and M staging, were both also predictive of decreased survival in this study. A French study by Michel and colleagues[57] corroborated these findings and also found an improved survival for T1 and T2 disease, compared with advanced T3/T4 disease.

SUMMARY

The tremendous pathologic diversity among sinonasal and ventral skull base malignancies complicates the development of a uniform and prognostically relevant staging system. Moreover, because of the comparatively low incidence of these tumors, comprehensive evaluation and comparison of specific staging systems is difficult. Overall, the current AJCC TNM staging system for sinonasal malignancies is the most common and widely used system in current clinical practice. A variety of alternative systems have been proposed for use with individual histopathologic subtypes, including ENB, SNUC, and sinonasal mucosal melanoma. Many of these staging systems have been found to be of great utility and accurately predict patient survival. As strides in surgical and medical treatment of these malignancies continue, further research and adjustment of these current staging systems remains an important area of research.

REFERENCES

1. Dulguerov P, Jacobsen MS, Allal AS, et al. Nasal and paranasal sinus carcinoma: are we making progress? Cancer 2001;92(12):3012–29.
2. Turner JH, Reh DD. Incidence and survival in patients with sinonasal cancer: a historical analysis of population-based data. Head Neck 2011;34(6):877–85.
3. Llorente JL, López F, Suárez C, et al. Sinonasal carcinoma: clinical, pathological, genetic and therapeutic advances. Nat Rev Clin Oncol 2014;11(8):460–72.
4. Acheson ED, Cowdell RH, Hadfield E, et al. Nasal cancer in woodworkers in the furniture industry. BMJ 1968;2(5605):587–96.
5. Hernberg S, Westerholm P, Schultz-Larsen K, et al. Nasal and sinonasal cancer. Connection with occupational exposures in Denmark, Finland and Sweden. Scand J Work Environ Health 1983;9(4):315–26.
6. Luce D, Gérin M, Morcet JF, et al. Sinonasal cancer and occupational exposure to textile dust. Am J Ind Med 1997;32(3):205–10.
7. Barnes L, Eveson J, Reichart P. Pathology and genetics of head and neck tumours. Lyon (France): Oxford University Press; 2005.
8. Khademi B, Moradi A, Hoseini S, et al. Malignant neoplasms of the sinonasal tract: report of 71 patients and literature review and analysis. Oral Maxillofac Surg 2009;13(4):191–9.

9. Öhngren G. Malignant disease of the upper jaw: (Section of Laryngology and Section of Otology). Proc R Soc Med 1936;29(11):1497–514.
10. Cuccurullo V, Mansi L. AJCC cancer staging handbook: from the AJCC cancer staging manual (7th edition). Eur J Nucl Med Mol Imaging 2010;38(2):408.
11. Shah JP, Patel SG, Singh B. Jatin Shah's head and neck surgery and oncology: expert consult: online and print. Philadelphia (PA): Elsevier Science Health Science div; 2012.
12. Jackson RT, Fitz-Hugh GS, Constable WC. Malignant neoplasms of the nasal cavities and paranasal sinuses: (a retrospective study). Laryngoscope 1977;87(5):726–36.
13. Lund V. Malignant sinonasal tumors. Rhinology 2012;409–23.
14. Ho AS, Zanation A, Ganly I. Malignancies of the paranasal sinus. In: Flint PW, editor. Cummings otolaryngology. 6th edition. Philadelphia: Elsevier; 2015. p. 1176–201.
15. Cantù G, Bimbi G, Miceli R, et al. Lymph node metastases in malignant tumors of the paranasal sinuses. Arch Otolaryngol Head Neck Surg 2008;134(2):170.
16. Lloyd G, Lund VJ, Howard D, et al. Optimum imaging for sinonasal malignancy. J Laryngol Otol 2000;114(7):557–62.
17. Razek AAKA, Sieza S, Maha B. Assessment of nasal and paranasal sinus masses by diffusion-weighted MR imaging. J Neuroradiol 2009;36(4):206–11.
18. Svane-Knudsen V, Jørgensen K, Hansen O, et al. Cancer of the nasal cavity and paranasal sinuses: a series of 115 patients. Rhinology 1998;36(1):12–4.
19. Morita A, Ebersold MJ, Olsen KD, et al. Esthesioneuroblastoma. Neurosurgery 1993;32(5):706–15.
20. Bak M, Wein RO. Esthesioneuroblastoma. Hematol Oncol Clin North Am 2012; 26(6):1185–207.
21. Cohen ZR, Marmor E, Fuller GN, et al. Misdiagnosis of olfactory neuroblastoma. Neurosurg Focus 2002;12(5):1–6.
22. Bell D, Hanna EY, Weber RS, et al. Neuroendocrine neoplasms of the sinonasal region. Head Neck 2015;38(S1):E2259–66.
23. Collins BT, Cramer HM, Hearn SA. Fine needle aspiration cytology of metastatic olfactory neuroblastoma. Acta Cytol 1997;41(3):802–10.
24. Gore MR, Zanation AM. Salvage treatment of late neck metastasis in esthesioneuroblastoma. Arch Otolaryngol Head Neck Surg 2009;135(10):1030.
25. de Gabory L, Abdulkhaleq HM, Darrouzet V, et al. Long-term results of 28 esthesioneuroblastomas managed over 35 years. Head Neck 2011;33(1):82–6.
26. Nalavenkata SB, Sacks R, Adappa ND, et al. Olfactory neuroblastoma: fate of the neck–a long-term multicenter retrospective study. Otolaryngol Head Neck Surg 2015;154(2):383–9.
27. Bell D, Hanna EY, Weber RS, et al. Neuroendocrine neoplasms of the sinonasal region. Head Neck 2015;38(S1):E2259–66.
28. Kadish S, Goodman M, Wang CC. Olfactory neuroblastoma: a clinical analysis of 17 cases. Cancer 1976;37(3):1571–6.
29. Levine PA, Gallagher R, Cantrell RW. Esthesioneuroblastoma: reflections of a 21-year experience. Laryngoscope 1999;109(10):1539–43.
30. Jethanamest D, Morris LG, Sikora AG, et al. Esthesioneuroblastoma. Arch Otolaryngol Head Neck Surg 2007;133(3):276.
31. Hyams V. Tumors of the upper respiratory tract and ear. In: Hyams V, Batsakis L, Michaels L, editors. Atlas of tumor pathology. Washington, DC: Armed Forces Institute of Pathology; 1988. p. 240–8.
32. Kaur G, Kane AJ, Sughrue ME, et al. The prognostic implications of Hyam's subtype for patients with Kadish stage C esthesioneuroblastoma. J Clin Neurosci 2013;20:281–6.

33. Malouf GG, Casiraghi O, Deutsch E, et al. Low- and high-grade esthesioneuro-blastomas display a distinct natural history and outcome. Eur J Cancer 2013; 49:1324–34.
34. Bell D, Saade R, Roberts D, et al. Prognostic utility of Hyams histological grading and Kadish–Morita staging systems for esthesioneuroblastoma outcomes. Head Neck Pathol 2015;9:51–9.
35. Dulguerov P, Allal AS, Calcaterra TC. Esthesioneuroblastoma: a meta-analysis and review. Lancet Oncol 2001;2(11):683–90.
36. Frierson HF, Mills S, Fechner R, et al. Sinonasal undifferentiated carcinoma: an aggressive neoplasm derived from schneiderian epithelium and distinct from olfactory neuroblastoma. Am J Surg Pathol 1986;10(11):771–9.
37. Chambers KJ, Lehmann AE, Remenschneider A, et al. Incidence and survival patterns of sinonasal undifferentiated carcinoma in the United States. J Neurol Surg B Skull Base 2015;76(2):94–100.
38. Reiersen DA, Pahilan ME, Devaiah AK. Meta-analysis of treatment outcomes for Sinonasal undifferentiated carcinoma. Otolaryngol Head Neck Surg 2012;147(1): 7–14.
39. Lin E, Sparano A, Spalding A, et al. Sinonasal undifferentiated carcinoma: a 13-year experience at a single institution. Skull Base 2009;20(02):061–7.
40. Kuan EC, Arshi A, Mallen-St Clair J, et al. Significance of tumor stage in Sinonasal undifferentiated carcinoma survival: a population-based analysis. Otolaryngol Head Neck Surg 2016;154(4):667–73.
41. Chang AE, Karnell LH, Menck HR. The national cancer data base report on cutaneous and noncutaneous melanoma. Cancer 1998;83(8):1664–78.
42. Gal TJ, Silver N, Huang B. Demographics and treatment trends in sinonasal mucosal melanoma. Laryngoscope 2011;121(9):2026–33.
43. Dauer E, Lewis J, Rohlinger A, et al. Sinonasal melanoma: a clinicopathologic review of 61 cases. Otolaryngol Head Neck Surg 2008;138(3):347–52.
44. Ballantyne AJ. Malignant melanoma of the skin of the head and neck. Am J Surg 1970;120(4):425–31.
45. Prasad ML, Patel SG, Huvos AG, et al. Primary mucosal melanoma of the head and neck. Cancer 2004;100(8):1657–64.
46. Thompson LDR, Wieneke JA, Miettinen M. Sinonasal tract and nasopharyngeal melanomas: a clinicopathologic study of 115 cases with a proposed staging system. Am J Surg Pathol 2003;27(5):594–611.
47. Shuman AG, Light E, Olsen SH, et al. Mucosal melanoma of the head and neck. Arch Otolaryngol Head Neck Surg 2011;137(4):331.
48. Koivunen P, Bäck L, Pukkila M, et al. Accuracy of the current TNM classification in predicting survival in patients with sinonasal mucosal melanoma. Laryngoscope 2012;122(8):1734–8.
49. Malempati S, Hawkins DS. Rhabdomyosarcoma: review of the children's oncology group (COG) soft-tissue sarcoma committee experience and rationale for current COG studies. Pediatr Blood Cancer 2012;59(1):5–10.
50. Radzikowska J, Kukwa W, Kukwa A, et al. Rhabdomyosarcoma of the head and neck in children. Contemp Oncol (Pozn) 2015;19(2):98–107.
51. Christ W, Anderson J, Meza J. Intergroup rhabdomyosarcoma study-IV: results for patients with nonmetastatic disease. J Clin Oncol 2001;19(12):3091–102.
52. Dutta R, Dubal PM, Svider PF, et al. Sinonasal malignancies: a population-based analysis of site-specific incidence and survival. Laryngoscope 2015;125(11): 2491–7.

53. Bhattacharyya N. Cancer of the nasal cavity: survival and factors influencing prognosis. Arch Otolaryngol Head Neck Surg 2002;128(9):1079–83.
54. Myers LL, Nussenbaum B, Bradford CR, et al. Paranasal sinus malignancies: an 18-year single institution experience. Laryngoscope 2002;112(11):1964–9.
55. McKay SP, Gregoire L, Lonardo F, et al. Human papillomavirus (HPV) transcripts in malignant inverted papilloma are from integrated HPV DNA. Laryngoscope 2005;115(8):1428–31.
56. Ansa B, Goodman M, Ward K, et al. Paranasal sinus squamous cell carcinoma incidence and survival based on surveillance, epidemiology, and end results data, 1973 to 2009. Cancer 2013;119(14):2602–10.
57. Michel J, Fakhry N, Mancini J, et al. Sinonasal squamous cell carcinomas: clinical outcomes and predictive factors. Int J Oral Maxillofac Surg 2014;43(1):1–6.

Endoscopic Resection of Sinonasal and Ventral Skull Base Malignancies

Ghassan Alokby, MD[a], Roy R. Casiano, MD[b],*

KEYWORDS

- Transnasal endoscopic • Anterior skull base • Tumors • Sinonasal tumors
- Endoscopic anterior skull base resection • Paranasal sinus

KEY POINTS

- Ventral skull base tumors are rare head and neck tumors that present with nonspecific symptoms.
- The principles of endoscopic skull base surgery involve extensive surgical planning and a multidisciplinary approach.
- Preoperative assessment is essential to guide surgical approach.
- Transnasal endoscopic resection (TER) is a safe and effective surgical option in appropriately selected cases in the presence of an experienced surgical team.

 Video content accompanies this article at http://www.oto.theclinics.com.

INTRODUCTION

Sinonasal and ventral skull base malignancies represent 3% of all head and neck cancers.[1] Their incidence is 0.83 per 100,000 patients.[2] They usually present with nonspecific symptoms, such as nasal obstruction, epistaxis, and facial pain.

Contemporary management of sinonasal and ventral skull base tumors involves an oncologically sound and multidisciplinary approach. When surgery is indicated, open surgical approaches have long been considered the standard of care. These approaches have been associated, however, with multiple morbidities, including external surgical scarring, wound complications, prolonged brain retraction with all its sequelae, and long postoperative recovery times, resulting in extended hospital length of stays. Postoperative complications with external surgical approaches

Conflict of Interest/Disclosures: The authors have nothing to disclose.
[a] Division of Rhinology and Endoscopic Skull Base Surgery, Department of Otolaryngology- Head and Neck Surgery, Prince Sultan Military Medical City, Riyadh, Saudi Arabia; [b] Rhinology and Endoscopic Skull Base Program, Department of Otolaryngology, Miller School of Medicine, University of Miami, Clinical Research Building, 5th Floor, 1120 Northwest 14th Street, Miami, FL 33136, USA
* Corresponding author.
E-mail address: RCasiano@med.miami.edu

Otolaryngol Clin N Am 50 (2017) 273–285
http://dx.doi.org/10.1016/j.otc.2016.12.005
0030-6665/17/© 2016 Elsevier Inc. All rights reserved.

oto.theclinics.com

have been reported as high as 50%, with postoperative mortality at approximately 4% in most published series.[3] This has led to an interest in alternative surgical approaches that would give similar results with less morbidity and in a minimally invasive manner.

Interest in the endonasal approach for management of skull base tumors goes back to the late nineteenth century.[4] In the 1990s, endoscopic-assisted craniofacial resection (CFR) was described.[5] Similar to a traditional CFR, the tumor is approached superiorly through a bicoronal frontal craniotomy, but the sinonasal surgical component is approached inferiorly through a transnasal endoscopic approach. Although somewhat controversial, some investigators have advocated total endoscopic control of tumors (gross tumor removal without microscopic margins), short of a significant dural resection but combined with adjuvant stereotactic radiosurgery.[6]

Over the past 2 decades, the management of chronic sinus disease has shifted from using the open approaches, or transnasal microscopes, to the use of the endoscopes. The wide adaptation of this technique resulted from improved comfort endoscopically navigating the complex anatomy of the paranasal sinuses, orbit, and skull base. In addition, new technologies, such as intraoperative navigation, have led to the expansion of endoscopic sinus surgery to include the management of neoplasms.[7] Furthermore, improvement in skull base reconstruction techniques, such as using the pedicled nasoseptal flap as well as alloplastic graft techniques, has improved clinical outcomes from endoscopic skull base surgery with a reduction in hospitalization.[8]

The endoscopic approach had been criticized initially for what was perceived as a non–en bloc resection with piecemeal tumor removal that may theoretically result in tumor seeding.[4] Subsequent studies have shown, however, that positive resection margins, and not en bloc resection, is the most significant risk factor for tumor recurrence.[9–11] It has been shown in different studies that endoscopic transnasal resections carries comparable rates of negative margins to open CFR.[11–13]

Casiano and colleagues[14] reported the first purely TER of the anterior skull base (ASB) for esthesioneuroblastoma that included resection of the entire anterior ventral skull base (as described in the traditional CFR) with overlying dura. Since then, several studies have compared endoscopic with open approaches in the management of different sinonasal tumors.[12,13,15] Although many of these studies are limited due to selection bias in that more advanced and aggressive tumors are more likely to have been treated with an open approach, it shows a growing body of evidence that the TER method is as safe and effective as open approaches in appropriately selected patients and in experienced hands as long as oncologic principles are adhered to. This article presents Dr Casiano's technique of endoscopic anterior ventral skull base resection and reconstruction.[16,17]

PREOPERATIVE IMAGING

Imaging studies should be carefully reviewed with a neuroradiologist, who is an important part of the multidisciplinary team. MR imaging usually helps demonstrates the relationship of the tumor to the surrounding soft tissue and neural structures. CT scan and CT angiogram are used to evaluate bony involvement and vascular relationships, respectively.[18] Intraoperative navigation with CT and MR imaging fusion may be used for more extended ASB resections posteriorly adjacent to the internal carotid artery or optic nerves. Intraoperative navigation is not routinely used, however, by Dr Casiano for ASB resection.

CONTRAINDICATIONS AND LIMITATIONS

The key principle in choosing an approach for resection of sinonasal and ventral skull base malignancies is finding the most direct route with the least manipulation of neural and vascular structures. If a crucial neurovascular structure is found ventral or medial to the target structure, a transnasal approach should be reconsidered and the benefits and risks weighed against other approaches.[19]

Some of the contraindications of purely endoscopic procedures are infiltration of nasal bones, massive involvement of the superior or lateral recesses of the frontal sinus, massive involvement of the lacrimal system or orbital structures, or involvement of the lateral recesses or anterior walls of the maxillary sinus. A combined approach (even with more limited external incisions) should be considered when there is extensive tumor infiltration of the dura over the orbital roof or when tumor extends significantly into the brain parenchyma.[20] An external approach may be necessary during the course of TER if surgical margins cannot be cleared due to lack of adequate visualization or access. Therefore, careful preparation is necessary to anticipate all potential intraoperative eventualities. Neurosurgical support must be available in all cases where an open craniotomy may become necessary.[19]

PREOPERATIVE SURGICAL CONSIDERATIONS

A complete head and neck examination is performed. Any abnormalities that may affect the surgery should be noted. For example, the presence of a septal perforation or tumor involvement, may affect the use of a nasoseptal flap, and alternative reconstruction technique should be planned. The management plan should be discussed carefully with the patient.

Prophylactic antibiotics are administered perioperatively.[15,21] Acute sinonasal infection may be treated preoperatively with antibiotics.[22] Chronic inflammatory sinus disease can be addressed, however, at the time of the skull base procedure. In a series of 250 cases who had skull base surgery, 20 patients had chronic rhinosinusitis addressed during their ventral skull base surgery. None of the patients in this series had an acute purulent sinusitis. None developed intracranial infections.[22]

ENDOSCOPIC SURGICAL PROCEDURE

The ASB is formed by the frontal, sphenoid, and ethmoid bones. The posterior table of the frontal sinus forms the anterior limits of the ASB resection. The ethmoid bone, in the midline, gives rise to the cribriform plate, the perpendicular plate of the septum, and the fovea ethmoidalis with ethmoidal septations (anterior and posterior). It articulates anteriorly with the posterior wall of the frontal bone. The olfactory fibers pass from the intracranial cavity to the nasal cavity, forming a pathway that tumors can spread into the nose or intracranially, depending on where they originate.[23] The anterior and posterior ethmoid arteries pass from the orbit to the lateral lamella of the cribriform plate in their corresponding canals. These arteries should be identified and cauterized during surgery.

Traditional oncologic principles should be followed for endoscopic resection of the ASB. The final resection includes bilateral olfactory bulbs, cribriform plates, adjacent dura, and crista galli. The extension of the tumor dictates which additional structures are removed to achieve a negative resection margin.

Endoscopic Technique

- The intranasal component of the malignancy is debulked and its origin (epicenter) is identified to plan the extent of resection (Video 1). This is done with a microdébrider to expose the nasal septum, lateral nasal wall, and posterior choana. The remaining parts of the procedure are performed mainly with nonbiting forceps to assure adequate mucosal stripping and to yield adequate tissue for final (permanent) pathologic analysis and mapping of involved areas. A suction filter (sock) is used to collect the tissue debris removed by the micro-débrider and is labeled carefully for each side of the nose.

- Sinuses are opened and landmarks identified. This include a Draf III (Lothrop) procedure and an extended sphenoid sinusotomy, removing the sphenoid rostrum and intersinus septum along with the mucosa. The optic nerves and ca-rotid arteries are identified. An endoscopic medial maxillectomy is performed if the tumor appears to involve the ethmoid sinus and extends to the medial maxilla (middle meatal wall or inferior turbinate). This involves the systematic removal of the ipsilateral inferior and middle turbinate, medial maxillary wall with nasolacri-mal duct, a total ethmoidectomy without mucosal preservation, and removal of the lamina papyracea, throughout the length of the ethmoid cavity. A total eth-moidectomy, without mucosal preservation, and a middle meatal antrostomy are performed also on the contralateral side, mainly if the tumor appears to extend beyond the confines of the olfactory cleft to the contralateral side, if the biologic nature of the neoplasm warrants bilateral ASB resection or if there is any radiologic evidence of disease on the contralateral side. In select neoplasms where contralateral extension is not evident, a unilateral hemi-ASB resection may be a viable option. In these cases, the contralateral mucoperichondrium of the nasal septum and falx cerebri (with olfactory bulb) is preserved. The long-term olfactory function with this procedure, however, is unknown.
- The nasal septum is resected inferior to the area of tumor involvement from pos-terior wall of the frontal sinus to the rostrum of the sphenoid bone. Margins from the nasal septal mucosa are sent for frozen section analysis bilaterally.
- If the septal mucosa is not involved by the tumor, a septal flap can be harvested for reconstruction prior to the septectomy.
- The posterior table of the frontal sinus and the planum sphenoidale are identified in the course of performing the Draf III (extended) frontal and extended sphenoid sinusotomy (discussed previously). These structures form the anterosuperior and posteroinferior limits of the resection.
- The sphenopalatine foramen is identified and cauterized bilaterally if a nasosep-tal flap is not used. Otherwise, it is preserved on the ipsilateral side of the flap. The crista galli is removed between the 2 leaves of falx cerebri (dura), by first dril-ling with a diamond bur and then dissecting it free with a small dural elevator. The fovea ethmoidalis and sphenoid rostrum anterior to the optic chiasm are thinned with a large cutting and/or diamond bur or ultrasonic bone emulsifier to an eggshell thickness (**Fig. 1**), and the bone is removed piecemeal with a Kerrison bone rongeur, to expose the underlying dura circumferentially around the re-maining perpendicular plate of the nasal septum, the middle and superior turbi-nate remnants, and the olfactory cleft bilaterally. The anterior and posterior ethmoidal arteries are cauterized with a bipolar or monopolar cautery. This cre-ates a floating ASB, which pulsates and is easily moved with a suction tip.
- The dura is elevated off the orbital roof in a lateral direction to facilitate further resec-tion and sampling of dural margins as well as placement of the graft during recon-struction. A wide margin of dura is resected, extending from the posterior wall of the frontal sinus to the anterior planum sphenoidale. Fine skull base microscissors may be use to cut the dura. Dr Casiano, however, prefers a small Thru-Cut Forceps to make the cuts as well as sample dural margins simultaneously. Laterally, the dural

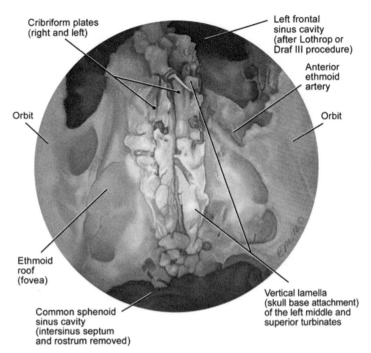

Fig. 1. Artistic depiction of the anterior ventral skull base after initial exposure prior to endoscopic craniotomy. (*From* Casiano RR, editor. Endoscopic sinonasal dissection guide. New York: Thieme Medical Publishers; 2011; with permission.)

margin initially is resected a few millimeters medial to the junction of the orbital wall and the ethmoid roof. The dura, bilateral cribriform plate with olfactory bulbs, middle and superior turbinate remnants, and superior perpendicular plate remnant of the septum are removed en bloc through the nose as a final specimen.

- Adjacent brain parenchyma is inspected for the presence of neoplasm and frozen sections are sent circumferentially from the dural margins, olfactory nerve endings, septum, and nasopharynx. Additional margins are sent as needed. Brain parenchyma involvement can be systematically removed through a gentle suction traction technique, cauterizing any feeding vessels with bipolar cautery (**Fig. 2**).
- In cases of no ventral skull base erosion or thinning, the dura generally is kept intact after thorough bone removal, unless tumor histology dictates dural removal as well. The bone is left undisturbed if the tumor does not extend to the skull base with a clear aerated space between the tumor and the ethmoid roof.
- Endoscopic marsupialization of the lacrimal duct remnant and inferior lacrimal sac is performed with a cutting forceps or powered instruments to minimize the chance of subsequent stenosis and secondary epiphora.

Fig. 3 shows the preoperative and postoperative CT scans of a patient with a left-sided esthesioneuroblastoma who underwent a typical endoscopic anterior ventral skull base resection.

Endoscopic Anterior Skull Base Reconstruction

Dr Casiano has had success reconstructing large skull base defects using cadaveric alloplastic tissue, AlloDerm (LifeCell Corp, Woodlands, Texas). Acellular dermal allograft

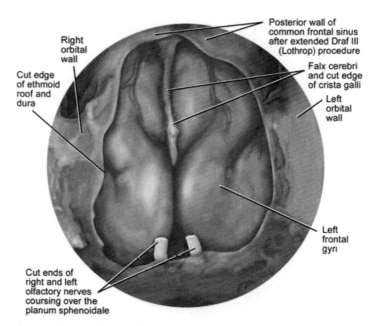

Right orbital wall

Cut edge of ethmoid roof and dura

Posterior wall of common frontal sinus after extended Draf III (Lothrop) procedure

Falx cerebri and cut edge of crista galli

Left orbital wall

Left frontal gyri

Cut ends of right and left olfactory nerves coursing over the planum sphenoidale

Fig. 2. Artistic depiction of the undersurface of the brain after endoscopic craniotomy and resection of the anterior ventral skull base. (*From* Casiano RR, editor. Endoscopic sinonasal dissection guide. New York: Thieme Medical Publishers; 2011; with permission.)

is cadaveric dermis that has been processed to remove cellular elements. A medium-thickness graft approximately 1 mm in thickness is typically used. If the graft is too thick, it is nonpliable and difficult to bend and conform to the bony irregularities of the skull base circumferentially. If it is too thin, then it is too pliable and difficult to work with.

The final dural defect is measured, and 2 cm are added on each side to calculate the desired graft size. For example, a 3-cm × 4-cm defect needs a 7-cm × 8-cm graft. The graft is placed in a manner so that the acellular dermal allograft doubles back on itself over the orbit, behind the posterior wall of the common frontal sinus, and over the planum sphenoidale, thus creating a pocket circumferentially. Oxidative cellulose, Surgicel (Ethicon, Somerville, New Jersey), is wrapped around a plug of dry Gelfoam (Pfizer, New York, New York), like a cigarette, and used as wedges into these pockets to keep the graft it in place and maintain a circumferential water-tight seal around the bony defect. The intranasal ends of the graft are allowed to fold back and make contact with bone circumferentially. This creates a hammock-like structure that supports the skull base and is anchored circumferentially by these wedges of surgical/gel foam

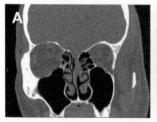
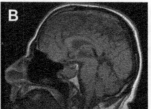
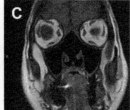

Fig. 3. (*A*) Preoperative coronal and postoperative (*B*) sagittal and (*C*) coronal noncontrast CT scan of a patient with a left-sided esthesioneuroblastoma.

plugs. Care is taken to compress the graft on the bony surfaces, so that no blood or air collection is present between the graft and bony wall of the defect circumferentially (**Fig. 4**). Over the ensuing 6 months postoperatively, granulation tissue, fibrosis, and then mucosal migration occur from the periphery of the defect to the center, creating a thick fibrotic wall separating the intracranial cavity and brain from the nasal cavity. Any granulations or partial extrusion of graft material may be systematically trimmed with Thru-Cut Forceps to minimize crusting and facilitate healing and remucosalization.

If a nasoseptal flap is used, then it is positioned over the grafted ventral skull base defect at this time.[24–28] A wet compressed Gelfoam is carefully placed over the reconstructed cavity, followed by 1 to 2 nasal tampons, Merocel 2000 8 cm (Medtronic Xomed Surgical Products, Jacksonville, Florida). A nasoseptal flap is not critical to achieve a water-tight seal. It does, however, provide more rapid remucosalization of the anterior ventral skull base. Another Merocel packing is placed across the nasal cavity with the ends positioned in the maxillary sinuses bilaterally to help keep the more superiorly positioned Merocel in place. The packing is left in the nose for 7 to 10 days and removed in the clinic. Prophylactic antibiotics are used while packing is in place.[29,30]

LITERATURE REVIEW

In a retrospective analysis of ventral skull base defects repair at the University of Miami, 30 patients with different-sized defects had repair with acellular dermal allograft. The success rate (no postoperative cerebrospinal fluid [CSF] leak with complete

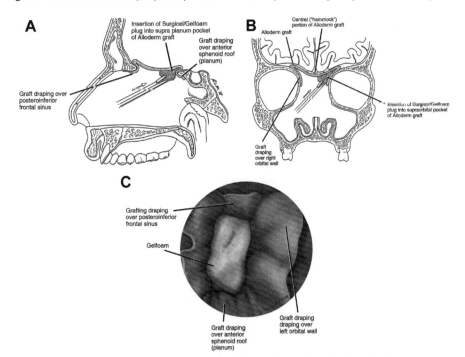

Fig. 4. (*A*) Sagittal and (*B*) coronal depiction of the acellular dermal allograft placement during endoscopic ventral skull base reconstruction (*C*) Endoscopic view of the skull base defect after repairing it with acellular dermal graft. (*From* Germani RM, Vivero R, Herzallah IR, et al. Endoscopic reconstruction of large anterior skull base defects using acellular dermal allograft. Am J Rhinol 2007;21(5):615–8; with permission.)

healing) was 97% compared with 92% for the control group who had different material method. No significant differences were observed in postoperative complications. As far as defect size, 29% of the repaired defects were classified as large (>2 cm).[30]

Since the introduction of the TER for sinonasal and ventral skull base tumors, there have been several studies to compare the result to traditional open approaches.[31] Casiano and colleagues[32] published a series of select patients who underwent purely TER for ASB tumors. The patients were followed for a mean of 34.3 months. There were 17 malignant lesions. One patient recurred locally, resulting in an overall local control rate of 94.7%.[32]

In a subsequent study, Dr Casiano published a retrospective analysis of 82 patients who underwent ASB resection between 1997 and 2011. The follow-up periods were 30 and 31 months, respectively. After accounting for stage and type of neoplasm, TER patients had shorter operating room times, lower intraoperative blood loss, shorter ICU stays, and shorter hospital stays. There were no differences for the rates of true en bloc resection (minimally ascertainable in either group), negative margins, or disease-specific mortality. CFR patients were more likely, however, to have disease present within the first year postoperatively than the TER group. This was a reflection of the more advanced tumor stage or more aggressive pathology at the time of surgery in the CFR group. Subanalysis was performed to obtain a median follow-up of 5 years for both the TER and CFR groups. There were no significant differences in disease-specific mortality or recurrences in this group. There was no statistical difference in major complications between the 2 groups. There were 3 major complications in 2 of the patients who had TER. One patient developed hemorrhage that resulted in stroke and death on postoperative day 10. It resulted from a ruptured aneurysm seen on CT scan. It was not possible to determine whether this was a complication of the operation or a separate disease process that occurred during hospitalization. The other major complication was anterior ethmoid artery bleeding resulting in an orbital hematoma. The patient had to be taken to the operating room for orbital decompression. No long-term visual deficit resulted. The same patient developed an unplanned CSF leak that was successfully repaired endoscopically.[13]

One of the largest series was published by Nicolai and colleagues.[15] In this retrospective analysis, TER was performed on 134 patients whereas 50 patients underwent an endoscopically assisted open CFR (cranioendoscopic approach [CEA]). The patients were followed for a mean of 34.1 months. There were 5 major complications in the TER group. Four of these complications were postoperative CSF leak and the fifth patient developed meningitis. The 5-year disease-specific survival rates were 91.4% ± 3.9% and 58.8% ± 8.6% (P = .0004) for the TER and CEA groups, respectively. Again, there was tumor histology and stage selection bias between the 2 groups that accounted for these observed differences. At the least, however, TER was as effective as open approaches when comparing similar tumors and stages.

Hanna and colleagues[12] published a series of 120 patients; 93 underwent TER and 27 underwent CEA. The mean follow-up was 37 months. There was no statistically significant difference in disease-specific (P = .92) or overall survival (P = .79) between the 2 groups.

These studies reach a common conclusion that TER of ASB neoplasms, when properly planned and in expert hands, is a valid alternative to standard surgical approaches for management of malignancies of the sinonasal tract. The studies are summarized in **Table 1**. **Table 2** provides a literature review showing studies reporting purely endoscopic resection of sinonasal/ventral skull base malignancy.

Several studies have evaluated the quality of life of patients undergoing endoscopic ventral skull base resection.[33,34] Abergel and colleagues[33] did a retrospective analysis

Table 1
Studies that reviewed the out come of surgical resection of sinonasal/ventral skull base tumors by transnasal endoscopic or open approach

	Pathology (n)	Stage (n)
Dave et al,[32] 2007[a]	Esthesioneuroblastoma (10)	KA (5), KB (2), KC (2)
	Sarcomatous meningioma (1)	T1 (2), T2 (1), T3 (2), T4 (2)
	Hemangiopercytoma (1)	
	Other neoplasms (5)	

	Pathology	TER	CFR	Stage	TER	CFR	P
Wood et al,[13] 2012[a]	ACC	3	8	T1	10	3	.006
	Adenocarcinoma	2	4	T2	8	2	.008
	BCC	0	1	T3	6	11	.595
	Sarcoma	0	1	T4	10	32	.002
	Hemangiopericytoma	5	0				
	Esthesioneuroblastoma	15	4				
	Mucosal melanoma	1	2				
	NEC	4	0				
	SNUC	2	2				
	SCC	1	25				
Nicolai et al,[15] 2008	Adenocarcinoma	44	24	T1	49	3	
	SCC	16	9	T2	25	1	
	Esthesioneuroblastoma	19	3	T3	20	12	
	Mucosal melanoma	14	3	T4	12	23	
	ACC	12	1				
	Hemangiopericytoma	8	0				
	Lymphoproliferative	6	1				
	SNUC	2	3				
	Chondrosarcoma	3	0				
	Ewing sarcoma	1	1				
	NEC	1	1				
	Triton tumor	2	0				
	Ectomesenchymoma	0	1				
	Fibrosarcoma	0	1				
	Giant cell tumor	1	0				
	Leiomyosarcoma	0	1				
	Malignant schwannoma	0	1				
	Myofibrosarcoma	1	0				
	Oncocytic carcinoma	1	0				
	Osteosarcoma	1	0				
	Secondary tumor	1	0				
	Synovial sarcoma	1					
Hanna et al,[12] 2009	Esthesioneuroblastoma	17		T1	32	25	
	Adenocarcinoma	14		T2	31	25	
	Melanoma	14		T3	17	21	
	SCC	13		T4	20	29	
	ACC	7					
	NEC	4					
	SNUC	2					
	Sarcoma	15[b]					

Abbreviations: ACC, adenoid cystic carcinoma; BCC, basal cell carcinoma; K, Kadish staging for esthesioneuroblastoma; NEC, neuroendocrine carcinoma; SCC, squamous cell carcinoma; SNUC, sinonasal undifferentiated carcinoma.
[a] Overlapping studies.
[b] No significant difference in the distribution of pathologies between the 2 groups (P = .22).

Table 2
Studies that reviewed the out come of Transnasal Endoscopic Resection of sinonasal/ventral skull base tumors

	N	Pathology	Stage (n)	Follow-up (mo)	Local Recurrence (%)
Unger et al,[36] 2005	14	Esthesioneuroblastoma	KB (5), KC (9)	59.8	3
Poetker et al,[37] 2005	14	Esthesioneuroblastoma (4)	KA (1), KB (2), KC (1)	51.5	21.4
		SCC (4)	T1 (3), T2 (4)		
		Hemangiopericytoma (1)	NR		
		Chondrosarcoma (1)	Grade 2		
		Adenocarcinoma (2)	T1 (2)		
		ACC (1)	T2 (1)		
		Malignant melanoma (1)	T2 (1)		
Suriano et al,[38] 2007	9	Esthesioneuroblastoma	KA (3), KB (6)	42.8	0
Lund et al,[39] 2007	49	Adenocarcinoma (15)	For all the histopathologies	36	22
		malignant melanomas (11)	T1 (21), T2 (16), T3 (12)		
		Esthesioneuroblastoma (11)			
		SCC (3)			
		Chondrosarcoma (3)			
		Hemangiopericytoma (2)			
		Malignant schwannoma (1)			
		ACC (1)			
		SNUC (1)			
		TC (1)			
De Bonnecaze et al,[40] 2014	8	Esthesioneuroblastoma	A (1), B (3), C (4)	95	25
Jardeleza et al,[41] 2009	12	Adenocarcinoma	T2 (6), T3 (5), T4 (1)	42	16.6
Revenaugh et al,[42] 2011	6	SNUC	T4 (5), T1 (1)	32	14
Antognoni et al,[43] 2015	27	Adenocarcinoma	NR	48	14
Lombardi et al,[44] 2016	47	Malignant melanoma	T3 (26), T4a (14), T4b (7)	20	61 (local, regional, or distal relapse)

Abbreviations: ACC, adenoid cystic carcinoma; K, Kadish staging for esthesioneuroblastoma; NR, not reported; SCC, squamous cell carcinoma; SNUC, sinonasal undifferentiated carcinoma; TC, transitional carcinoma.

to compare the quality of life of 78 patients who underwent resection of skull base neoplasms using TER or an open approach. The Anterior Skull Base Surgery Questionnaire, the reliability and validity of which have been described previously, was used.[35] The data showed a significant advantage in favor of the TER on the psychosocial, functional, and emotional status of patients undergoing skull base tumor resection. This significant difference continued when controlling for other variable affecting the outcome, including malignancy.[33]

SUMMARY

The TER of anterior ventral skull base lesions has shown a safe and effective method for the surgical management of sinonasal and skull base malignancies in select cases. Oncological principles are the same as for historical open approaches, in that the goal should be to achieve complete removal of all tumor with negative resection margins. Careful selection of cases, along with the presence of an experienced surgeon and a fully involved multidisciplinary skull base team trained in the management of ventral skull base neoplasms, are essential for excellent outcomes.

SUPPLEMENTARY DATA

Supplementary data related to this article can be found online at http://dx.doi.org/10.1016/j.otc.2016.12.005.

REFERENCES

1. Kaplan DJ, Kim JH, Wang E, et al. Prognostic indicators for salvage surgery of recurrent sinonasal malignancy. Otolaryngol Head Neck Surg 2016;154(1):104–12.
2. Dutta R, Dubal PM, Svider PF, et al. Sinonasal malignancies: a population-based analysis of site-specific incidence and survival. Laryngoscope 2015;125(11):2491–7.
3. Krischek B, Godoy BL, Zadeh G, et al. From craniofacial resection to the endonasal endoscopic approach in skull base surgery. World Neurosurg 2013;80(1–2):56–8.
4. Rawal RB, Gore MR, Harvey RJ, et al. Evidence-based practice: endoscopic skull base resection for malignancy. Otolaryngol Clin North Am 2012;45(5):1127–42.
5. Yuen AP, Fung CF, Hung KN. Endoscopic cranionasal resection of anterior skull base tumor. Am J Otolaryngol 1997;18(6):431–3.
6. Walch C, Stammberger H, Anderhuber W, et al. The minimally invasive approach to olfactory neuroblastoma: combined endoscopic and stereotactic treatment. Laryngoscope 2000;110(4):635–40.
7. Wagenmann M, Schipper J. The transnasal approach to the skull base. From sinus surgery to skull base surgery. GMS Curr Top Otorhinolaryngol Head Neck Surg 2011;10:Doc08.
8. Hosemann W, Schroeder HW. Comprehensive review on rhino-neurosurgery. GMS Curr Top Otorhinolaryngol Head Neck Surg 2015;14:Doc01.
9. Feiz-Erfan I, Suki D, Hanna E, et al. Prognostic significance of transdural invasion of cranial base malignancies in patients undergoing craniofacial resection. Neurosurgery 2007;61(6):1178–85 [discussion: 1185].
10. Wellman BJ, Traynelis VC, McCulloch TM, et al. Midline anterior craniofacial approach for malignancy: results of en bloc versus piecemeal resections. Skull Base Surg 1999;9(1):41–6.

11. Ganly I, Patel SG, Singh B, et al. Complications of craniofacial resection for malignant tumors of the skull base: report of an International Collaborative Study. Head Neck 2005;27(6):445–51.
12. Hanna E, DeMonte F, Ibrahim S, et al. Endoscopic resection of sinonasal cancers with and without craniotomy: oncologic results. Arch Otolaryngol Head Neck Surg 2009;135(12):1219–24.
13. Wood JW, Eloy JA, Vivero RJ, et al. Efficacy of transnasal endoscopic resection for malignant anterior skull-base tumors. Int Forum Allergy Rhinol 2012;2(6): 487–95.
14. Casiano RR, Numa WA, Falquez AM. Endoscopic resection of esthesioneuroblastoma. Am J Rhinol 2001;15(4):271–9.
15. Nicolai P, Battaglia P, Bignami M, et al. Endoscopic surgery for malignant tumors of the sinonasal tract and adjacent skull base: a 10-year experience. Am J Rhinol 2008;22(3):308–16.
16. Casiano RR, Herzallah IR, Anstead A, et al. Advanced endoscopic sinonasal dissection. In: Casiano RR, editor. Endoscopic sinonasal dissection guide. New York: Thieme Medical Publishers Inc; 2012. p. 59–99.
17. Eloy JA, Tessema B, Casiano RR. Surgical approaches to the anterior cranial fossa. In: Kennedy DW, Hwang PH, editors. Rhinology: diseases of the nose, sinuses, and skull base. New York: Thieme Medical Publishers Inc; 2012. p. 605–14.
18. Gardner PA, Kassam AB, Rothfus WE, et al. Preoperative and intraoperative imaging for endoscopic endonasal approaches to the skull base. Otolaryngol Clin North Am 2008;41(1):215–30, vii.
19. Snyderman CH, Pant H, Carrau RL, et al. What are the limits of endoscopic sinus surgery?: the expanded endonasal approach to the skull base. Keio J Med 2009; 58(3):152–60.
20. Castelnuovo P, Battaglia P, Turri-Zanoni M, et al. Endoscopic endonasal surgery for malignancies of the anterior cranial base. World Neurosurg 2014;82(Suppl 6): S22–31.
21. Brown SM, Anand VK, Tabaee A, et al. Role of perioperative antibiotics in endoscopic skull base surgery. Laryngoscope 2007;117(9):1528–32.
22. Nyquist GG, Rosen MR, Friedel ME, et al. Comprehensive management of the paranasal sinuses in patients undergoing endoscopic endonasal skull base surgery. World Neurosurg 2014;82(Suppl 6):S54–8.
23. Pinheiro-Neto CD, Fernandez-Miranda JC, Wang EW, et al. Anatomical correlates of endonasal surgery for sinonasal malignancies. Clin Anat 2012;25(1):129–34.
24. Eloy JA, Patel AA, Shukla PA, et al. Early harvesting of the vascularized pedicled nasoseptal flap during endoscopic skull base surgery. Am J Otolaryngol 2013; 34(3):188–94.
25. Eloy JA, Kuperan AB, Choudhry OJ, et al. Efficacy of the pedicled nasoseptal flap without cerebrospinal fluid (CSF) diversion for repair of skull base defects: incidence of postoperative CSF leaks. Int Forum Allergy Rhinol 2012;2(5):397–401.
26. Eloy JA, Choudhry OJ, Friedel ME, et al. Endoscopic nasoseptal flap repair of skull base defects: Is addition of a dural sealant necessary? Otolaryngol Head Neck Surg 2012;147(1):161–6.
27. Kassam AB, Thomas A, Carrau RL, et al. Endoscopic reconstruction of the cranial base using a pedicled nasoseptal flap. Neurosurgery 2008;63(1 Suppl 1): ONS44–52 [discussion: ONS52–43].
28. Liu JK, Schmidt RF, Choudhry OJ, et al. Surgical nuances for nasoseptal flap reconstruction of cranial base defects with high-flow cerebrospinal fluid leaks after endoscopic skull base surgery. Neurosurg Focus 2012;32(6):E7.

29. Gaynor BG, Benveniste RJ, Lieberman S, et al. Acellular dermal allograft for sellar repair after transsphenoidal approach to pituitary adenomas. J Neurol Surg B Skull Base 2013;74(3):155–9.
30. Germani RM, Vivero R, Herzallah IR, et al. Endoscopic reconstruction of large anterior skull base defects using acellular dermal allograft. Am J Rhinol 2007; 21(5):615–8.
31. Eloy JA, Vivero RJ, Hoang K, et al. Comparison of transnasal endoscopic and open craniofacial resection for malignant tumors of the anterior skull base. Laryngoscope 2009;119(5):834–40.
32. Dave SP, Bared A, Casiano RR. Surgical outcomes and safety of transnasal endoscopic resection for anterior skull tumors. Otolaryngol Head Neck Surg 2007; 136(6):920–7.
33. Abergel A, Cavel O, Margalit N, et al. Comparison of quality of life after transnasal endoscopic vs open skull base tumor resection. Arch Otolaryngol Head Neck Surg 2012;138(2):142–7.
34. Castelnuovo P, Lepera D, Turri-Zanoni M, et al. Quality of life following endoscopic endonasal resection of anterior skull base cancers. J Neurosurg 2013; 119(6):1401–9.
35. Gil Z, Abergel A, Spektor S, et al. Development of a cancer-specific anterior skull base quality-of-life questionnaire. J Neurosurg 2004;100(5):813–9.
36. Unger F, Haselsberger K, Walch C, et al. Combined endoscopic surgery and radiosurgery as treatment modality for olfactory neuroblastoma (esthesioneuroblastoma). Acta Neurochir (Wien) 2005;147(6):595–601 [discussion: 601–592].
37. Poetker DM, Toohill RJ, Loehrl TA, et al. Endoscopic management of sinonasal tumors: a preliminary report. Am J Rhinol 2005;19(3):307–15.
38. Suriano M, De Vincentiis M, Colli A, et al. Endoscopic treatment of esthesioneuroblastoma: a minimally invasive approach combined with radiation therapy. Otolaryngol Head Neck Surg 2007;136(1):104–7.
39. Lund V, Howard DJ, Wei WI. Endoscopic resection of malignant tumors of the nose and sinuses. Am J Rhinol 2007;21(1):89–94.
40. De Bonnecaze G, Chaput B, Al Hawat A, et al. Long-term oncological outcome after endoscopic surgery for olfactory esthesioneuroblastoma. Acta Otolaryngol 2014;134(12):1259–64.
41. Jardeleza C, Seiberling K, Floreani S, et al. Surgical outcomes of endoscopic management of adenocarcinoma of the sinonasal cavity. Rhinology 2009;47(4): 354–61.
42. Revenaugh PC, Seth R, Pavlovich JB, et al. Minimally invasive endoscopic resection of sinonasal undifferentiated carcinoma. Am J Otolaryngol 2011;32(6):464–9.
43. Antognoni P, Turri-Zanoni M, Gottardo S, et al. Endoscopic resection followed by adjuvant radiotherapy for sinonasal intestinal-type adenocarcinoma: retrospective analysis of 30 consecutive patients. Head Neck 2015;37(5):677–84.
44. Lombardi D, Bottazzoli M, Turri-Zanoni M, et al. Sinonasal mucosal melanoma: a 12-year experience of 58 cases. Head Neck 2016;38(Suppl 1):E1737–45.

Transfacial and Craniofacial Approaches for Resection of Sinonasal and Ventral Skull Base Malignancies

CrossMark

Elizabeth L. Perkins, MD[a], Bryan M. Brandon, MD[a],
Satyan B. Sreenath, MD[a], Dipan D. Desai, BS[a],
Brian D. Thorp, MD[a], Charles S. Ebert, MD, MPH[a],
Adam M. Zanation, MD[a,b],*

KEYWORDS

- Ventral skull base surgery • Craniofacial approach • Transfacial approach
- Sinonasal malignancy • Skull base • Open resection

KEY POINTS

- A transfacial or craniofacial approach allows for wide, potentially en bloc resection and is ideal for tumors that involve surrounding soft tissue, the palate, anterolateral frontal sinus, and dura.
- Regardless of an open versus combined approach, a complete resection with negative margins should be the primary goal.
- The transfacial approach can be gradual and stepwise depending on the extent of the disease and often begins with a lateral rhinotomy to gain access to facial and orbital regions.
- Craniofacial approaches combine the traditional transfacial approaches with a bifrontal or subfrontal craniotomy to provide greater exposure to the ventral skull base.
- Transfacial and craniofacial approaches have been greatly refined since their initial descriptions, but now are mostly reserved for advanced lesions not amenable to endoscopic removal.

[a] Department of Otolaryngology—Head and Neck Surgery, University of North Carolina at Chapel Hill, 170 Manning Drive, CB #7070, Physician's Office Building Room G-190, Chapel Hill, NC 27599, USA; [b] Department of Neurosurgery, University of North Carolina at Chapel Hill, 170 Manning Drive, CB #7070, Physician's Office Building Room G-190, Chapel Hill, NC 27599, USA
* Corresponding author. Department of Otolaryngology—Head & Neck Surgery, University of North Carolina at Chapel Hill, 170 Manning Drive, CB #7070, Physician's Office Building Room G-190, Chapel Hill, NC 27599.
E-mail address: adam_zanation@med.unc.edu

Otolaryngol Clin N Am 50 (2017) 287–300
http://dx.doi.org/10.1016/j.otc.2016.12.006
0030-6665/17/© 2016 Elsevier Inc. All rights reserved.

INTRODUCTION

Malignancies of the paranasal sinuses present unique challenges to physicians given their late presentation, diverse histology, and involvement of complex anatomic structures. Surgical resection with sound oncologic principles and reconstruction can restore function and prolong meaningful life. Small tumors of the anterior ventral skull base, such as T1 or T2, can often be managed solely by endoscopic resection. Larger tumors involving complex neurovascular or intraorbital structures often necessitate open transfacial or craniofacial resection. The decision to proceed with endoscopic versus open versus a combined approach should be made based on tumor location, reconstruction options, and surgeon experience. The preoperative planning, surgical steps, postoperative care, and clinical results from the literature are discussed in this article.

PREOPERATIVE PLANNING

The evaluation of every patient with concerns for a sinonasal and ventral skull base malignancy should begin with a thorough clinical history, review of systems and physical examination. With careful attention made to the ocular and cranial nerve examination, the extent and spread of tumor can be predicted. Sinonasal endoscopy is performed for further tumor characterization and to exclude any underlying infection. Imaging is essential to diagnosis and preoperative planning. A combination of computed tomography (CT) and MRI is invaluable for determining the extent of tumor involvement, orbital invasion, and intracranial extension (**Fig. 1**). Although CT is superior to MRI in evaluating bony detail (particularly the skull base), MRI is beneficial for evaluating the soft tissues, perineural and dural involvement, and intracranial extension (see **Fig. 1**). Contraindications to surgical management of ventral skull base lesions include significant gross brain invasion, bilateral invasion of the optic nerve or optic chiasm, carotid artery invasion, and distant metastasis.[1]

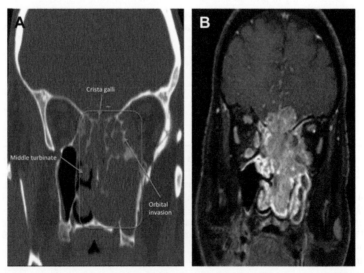

Fig. 1. Coronal CT (*A*) and T1-weighted MRI (*B*) show highly infiltrative sinonasal carcinoma centered within the left nasal cavity with extensions to the orbit, anterior cranial fossa, soft tissue of the nose, and pterygoid fossa.

A preoperative evaluation is not complete without a histologic diagnosis by the way of tissue biopsy. Biopsy can often be performed in a clinical setting, but if there is any concern that excessive bleeding may be encountered, biopsy should be performed in the operating room. Before biopsy, imaging should be obtained to exclude an encephalocele or hypervascular tumor. Once a tissue diagnosis has been made, the correct oncologic resection and possible need for multimodality therapy can be planned. Additionally, it is recommended that the patient be presented at a multidisciplinary tumor board to facilitate multimodality management planning.

The role of PET/CT with diagnosis and management of sinonasal and ventral skull base malignancies is ideal for identification of distant metastasis, rather than localization of a primary tumor. PET/CT should be obtained when there is concern for spread beyond the paranasal sinuses, especially for tumors that have a propensity for distant metastasis, such as adenoid cystic carcinoma, lymphoma, mucosal melanoma, and sinonasal undifferentiated carcinoma.

Transfacial and open craniofacial resection are indicated for any benign or malignant tumor of the anterior ventral skull base. Open approaches allow for wide, potentially en bloc resection and are ideal for tumors that involve surrounding facial soft tissue, the palate, anterolateral frontal sinus, and dural involvement lateral to the midpupillary line. An endoscopic endonasal approach can be ideal for smaller, midline tumors, and a combined approach may be beneficial. Regardless of the approach chosen, the goal should always be for complete tumor resection with negative margins while balancing optimal cosmetic and functional outcome. Additionally, the surgeon should feel comfortable with reconstruction of the ventral skull base, which often involves local flaps and free tissue transfer.

OPERATIVE SETUP

All of the following procedures are performed under general anesthesia with endotracheal intubation. Of note, preprocedural tracheostomies before tumor extirpation are not routinely performed unless there is extensive pharyngeal or palatal involvement or if microvascular free flap reconstruction is planned. Constant communication between the surgeon and the anesthesiologist is crucial for any operative case and should not be dismissed. The patient is rotated 180° from anesthesia equipment and both arms tucked at the patient's side. Perioperative antibiotics, such as a third-generation cephalosporin, are administered 30 minutes before incision. If anterior craniofacial resection is planned, the patient's head is secured on a horseshoe head holder in a neutral position. If endoscopic assistance will be used, the navigation system is registered. Temporary unilateral or bilateral tarsorrhaphies are performed, and the planned incision is marked and injected with 1% 1:100,000 lidocaine with epinephrine. The skin is then prepared in the usual sterile fashion.

SURGICAL TECHNIQUE
Transfacial Approach

The transfacial approach is ideal for low-lying tumors involving the anterior nasal cavity, inferior maxilla, and hard palate. The approach and incision can be gradual and stepwise, depending on the extent of the disease. The basic incision begins with a lateral rhinotomy and is extended to a Weber-Ferguson incision if required. The lateral rhinotomy is often combined with a medial, subtotal, or total maxillectomy depending on tumor size and location.

Lateral Rhinotomy and Midfacial Degloving

The lateral rhinotomy incision begins at the level of the medial canthus extending inferiorly along the nasal sidewall, around the nasal ala, and into the nasal cavity (**Fig. 2**). The approach may be extended to a lynch incision for tumors that involve the medial orbit by continuing the incision superiorly to the medial eyebrow. If access to the orbital floor is needed, the rhinotomy incision is carried 90° laterally with a subciliary incision through the lower eyelid crease. A Weber-Ferguson incision and upper lip split can also be included for access to the hard palate and alveolar ridge (see **Fig. 2**). The vertical upper lip incision is made on the ipsilateral side of the philtrum for optimal cosmetic result and scar camouflage.

The incision medial to the eye is deepened and the angular vessels identified and ligated. The periosteum and soft tissue are elevated off the anterior wall of the maxilla, nasal bones, and inferior orbital rim, with careful attention being made to preserve the infraorbital nerve. The periosteum is elevated off the lamina papyracea dislocating the lacrimal sac from the lacrimal fossa. The medial canthal tendon is transected and tagged for future repair. The lacrimal duct is transected sharply without electrocautery to allow further dissection of the medial orbit. The periorbita is elevated, and the anterior and posterior ethmoidal arteries are identified and ligated. A curved osteotome can be used to make a nasal bone osteotomy through the frontal process of the

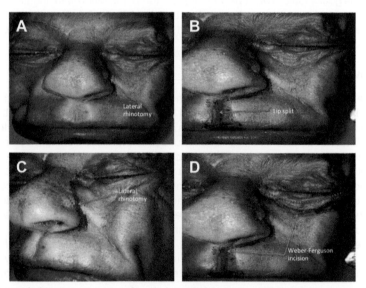

Fig. 2. Lateral rhinotomy incision (*A, C*), lateral rhinotomy with lip split incision (*B*), and Weber-Ferguson modification incision (*D*). Several modifications of the incisions can be made: (*B*) is a lip-splitting extension with dart. The dart provides some potential benefits for lip notching. (*A, C*) is the senior author's preferred lateral rhinotomy incision (*dotted red line*) where instead of being in the nasolabial crease (*purple marking*), the incision is carried up onto the nose at the junction of the dorsum and the lateral nasal wall. This method has potential cosmetic benefits as well, placing the incision over the nasal bones, an area that will have less contact with the intranasal air containing spaces. (*D*) is a subciliary or transconjunctival incision (*dotted red line*) periocular extension that would be preferred in a younger patient compared with the standard incision at the inferior orbital rim (*purple marking*).

maxilla then medially across the nasal dorsum to allow for medial retraction of the nasal bones and nose.

Midfacial degloving is an alternative to the lateral rhinotomy approach to the nasal cavity, ventral skull base, and infratemporal fossa. The approach involves the release of the soft tissues overlying the nasal skeleton. Its major advantage over the lateral rhinotomy is the lack of external facial incisions and visible scarring. The major limitation is limited visualization of the orbital floors, as the flap is tethered inferiorly by the inferior alveolar nerve. The procedure begins with a full transfixion incision of the columella followed by an intercartilaginous incision that extends past the piriform aperture. A circumvestibular release is completed by carrying the incision down to the periosteum laterally and then curving medially to the nasal cavity floor to meet the transfixion incision. Finally, dissection is carried in the submucoperichondrial plane over the upper lateral cartilages and to the nasal bones. At this time, attention is turned to the oral cavity in which bilateral sublabial incision is made from the first molar on one side to the first molar on the contralateral side leaving a 1-cm cuff of tissue to allow for closure. This incision is carried down to the periosteum of the maxilla, which is then elevated to the level of the inferior orbital rim, piriform aperture medially, and the pterygomaxillary suture posteriorly. This method effectively connects the intraoral component of the approach with the circumvestibular incision to elevate the soft tissue of the middle third of the face and expose essentially the entire maxillary bone bilaterally.[2]

MEDIAL MAXILLECTOMY

The medial maxillectomy first begins with an osteotomy made in the anterior-posterior direction in the inferior meatus, the most inferior portion of the medial maxillary sinus. The cut begins at the pyriform rim and extends posteriorly to the posterior maxillary wall. A second cut is made in the anterior-posterior direction through the medial orbit just below the fronto-ethmoidal suture line and anterior ethmoidal artery. A third cut is made through the orbital floor just medial to the infraorbital nerve and foramina, releasing the lamina papyracea and joining the second cut posteriorly. Heavy mayo scissors are then used along the previously made osteotomies and to release the posterior soft tissue attachments. A gentle rocking motion can be applied with one finger inside the nasal cavity and the other in the maxillary sinus to fracture the remaining posterior bony attachments of the palatine bone. Any remaining bony remnants can be removed with Blakesley and Takahashi forceps. Remaining ethmoid mucosa is removed to prevent mucocele formation and final margins are collected. The specimen is removed anteriorly and sent to pathology, and hemostasis is obtained.

Closure first begins with either stenting of the nasolacrimal duct or, more often, marsupialization. The medial canthal ligament is sutured back to the nasal bone with nonabsorbable suture. Any lacerations in the periorbita should be repaired with absorbable suture. The wound is copiously irrigated and closed in a 2-layer fashion.

SUBTOTAL AND TOTAL MAXILLECTOMY

A subtotal maxillectomy is an extension of the medial maxillectomy to include removal of the alveolar ridge, hard palate, or the entire maxilla if necessary. A total maxillectomy includes the orbital floor. Ohngren line, an imaginary line drawn from medial canthus to the angle of the mandible divides the maxillary sinus into infrastructural and suprastructural lesions (Fig. 3).[3] Infrastructural lesions are associated with an earlier presentation and more complete resection, whereas suprastructural lesions present at more advantaged tumor stages and are more difficult to resect carrying a poorer prognosis.

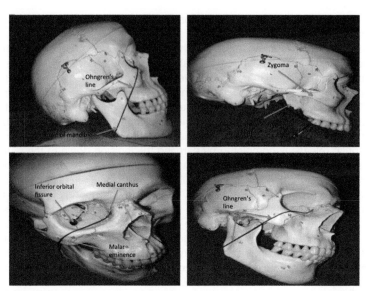

Fig. 3. Skull model demonstrating Ohngren line, an imaginary line extending from the medial canthus to the angle of the mandible, which divides the maxillary sinus into infrastructural and suprastructural lesions. Use of this line and a thorough understanding of key bony and neurovascular landmarks assist in subtotal and total maxillectomies as part of transfacial approaches.

A subtotal maxillectomy begins with a lateral rhinotomy and a modified Weber-Ferguson incision as described previously. A cheek flap is elevated off the anterior maxilla, and the inferior orbital nerve is identified. The cheek flap is carried 1 cm lateral to the lateral canthus. The orbicularis oculi and periorbita are elevated off the orbital rim along the orbital floor posteriorly to the orbital apex. Medial elevation is done above the fronto-ethmoid suture line, identified superior to the anterior and posterior ethmoid arteries. At this point, the surgeon can thoroughly inspect the orbit for tumor involvement. If the tumor involves the periorbita, then an orbital dissection or possibly exenteration is indicated as described in further detail below.

Next, the lacrimal fossa, lamina, and lacrimal duct are identified, and the duct is transected and marsupialized. The attachment of the masseter to the zygoma is divided, and attention is then turned to the intraoral part of the procedure. First, an incision is made within the ipsilateral gingivobuccal sulcus. Next, another incision is made between the ipsilateral lateral incisor and canine and is carried posteriorly and just ipsilateral (2–3 mm) to the midline of the hard palate. At the junction of the hard and soft palate, the incision is turned 90° laterally to join the gingivobuccal incision around the maxillary tubercle. Next, the trimalar suture, floor of the orbital, medial orbital wall (2 mm below the fronto-ethmoid suture line), and palate are cut using a rongeur, osteotome, or high-speed cutting drill. The palate osteotomy should be made through the lateral incisor tooth socket along with preservation of the nasal septum and as much palatal mucosa as possible to aid in reconstruction. A large curved osteotome is used to free the maxilla from the pterygoid plates, and any remaining soft tissue attachments are transected with heavy mayo scissors.

Lastly, the specimen is removed en bloc and sent for final pathology testing. Brisk bleeding may be encountered, most likely from the internal maxillary artery, which can initially be controlled with packing and ligation, once the artery is identified. The cheek skin flap is lined with a split-thickness skin graft, and the cavity is packed with anti-biotic impregnated gauze. At this point, a prosthesis is set in place and secured with lag screws. The posterior prosthesis can be sutured to the soft palate to aid in speech and swallowing. If the remaining defect is large, local or free tissue transfer may be required. Once again, careful attention is made to reapproximate the medial canthal tendon to the lacrimal crest, and the incision is meticulously closed in a 2-layer fashion.

ORBITAL EXENTERATION

Orbital exenteration is indicated when tumor invades the periorbita, extraocular mus-cles, or orbital fat. Preoperatively, this is best determined by physical examination and close evaluation of MRI. Sometimes this cannot be determined preoperatively, and the patient should be educated and counseled that this may be a decision made intraoperatively.

The approach for orbital exenteration is performed by extending the lateral rhinot-omy and modified Weber-Ferguson incision superiorly and then laterally from medial to lateral canthi. If the orbital septum is known to be free of tumor invasion, the incision can be made through either the upper or lower conjunctiva. Skin flaps are raised from the orbicularis oculi and the periorbital periosteum is incised. A circumferential sub-periosteal dissection is carried posteriorly to the orbital apex, sparing the quadrant to be included in the maxillectomy specimen. Next the extraocular muscles are divided, allowing for cauterization of the optic vessels and nerve using bipolar cautery. Next the planned osteotomies can be made to facilitate the maxillectomy portion of the procedure. The upper and lower lid, if not included in the specimen, can be denuded of epithelium and sutured shut and the remaining defect lined with a split thickness skin graft.

RECONSTRUCTION

The goal for reconstruction after subtotal and total maxillectomy is to restore separa-tion of the nasal and oral cavity. This reconstruction aids in speech and swallowing and prevents velopharyngeal insufficiency. Options for reconstruction of the defect include a temporary obturator and local flap, followed by microvascular free tissue reconstruction (**Fig. 4**). If a defect is too large to be reconstructed with an obturator, free tissue transfer allows for an immediate and functional reconstruction at the time of ablation. Many free tissue flap options exist to reconstruct the palate and include the parascapular flap, rectus abdominis flap, anterolateral thigh flap, thoraco-dorsal artery perforator, and radial forearm free flap.[4] Osseous flap options include fib-ula, iliac crest, and scapula. Osseous flaps can re-create the palate and nasal floor while also providing a bone scaffold for future dental implants. Choosing a flap with a long vascular pedicle, such as the radial forearm free flap, are advantageous when reconstructing a more cephalic defect of the anterior ventral skull base.[5] Overall, reconstruction with free tissue transfer has been successful in restoring swallowing and speech. Patients report high satisfaction rates with low donor site morbidity.[4] In general, the cosmetic and functional sequelae of total maxillectomy is well tolerated by patients.[6]

POSTOPERATIVE CARE

Immediately postoperatively patients should be monitored closely in a step-down unit, at minimum. If free tissue transfer was used for reconstruction, overnight stay in a

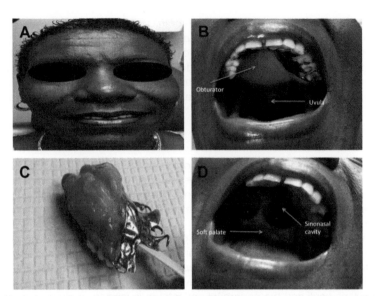

Fig. 4. Healed complete maxillectomy defect with obturator reconstruction. (*A*) Healed frontal view of a 5-year postoperative patient after a Weber-Ferguson incision and complete maxillectomy. Note the good alignment of the nose and lip and the dental rehabilitation that the final obturator gives. (*B*) Intraoral view of the same patient with the obturator in place. (*C*) View of the actual obturator ex vivo. (*D*) Intraoral view of complete maxillectomy defect with obturator removed.

surgical intensive care unit may be necessary for routine flap monitoring and tracheostomy care. After the immediate postoperative phase, oral saline irrigations should be completed daily and postprandial. Frequent jaw exercises are helpful in preventing trismus. On postoperative day 5 to 7, the temporary obturator and packing is removed. Routine close follow-up with the prosthodontist is important for restoring palatal function to avoid velopharyngeal insufficiency.

CRANIOFACIAL RESECTION

Anterior craniofacial resection combines extracranial and intracranial exposures using a bifrontal craniotomy in tandem with transfacial exposure of the nasal cavity, ethmoid, maxillary, and orbital areas. The transfacial exposures are usually performed by modifications of either the lateral rhinotomy or midfacial degloving. A bifrontal craniotomy allows for superior access and visualization of the anterior ventral skull base including the cribriform plates, orbital roofs, and lateral planum sphenoidale not often provided by transfacial approaches without endoscopic assistance alone (**Fig. 5**).[2] Craniofacial resection allows for resection of dural and intracranial involvement and the appropriate reconstruction. Like many of the aforementioned procedures, a craniofacial resection may be combined with a transfacial or endoscopic approach to allow for complete resection and reconstruction.

The procedure first begins with a bicoronal incision from preauricular ear tragus to contralateral ear tragus following a coronal plane behind the hairline and is carried down through the subcutaneous tissue. Dissection is carried anteriorly in the subgaleal plane, which is a relatively avascular plane, to preserve the pericranium for reconstructive purposes. The anterior skin flap is elevated to the level of the supraorbital rim,

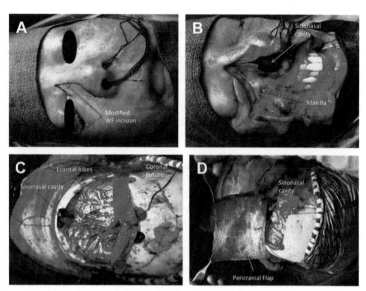

Fig. 5. Intraoperative photos of the craniofacial approach and pericranial flap reconstruction. (*A*) Planned transfacial incisions with Weber Ferguson modification. (*B*) Transfacial partial maxillectomy and sinonasal tumor dissection. (*C*) Bifrontal craniotomy to allow for dissection and clearance of dural and intracranial margins. (*D*) Anterior based pericranial flap after primary dural reconstruction with dura repair substitute.

taking great care not to injure the supraorbital or supratrochlear neurovascular bundles because the pericranial flap is based off of these vessels. Once the supraorbital foramen (or notch) is encountered, an elevator is used to isolate the neurovascular bundle. If a true foramen exists, a 2-mm osteotome is used to fracture the inferior portion of the foramen to free the pedicle and allow it to be mobilized with the rest of the pericranial flap. Posteriorly, the dissection should continue far enough to allow for an adequate amount of pericranium for reconstruction. Laterally, dissection should be carried deep to the superficial layer of the deep temporal fascia. Further laterally, dissection into or deep to the temporal fat pads is necessary to protect the facial nerve. The frontal branch of the facial nerve courses along in the temporoparietal fascia just superficial to the zygoma. By remaining in the plane of the deep layer of the deep temporal fascia, the temporal fat pad along with the superficial fascia will be elevated and thus protect the nerve.

Completion of the exposure is followed by a bicoronal craniotomy (see **Fig. 5**). Bur holes are drilled bilaterally near the midline just anterior to the coronal suture. Two additional bur holes are placed laterally, posterior to the frontozygomatic suture. These are connected using a guarded craniotome through the frontal bone and anterior table of the frontal sinus. The lower horizontal bone cut is placed approximately 1 to 2 cm above the supraorbital rim to reduce need for frontal lobe retraction. The underlying dura is then elevated with great care particularly taken in elevating the dura from the underlying cranial sutures and superior sagittal sinus, where the dura may be more adherent.

A subfrontal approach may also be used when the anterior osteotomy includes the superior orbit, glabella, nasal root, and nasal bones. This approach allows for minimal retracting on the frontal lobes while providing more direct access to the anterior ventral skull base up to the planum sphenoidale. After the bicoronal flap is raised to the inferior border of the nasal bones, 2 burr holes are created at the level of the supraorbital foramen above the glabella and medial to the supraorbital foramina bilaterally and at the superior extent of the frontal sinus bilaterally. Dura is elevated over the planned osteotomies, which are then created connecting the 4 burr holes. The osteotomies are then carried inferiorly from the supraorbital foramina anterior to the lacrimal crest and insertion of the medial canthal ligament. At this point, the upper lateral cartilages can be disarticulated from the nasal bones, or a horizontal osteotomy can be created 3 to 5 mm superior to their junction to connect to the contralateral side. Finally, a posterior osteotomy is created with an osteotome separating the bone flap from the crista galli.

After the bone flap is removed, the frontal lobes are mechanically retracted and protected with malleable retractors. The frontal sinus is cranialized, and the dura is opened and divided from the anterior ventral skull base by sharply dividing the dural attachments at the crista galli. The olfactory bulb is transected at the cribriform plate. Dural elevation continues exposing the orbital roofs, planum sphenoidale, and optic chiasm to obtain complete dural margins. In cases in which there is gross involvement of the orbit, this approach can be extended to include orbital exenteration. At this point, the intracranial portion of the procedure is complete and can be combined with the previously described transfacial approaches to provide optimal exposure.

RECONSTRUCTION

A primary concern of reconstruction after craniofacial approaches to the anterior ventral skull base is minimizing the risk of cerebrospinal fluid (CSF) leak and thereby meningitis by providing a watertight closure of the dura. Risk of reconstructive failure is greatly reduced if the original repair is performed with a vascularized flap.[7] Larger defects typically require a dural patch. Potential sources include temporal fascia, fascia lata, or dural substitutes. The defect created in the anterior cranial fossa floor will then be reconstructed using the pedicled pericranial flap, which is based on the supraorbital/supratrochlear neurovascular bundles (see **Fig. 5**). The flap is elevated from the previously developed anterior skin flap and is carried down to the level of the glabella as previously described. This flap is then rotated intracranially but kept extradural and secured to the dura over the planum sphenoidale. This provides a vascularized barrier separating the dura and the nasal cavity. Free bone grafts used to span the defect and support the brain are usually not required and have been found to increase the risk of osteoradionecrosis and infection. It is also unnecessary to place a skin graft along the inferior surface of the flap in the nasal cavity, as this tissue rapidly mucosalizes. The pericranial flap will traverse the frontal sinus outflow tract; therefore, it is important to fully cranialize the sinus to prevent mucocele formation. This procedure can be performed by stripping all of the mucosa from the frontal sinus and the nasofrontal ducts with placement of fat or free muscle to obliterate dead space inferiorly. The bone flap is then replaced and secured with miniplates and burr hole covers, and the scalp incision is closed in the usual 2-layered fashion.

POSTOPERATIVE CARE, REHABILITATION, AND RECOVERY

Patients are typically admitted to the intensive care unit with a dedicated critical care team for close neurologic monitoring including hourly neurologic checks and continuous cardiopulmonary monitoring with continuous electrocardiogram, blood pressure with arterial line, and pulse oximetry. Fluid status is also closely tracked to maintain normal cardiac output and cerebral blood flow. Electrolyte abnormalities are adequately corrected to prevent confounding factors that may impair the ability to assess mental status.

Prophylactic broad-spectrum antibiotics are routinely given perioperatively and while nasal packing remains in place. If significant frontal lobe manipulation (excessive retraction) was required, the patient is also typically started on anticonvulsant therapy. Deep venous thrombosis prophylaxis includes the sequential compression devices, early mobilization of patients who are typically "up out of bed" by postoperative day 1, and prophylactic subcutaneous heparin by postoperative day 2.

Postoperative imaging when the cranial vault is entered includes CT scan obtained within the first 12 hours postoperatively as a baseline for future studies and to assess for any possible intracranial complication. Additionally an early MRI is obtained to evaluate for completeness of the oncologic resection.

COMPLICATIONS AND MANAGEMENT

Complications of anterior ventral skull base resection include brain contusion, edema, stroke, Syndrome of Inappropriate Antidiuretic Hormone Secretion, CSF leakage, pneumocephalus, meningitis, intracranial abscess, and osteomyelitis with the most serious complications being related to the brain. Decreasing excess brain manipulation by reducing retraction and by maximizing exposure can greatly reduce the risk of many of the brain-related complications.[8] Intraoperative bleeding is a significant risk as well and can occur when the ethmoidal or sphenopalatine arteries fail to be sufficiently addressed.

Pneumocephalus may occur as a result of air leak from the sinonasal tract into the cranial cavity. This condition may occur as a result of a patient blowing his or her nose, which drives air through the dural closure or via a siphoning effect created by lumbar spinal drains. A change in a patient's mental status should alert the clinician to the possibility of this complication and should be evaluated immediately with CT scan. Small amounts of air may be treated with continued observation, but larger volumes of air should be evacuated. Preventative measures are key, and it may be helpful to keep a patient intubated or with tracheotomy until they can follow commands.

CSF leak is also a common complication and is significant because of the increased risk of meningitis. CSF leak typically presents as clear rhinorrhea or as a salty/metallic taste in the back of the patient's throat. Small or low-flow leaks may be managed conservatively with continued lumbar CSF drainage, but high-flow or persistent leaks require operative repair.

Central nervous system infections, such as meningitis and intracranial abscess, are also a major source of postoperative morbidity and mortality in patients who have undergone craniofacial resections. The risk of these complications can be significantly mitigated with the use of sterile technique, vascularized reconstruction to separate the sinonasal mucosa from the intracranial compartment, and with appropriate perioperative prophylactic antibiotics.

Ocular complications such as vision loss and epiphora can occur with inadequate corneal protection, failure to preserve lacrimal drainage, or excessive dissection in the orbit. Scarring and stenosis of the nasolacrimal duct may also lead to epiphora. Restriction of extraocular movement may occur secondary to entrapment of an extraocular muscle during reconstruction.

CLINICAL RESULTS

Craniofacial resection was first described in 1963[9] but it was associated with significant morbidity because of cranial bone manipulation, brain retraction, and protracted recovery times. In fact, Ketcham and Van Buren[10] reported a 54% overall complication rate in their first 89 patients. However, with improvements in surgical techniques and reconstruction, technologic advances, and increased use of multidisciplinary teams, it quickly became the gold standard for resection of anterior ventral skull base tumors. Over the next 2 decades, reported complication rates of craniofacial resection ranged from 25% to 49%[11-14] with hospital mortality rates ranging from 4% to 5%.[13]

The International Collaborative Study Group[15] reviewed 1193 patients who underwent craniofacial resection from 1970 to 2000. They found the postoperative mortality rate to be 4.7%. The overall complication rate was 36.3%, with wound complications occurring in 19.8% of patients, central nervous system–related complications in 16.2%, orbital complications in 1.7%, and systemic complications in 4.8% of patients. Further subdivision of this patient cohort included 334 patients who underwent craniofacial resection for paranasal sinus malignancy. Five-year overall, disease-specific, and recurrence-free survival rates were 48.3%, 53.3%, and 45.8%, respectively.[16] Postoperative complications occurred in 32.9% and the postoperative mortality rate was 4.5%. The authors concluded that craniofacial resection was a safe surgical treatment for malignancies of the paranasal sinuses but not without significant morbidity.[15]

Larger resections have long been known to predispose to higher complications, as early studies found that extent of intracranial extension to be the largest predictor of postoperative complication and that surgical involvement of more than one skull base site is significantly associated with postoperative complications.[17,18] Independent predictors of overall, disease-specific, and recurrence-free survival have been found to be the status of surgical margins, histologic findings of the primary tumor, and intracranial extent.[15,19]

Significant advancements in intraoperative image guidance, endoscopic instrumentation, and understanding of anatomic relationships were made starting in the 1980s and resulted in a paradigm shift toward the treatment of ventral skull base malignancies with endoscopic resection. Anatomic sites that were formerly reserved for open procedures can now be accessed endoscopically, and thus the indications for open approaches to the skull base have decreased dramatically.[20-25] Recently, the remaining indications for use of open approach to the ventral skull base were proposed to include lesions necessitating larger resections of more morbid disease with greater intracranial extension and more firm tumor consistency, and increased proximity or encasement of vital structures.[26]

Lastly, although rapid advancement in endoscopic technology has opened new surgical corridors to the ventral skull base, it is critical to appreciate outcome differences and biases in the literature with regard to tumor stage between endoscopic and open craniofacial approaches. In 2 separate meta-analyses of 23 and 47 studies each, comparing surgical outcomes for endoscopic and open craniofacial resections of esthesioneuroblastomas, the endoscopic group in comparison to the open group had significantly higher overall survival rates, lower rates of local recurrence, and lower regional metastases rates.[27,28] However, although these results evidently support the endoscopic approach over open craniofacial techniques, neither of these studies controlled for tumor stage or grade, which are often key predictors of overall outcome. Additionally, it is generally understood that most patients undergoing an open approach compared with those underdoing purely endoscopic surgery will likely have a more advanced-stage tumor, which is necessitating open craniofacial techniques for tumor resection.

In Fu and colleagues,[29] multivariate and subgroup analyses were carried out that controlled for tumor stage and adjuvant therapy when comparing the endoscopic and open approaches, which continued to show improved overall survival in the endoscopic group but no significant difference in locoregional control or metastasis-free survival. In Miller and colleagues,[30] 465 patients at a single institution who underwent either open or endoscopic approaches for resection of anterior skull base tumors, were reviewed for postoperative outcomes and complications. Although there was a higher rate of postoperative infection and systemic complications in the open group, significant selection bias exists and may modestly increase the open group's complication profile, as higher stage and advanced tumors generally require an open approach for resection.[30] Thus, in the endoscopic era, higher complication rates seen in open craniofacial approaches when compared with endoscopic approaches must be interpreted with the caveat that tumor stage can dictate operative technique.

SUMMARY

Anterior ventral skull base tumors are anatomically complex, are histologically diverse, and provide surgeons with unique challenges in resection and reconstruction. The use of transfacial and craniofacial resection provides the surgeon with excellent exposure for possible en bloc resection but may come at a cost such as higher complication rates. Advances in endoscopic endonasal surgery have transformed the surgical approach for anterior ventral skull base tumors, but the utility and advantage of open resection remains invaluable for highly advanced tumors.

REFERENCES

1. Ho AS, Zanation AM, Ganly I. Malignancies of the Paranasal sinuses. In: Flint PW, Haughey BH, Lund V, et al, editors. Cummings otolaryngology head and neck surgery. 6th edition. Philadelphia: Saunders; 2015. p. 1176–201.
2. Pereira L, Carron MA, Mathog RH. Traditional craniofacial resection. Oper Tech Otolaryngology Head Neck Surg 2010;21(1):2–8.
3. Ohngren G. Malignant disease of the upper jaw. Proc R Soc Med 1936;29(11): 1497–514.
4. Thakker JS, Fernandes R. Evaluation of reconstructive techniques for anterior and middle skull base defects following tumor ablation. K Oral Maxillofac Surg 2014;72:198–204.
5. Fernandes R. Reconstruction of maxillary defects with the radial forearm free flap. Atlas Oral Maxillofacial Surg Clin N Am 2007;15:7–12.
6. Murphy J, Isaiab A, Wolf JS, et al. Quality of life factors and survival after total or extending maxillectomy for sinonasal malignancies. J Oral Maxillofac Surg 2015; 73:759–63.
7. Snyderman CH, Janecka IP, Sekhar LN, et al. Anterior cranial base reconstruction: role of galeal and pericranial flaps. The Laryngoscope 1990;100(6):607–14.
8. Eloy JA, Vivero RJ, Hoang K, et al. Comparison of transnasal endoscopic and open craniofacial resection for malignant tumors of the anterior skull base. The Laryngoscope 2009;119(5):834–40.
9. Ketcham AS, Wilkins RH, Vanburen JM, et al. A combined intracranial facial approach to the paranasal sinuses. Am J Surg 1963;106:698–703.
10. Ketcham AS, Van Buren JM. Tumors of the paranasal sinuses: a therapeutic challenge. Am J Surg 1985;150(4):406–13.
11. Richtsmeier WJ, Briggs RJ, Koch WM, et al. Complications and early outcome of anterior craniofacial resection. Arch Otolaryngol Head Neck Surg 1992;118(9): 913–7.

12. Kraus DH, Shah JP, Arbit E, et al. Complications of craniofacial resection for tumors involving the anterior skull base. Head Neck 1994;16(4):307–12.

13. Patel SG, Singh B, Polluri A, et al. Craniofacial surgery for malignant skull base tumors: report of an international collaborative study. Cancer 2003;98(6):1179–87.

14. Dias FL, Sa GM, Kligerman J, et al. Complications of anterior craniofacial resection. Head Neck 1999;21(1):12–20.

15. Ganly I, Patel SG, Singh B, et al. Complications of craniofacial resection for malignant tumors of the skull base: report of an International Collaborative Study. Head Neck 2005;27(6):445–51.

16. Ganly I, Patel SG, Singh B, et al. Craniofacial resection for malignant paranasal sinus tumors: report of an International Collaborative Study. Head Neck 2005; 27(7):575–84.

17. Irish JC, Gullane PJ, Gentili F, et al. Tumors of the skull base: outcome and survival analysis of 77 cases. Head Neck 1994;16(1):3–10.

18. Wornom IL 3rd, Neifeld JP, Mehrhof AI Jr, et al. Closure of craniofacial defects after cancer resection. Am J Surg 1991;162(4):408–11.

19. Bentz BG, Bilsky MH, Shah JP, et al. Anterior skull base surgery for malignant tumors: a multivariate analysis of 27 years of experience. Head Neck 2003;25(7):515–20.

20. Kassam A, Snyderman CH, Mintz A, et al. Expanded endonasal approach: the rostrocaudal axis. Part II. Posterior clinoids to the foramen magnum. Neurosurg Focus 2005;19(1):E4.

21. Kassam A, Snyderman CH, Mintz A, et al. Expanded endonasal approach: the rostrocaudal axis. Part I. Crista galli to the sella turcica. Neurosurg Focus 2005;19(1):E3.

22. Kassam AB, Gardner P, Snyderman C, et al. Expanded endonasal approach: fully endoscopic, completely transnasal approach to the middle third of the clivus, petrous bone, middle cranial fossa, and infratemporal fossa. Neurosurg Focus 2005;19(1):E6.

23. Kassam AB, Snyderman C, Gardner P, et al. The expanded endonasal approach: a fully endoscopic transnasal approach and resection of the odontoid process: technical case report. Neurosurgery 2005;57(1 Suppl):E213 [discussion: E213].

24. Kassam AB, Thomas AJ, Zimmer LA, et al. Expanded endonasal approach: a fully endoscopic completely transnasal resection of a skull base arteriovenous malformation. Childs Nerv Syst 2007;23(5):491–8.

25. Kassam AB, Vescan AD, Carrau RL, et al. Expanded endonasal approach: vidian canal as a landmark to the petrous internal carotid artery. J Neurosurg 2008; 108(1):177–83.

26. Zada G, Du R, Laws ER Jr. Defining the "edge of the envelope": patient selection in treating complex sellar-based neoplasms via transsphenoidal versus open craniotomy. J Neurosurg 2011;114(2):286–300.

27. Komotar RJ, Starke RM, Raper DM, et al. Endoscopic endonasal compared with anterior craniofacial and combined cranionasal resection of esthesioneuroblastomas. World Neurosurg 2013;80(1–2):148–59.

28. Devaiah AK, Andreoli MT. Treatment of esthesioneuroblastoma: a 16-year metaanalysis of 361 patients. The Laryngoscope 2009;119(7):1412–6.

29. Fu TS, Monteiro E, Muhanna N, et al. Comparison of outcomes for open versus endoscopic approaches for olfactory neuroblastoma: a systematic review and individual participant data meta-analysis. Head Neck 2016;38(Suppl 1):E2306–16.

30. Miller JD, Taylor RJ, Ambrose EC, et al. Complications of open approaches to the skull base in the endoscopic era. J Neurol Surg B 2016, in press.

Endoscopic Resection of Pterygopalatine Fossa and Infratemporal Fossa Malignancies

CrossMark

Gretchen M. Oakley, MD[a,b],*, Richard J. Harvey, MD, PhD[b,c,1]

KEYWORDS

- Pterygopalatine fossa • Infratemporal fossa • Sinonasal malignancy • Endoscopic
- Skull base

KEY POINTS

- The surgical approach should be sufficiently wide to allow the limits of dissection to be visualized and accessed easily with a 0° endoscope and straight instruments.
- Following fixed anatomic landmarks and finding normal boundaries are 2 principles that ensure safe surgery and complete resection in distorted anatomy.
- Rather than avoiding the internal carotid artery for fear of causing injury, it should be sought out and identified to ensure its safety and guide surgery.
- The junction of the vidian nerve and cartilaginous eustachian tube lies just anterior to the anterior genu of the petrous internal carotid artery and is an excellent surgical guide.
- The most common postoperative comorbidities are ipsilateral palate numbness, eustachian tube dysfunction (rather than effusion), and trismus.

INTRODUCTION

The pterygopalatine fossa (PPF) and infratemporal fossa (ITF) house complex and densely packed neurovascular anatomy. Surgery in this area is made possible by improved anatomic understanding of the complex ventral skull base anatomy, advances in endoscopic instrumentation, and improved ventral skull base reconstruction strategies.

Disclosure: R.J. Harvey is a consultant with Medtronic, Olympus, and NeilMed; Advisory Board for Sequiris; and has received grant support from ENTTech, Stallergenes, and NeilMEd. G.M. Oakley has no financial disclosures.
[a] Department of Otolaryngology – Head and Neck Surgery, University of California San Francisco, San Francisco, CA, USA; [b] Rhinology and Skull Base Research Group, Applied Medical Research Centre, University of New South Wales, Sydney, New South Wales, Australia; [c] Faculty of Medicine and Health Sciences, Macquarie University, Sydney, New South Wales, Australia
[1] 67 Burton Street, Darlinghurst, New South Wales 2010, Australia.
* Corresponding author. 2233 Post Street, San Francisco, CA 94115.
E-mail address: gmoakley@gmail.com

Otolaryngol Clin N Am 50 (2017) 301–313
http://dx.doi.org/10.1016/j.otc.2016.12.007
0030-6665/17/© 2016 Elsevier Inc. All rights reserved.

The transition from traditional craniofacial to endoscopic resections of sinonasal and ventral skull base malignancies initially brought on concerns about the appropriateness of the procedure. There was speculation that the lack of en bloc tumor resection in an endoscopic approach may compromise oncologic results. However, many clinicians are of the opinion that an en bloc resection of tumors in locations such as the skull base is rarely possible regardless of the approach used. The goal is always complete resection with negative margins regardless of technique. The endoscopic approach offers several additional advantages, including a shorter operation time, less morbidity, and a shorter hospital stay.[1,2] In addition, complication rates have been shown to be lower[3] and the reduction of quality of life likely less than in open resections.[4]

PREOPERATIVE PLANNING

If a portion of the tumor is accessible in the nasal or paranasal cavity, a tissue biopsy can be taken either in the office or in the operating room to gain further information as to the origin of the disorder for the purposes of treatment planning. A lesion extending anterior to the head of the middle turbinate that is without the clear appearance of a vascular neoplasm can safely be biopsied in a clinic setting. A bleeding tumor edge in the anterior nasal cavity can readily be managed with topical vasoconstriction and bipolar electrocautery with minimal discomfort to the patient. A problem posterior to this becomes more cumbersome and difficult for the patient to tolerate. However, tumors in the PPF or ITF often cannot be reached for biopsy without a surgical approach identical to that used for the endoscopic resection. In this scenario, imaging characteristics, location, involved structures, and tumor behavior are used to determine the most likely disorder, on which surgical planning is based. It is important also to prepare for any alterations to the plan that could occur if intraoperative diagnosis is different than expected. A metastatic work-up should also be completed before proceeding to the operating theater with either combined computed tomography (CT) and MRI or fluorodeoxyglucose PET.

Preoperative CT imaging for lesions of the PPF and ITF is useful to assess the surrounding bony anatomy, expansion versus erosion of the involved bone, and widening of adjacent foramina. T1 postcontrast MRI with fat suppression removes the fat signal of the ITF and the marrow of the bone of the skull base, and is vital for evaluating tumor margins, surrounding soft tissue detail, any tumor extension into the orbit, or involvement of adjacent nerves or dura. V2 should be followed from the roof of the maxillary sinus through the foramen rotundum, and V3 through the foramen ovale. Perineural spread associated with the vidian nerve is common, so it should be considered preoperatively as well. Particular attention should also be paid to perineural involvement in the cavernous sinus and the descending palatine nerve, because either of these could alter management. Involvement of the descending palatine nerve may indicate a need for some degree of hard palate resection. Any tumor extension through the inferior orbital fissure or intracranially must be noted as well. Direct extension through the middle cranial fossa will be apparent, so it is subtler dural enhancement, particularly adjacent to foramina, that is important to detect. Research has shown that 1 mm and greater than or equal to 2 mm of dural thickening correlate with a positive predictive value of dural invasion of 46.7% and 100%, respectively.[5] Tumor positioned laterally to the internal carotid artery (ICA) at its carotid foramen precludes a strictly endoscopic approach. An open approach, whether combined, staged, or on its own, is required to access this area. A checklist of important preoperative imaging evaluation steps is shown in **Box 1**.

Box 1
A checklist of important preoperative assessments for any sinonasal tumor by imaging study

CT

- Fine cut, bony windows, 3 view
  - Expansion versus erosion of bone
  - Widening of foramen rotundum and ovale
  - Adjacent normal bony anatomy
  - Involvement of hard palate

MRI

- T1, postgadolinium, fat suppression
  - Margins of tumor
  - Surrounding normal soft tissue
  - Orbital extension
    - Periorbita
    - Inferior orbital fissure
  - Intracranial extension
    - Direct through middle cranial fossa
    - Dural thickening or enhancement
    - Attention to foramen rotundum and ovale
  - Perineural spread
    - V2
    - V3
    - Vidian nerve
    - Descending palatine nerve
  - ICA
    - Intact flow
    - Tumor lateral to carotid foramen
  - Parapharyngeal disease
  - Inferior soft tissue extent

These imaging studies should be compatible with and used for image guidance during the procedure. Image guidance is a useful surgical adjunct to help surgeons confirm the location of vital structures when local anatomy is altered by tumor distortion or invasion and to verify the completeness of resection. However, it is simply a tool and does not replace the surgeon's knowledge of the local anatomy, and should have limited influence on the previously planned surgical resection.

Access to PPF and ITF malignancies should be decided preoperatively based on tumor pathology and stage. For resection of malignant tumors of the PPF or ITF, adequate access should not be compromised by efforts to keep the approach conservative or by concerns for subsequent sinonasal function. The approach should be sufficiently wide to allow the limits of dissection to be visualized and accessed with 0° instruments at all times.

SURGICAL TECHNIQUE
Preparation

Immediately following intubation, the patient's nose is packed with ten 75-mm by 12-mm (3-inch by 0.5-inch) patties soaked in a 10-mL mixture of 1% ropivacaine and 1:1000 adrenaline (5 mL each); clinicians should ensure they are in place for a minimum of 10 minutes before beginning the case so they may have a maximum topical vasoconstriction effect. The patient receives 1 g of intravenous ceftriaxone and has a Foley catheter and an arterial line placed for close monitoring. The image guidance is set up and registered to the patient with verification of accuracy. The bed should be in reverse Trendelenburg with the head elevated to 15° to decrease central venous pressure and maximize hemostasis and operative conditions. A solution of 1% ropivacaine with 1:100,000 adrenaline is injected locally, with particular attention to the root of the middle turbinate, the septum, the inferior turbinate, and the floor of the nose in this case. If the tumor burden in the nasal cavity is large enough to prevent adequate local injection in these areas, a greater palatine injection through the mouth is an effective alternative. Once the heart rate returns to a more bradycardic range, preferably under 70 beats/min, following the epinephrine effects from the local injection, the case is begun.

Lateral Access

Almost always, when addressing malignant disorders far lateral access into the ITF requires additional procedures beyond antrostomies. This requirement should be part of the surgical plan and performed outright rather than decided intraoperatively as a result of struggling with visualization and mobility. Any attempts at limited access almost certainly lead to loss of oncologic integrity in the tumor resection.

A modified medial maxillectomy is a standard part of accessing this region. However, a total rather than a modified medial maxillectomy can be used. In this case, the maxillary sinus is entered anterior to the nasolacrimal duct. If strictly lateral access is necessary, then this prelacrimal approach can remain low and the nasolacrimal duct can be cut cleanly, leaving the sac intact without the need for further reconstructive intervention (**Fig. 1**). If superior and lateral access is necessary, disruption of the nasolacrimal apparatus may include the nasolacrimal sac, in which case an

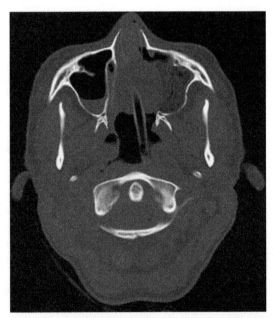

Fig. 1. Axial CT scan on postoperative day 1 following resection of a left sinonasal undifferentiated carcinoma that required a total medial maxillectomy to gain sufficient lateral access. Note the resection of the left nasolacrimal duct. The nasal cavity and maxillary sinus are filled with absorbable dressing and a Foley balloon as part of the reconstruction.

endoscopic dacryocystorhinostomy may be necessary to ensure adequate function postoperatively.

An endoscopic Denker maxillotomy is another option for lateral access. In this procedure, the entire medial buttress is removed with a drill (**Fig. 2**). The lacrimal apparatus is disrupted similar to a total medial maxillectomy. Complications related to the procedure include injury to the anterior superior alveolar nerve; potential transection of the canine root; and, importantly, loss of lateral support of the alar cartilage to the pyriform aperture. Alar retraction can occur when performed endoscopically but is usually less severe than when done open.[6]

The concept of transseptal access implies 2 meanings. A posterior septectomy allows for binostril, 2-surgeon, 4-handed operating, in addition to a more lateral reach within the ITF. Anterior transseptal approaches have been described to reach the anterior wall and zygomatic recess of the maxilla.[7] These approaches require reconstruction of anterior septum and are for anterolateral maxillary disease and not ITF disorder.

It has been shown that access lateral to the infraorbital nerve is possible with a maxillary antrostomy, modified medial maxillectomy, or total maxillectomy in 63.3% of cases, but this is improved to 97.6% when a transseptal approach is added.[7] A transseptal approach provides equivalent access to a Denker, with the average septal window being 1.56 cm from the columella to access the entire posterior maxillary sinus wall.[8] Surgeon should have a low threshold to use one of these extended procedures to ensure easy access to the lateral margin of the tumor and its adjacent normal tissue with use of a 0° endoscope and straight instruments. Ensuring comfortable maneuverability and easy visualization of the involved region maximizes the chances of complete resection and good postoperative surveillance.

Accessing the Pterygopalatine Fossa and Infratemporal Fossa

When operating in the PPF and ITF, it is necessary to first have good visualization of both the skull base and the orbit, which can be achieved beginning with a wide

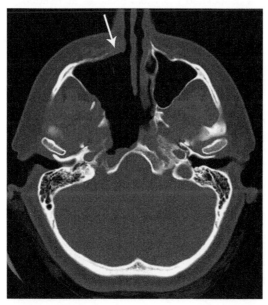

Fig. 2. Axial CT scan at 3 months after tumor resection showing what is resected for a Denker maxillotomy (*arrow*).

maxillary antrostomy and sphenoethmoidectomy using a 0° rigid endoscope and straight cutting instruments, a Kerrison rongeur, and a microdebrider. These procedures should not be considered complete unless there is easy visualization of the maxillary sinus roof, a smooth transition from roof to medial orbital wall, and the orbit can be followed all the way back to its apex in the sphenoid sinus (**Fig. 3**). A modified medial maxillectomy is then performed. The inferior turbinate is clamped just behind the head, then transected with curved iris scissors up to the anterior edge of the maxillary antrostomy leaving the clamped edge in situ to maintain hemostasis. The remainder of the inferior turbinate is cut back where it attaches to the medial maxillary wall and pushed into the nasopharynx. A mucosal flap from the nasal floor is preserved using the monopolar cautery and Cottle elevator and reflected medially out of the way, then ultimately laid back down on the nasal floor when dissection of this area is completed. The medial maxillary wall is resected posteriorly to the greater palatine canal and anteriorly to the level of the nasolacrimal duct using a Kerrison rongeur, Blakesley forceps, and a backbiter. The inferior turbinate is laid medially over the edge of the posterior wall for easy transection, leaving just the posterior stump, which is cauterized. It is important that the maxillectomy is taken down flush with the nasal floor using a drill with 15° 5-mm diamond burr to ensure that there is free movement of straight instruments through this area during the upcoming tumor dissection in the PPF or ITF (**Fig. 4**). Drilling is carried back through the descending palatine canal to the posterior maxillary sinus wall. The mucosa is elevated from the orbital process of the palatine bone to identify the crista ethmoidalis and the sphenopalatine artery exiting the sphenopalatine foramen posterior to it. The posterior wall of the maxillary sinus is removed using a Kerrison rongeur, exposing the PPF contents. At this point the internal maxillary artery must be identified, ligated, and displaced laterally (discussed later). The descending palatine artery and nerve are transected. The vertical portion of the palatine bone is drilled, posterior to which lies the medial pterygoid plate and muscle. Drilling can be extended laterally through the lateral pterygoid muscle with resection of the associated pterygoid muscles as needed. Hemostasis of the

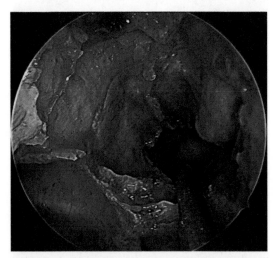

Fig. 3. Intraoperative endoscopic image showing a completed sphenoethmoidectomy in which the orbit can easily be visualized as it transitions from orbital floor to medial orbital wall and posteriorly to orbital apex.

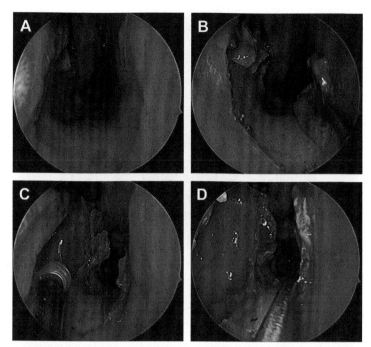

Fig. 4. Intraoperative endoscopic images of the steps of a modified medial maxillectomy appropriate for accessing a PPF or ITF tumor. The inferior turbinate is clamped and cut posterior to the anterior head and then reflected posteriorly out of the way before being ultimately resected (*A*). A nasal floor mucosal flap is preserved (*B*) and the medial wall of the maxillary sinus is resected with a Kerrison rongeur and high-speed diamond burr (*C*), until it is flush with the nasal floor (*D*).

pterygoid venous plexus may be necessary in this area. The pterygoid plates can be followed to their attachment to the middle cranial fossa. The infraorbital nerve can be seen as it traverses the roof of the maxillary sinus and followed posteriorly into the PPF. It enters the foramen rotundum in the middle cranial fossa. Posterior to the medial pterygoid plate in the nasopharynx is the eustachian tube. The vidian nerve and canal should also be identified at the inferolateral aspect of the sphenoid sinus floor at the junction of the sphenoid body and the pterygoid process (**Fig. 5**). Whether it is preserved or sacrificed, much like V2, depends on the extent of dissection needed, but in malignant resections of the PPF or ITF it typically needs to be sacrificed. The vidian nerve and eustachian tube together play a critical role in identifying the ICA, which is the most important step in any dissection of the infratemporal fossa.

Vascular Control

The sphenopalatine artery provides 90% of the blood supply for the nose and sinuses and commonly branches before exiting the sphenopalatine foramen,[9] and surgeons must be aware of these anatomic variations for effective vascular control. A standard sphenopalatine artery ligation is almost never sufficient. Most malignant cases need more lateral vascular control, which should be achieved with dissection of ITF fat and identification and ligation of the internal maxillary artery (**Fig. 6**). The prior lateral access facilitates this.

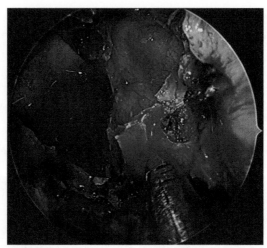

Fig. 5. Intraoperative endoscopic image of the opening of the vidian canal at the junction on the sphenoid body and pterygoid process.

Orientation Using Landmarks

Malignant tumors often invade, distort, or obliterate adjacent structures, which can frequently mean losing the normal anatomy that guides endoscopic surgery. Following fixed anatomic landmarks and finding the normal boundaries of the tumor are 2 principles that can help ensure safe surgery and complete resection in a difficult distorted field. The nasal floor, posterior choana, eustachian tube orifice, skull base, sella, and orbital wall are the fixed anatomic landmarks that aid in endoscopic surgery.[6] Unadulterated anatomy on the contralateral side may also be used for orientation. Finding normal landmarks around the periphery of the tumor is a critical element of

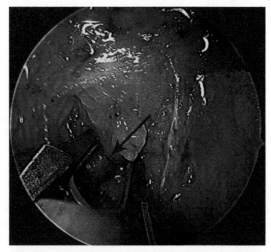

Fig. 6. The internal maxillary artery (*black arrow*) in its distal extent is identified in the pterygopalatine and infratemporal fossa fat. It is then clipped with a 5-mm endoscopic clip applier for lateral vascular control.

endoscopic resection of malignancies. In some cases, tumor debulking may be required to reveal the necessary anatomy.

Careful documentation of resection margins as they are taken is important in malignant tumor resections. It allows accurate reresection of any positive frozen-section margins, facilitates decision making, and guides postoperative radiation therapy field planning.

Identification and Management of the Internal Carotid Artery

The concept of following fixed anatomic landmarks for orientation and safe dissection is also the key to identifying the ICA, which is a critical step in any endoscopic resection of ITF disorder. Because of its complex course and multiple anatomic relationships, the ICA has previously been studied in segments (parapharyngeal, petrous, paraclival, parasellar, paraclinoid, and intradural),[10] with the petrous segment consisting of the vertical segment, posterior genu, horizontal segment, and anterior genu.[11] The eustachian tube[12–16] and vidian nerve[12,13,17] have been suggested in prior studies as landmarks to safely identify the petrous ICA. To accomplish this, the vidian canal is first located in the posterior PPF at the level of the sphenoid sinus floor and at the junction of the sphenoid body and the pterygoid process. Using a 15° 5-mm diamond burr, drilling then proceeds in a posterior direction along the medial and inferior borders of this canal (**Fig. 7**). As the pterygoid process and medial pterygoid plate are drilled away, the cartilaginous portion of the eustachian tube can be palpated and followed in the superolateral direction toward its attachment to the skull base. The point where the vidian nerve and the cartilaginous eustachian tube come together lies just anterior and inferior to the anterior genu of the petrous ICA (**Fig. 8**). As the vidian nerve is followed posteriorly a fibrocartilaginous tissue is identified, which marks the attachment to the foramen lacerum and the anterior border of the anterior genu of the ICA.[13,14] In a cadaveric study, the investigators showed the length of the vidian nerve from the PPF canal opening to its junction with the cartilaginous eustachian tube to be 17.4 ± 4.1 mm. The eustachian tube from its nasopharyngeal orifice to its junction with the vidian nerve was found to be 15.0 ± 3.6 mm. (Oakley GM, Ebenezer J,

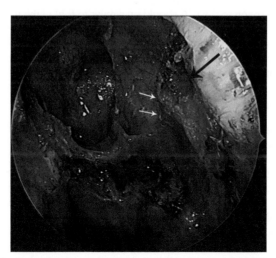

Fig. 7. The length of the vidian canal is shown following careful drilling along its medial and inferior borders (*white arrows*), beginning at its opening in the posterior PPF (*black arrow*).

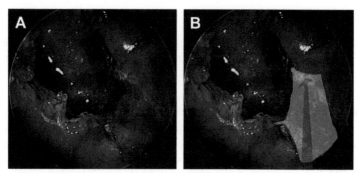

Fig. 8. The left ICA and vidian–eustachian tube junction is shown. The black star marks the vertical segment of the petrocavernous ICA as it nears the anterior genu and the thin black arrow marks the vidian canal (*A*). The eustachian tube from the nasopharyngeal orifice through its cartilaginous portion (*green shading*) as it tracks superolaterally toward the skull base (*blue arrow*) is shown (*B*).

Hamizan AW, et al: Finding the petrocavernous carotid artery: the vidian-eustachian junction as a reliable landmark. Int Forum Allergy Rhinol. Submitted for publication.) The horizontal and vertical segments and the anterior genu of the ICA are located posterior and superior to the vidian-eustachian junction point in all cases, and therefore this junction point acts as a fixed limit for dissection in these directions; however, superior to this point the medial-lateral position of the ICA is more variable. (Oakley GM, Ebenezer J, Hamizan AW, et al: Finding the petrocavernous carotid artery: the vidian-eustachian junction as a reliable landmark. Int Forum Allergy Rhinol. Submitted for publication.) From this point, the dissection can be extended superiorly to expose the vertical segment of the ICA, or medial to lateral to expose the horizontal segment. Resection of the cartilaginous portion of the eustachian tube, and following the line of the lateral pterygoid plate assist in exposing the entry point of the ICA to the petrous bone at the carotid foramen (posterior genu).[18]

The surgical approach to the ICA should be similar to that of the facial nerve in mastoid surgery. Instead of avoiding it for fear of causing injury, it should be sought out and identified to ensure its safety and guide surgery in the area. Having the ICA identified in the surgical field can give the surgeon confidence in the orientation and maximize the chance for a complete resection.

RECONSTRUCTION AND POSTOPERATIVE CARE

Any sinonasal resection requires some extra effort to ensure that the final cavity is optimized for healing and a return to normal function. This extra effort includes connecting natural ostia to the common cavity to prevent mucus recirculation, contouring the final resection cavity (and avoiding sumps), and good access for saline irrigations. Reconstruction following resection of PPF and ITF malignancy depends on involvement of the middle cranial fossa and ICA. Dural reconstruction has been shown to be successful[19] with free grafts and pedicled flaps[20–22] and is not discussed in detail here. The ICA is likely to be exposed to some degree following any malignant resection in the PPF or ITF. Although there are no clear guidelines as to how an exposed ICA in the sinonasal cavity should be managed long term, it seems prudent to at least add a covering over it in the form of a free mucosa graft or a biomaterial such as collagen matrix (**Fig. 9**). A free mucosa graft can be fashioned from a previously resected

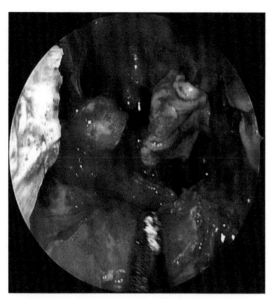

Fig. 9. Intraoperative image of a free mucosal graft being used to cover an exposed ICA following a left nasopharyngectomy for squamous cell carcinoma.

inferior or middle turbinate uninvolved with tumor that is filleted open and thinned by removing bone. Once the selected vascularized or free mucosa graft is positioned, absorbable gelatin sponge is used to cover the reconstruction and a removable bolster from either bismuth iodine paraffin–embedded gauze or a Foley balloon is used to keep the repair in place. To prevent adhesion formation in the nasal cavity, 0.5-mm Silastic sheets are placed between the inferior turbinate remnant and the septum bilaterally and secured with Prolene suture. Patients are placed on a standard postoperative management protocol that consists of at least 1 night in the intensive care unit with bed rest for 48 hours (if dural reconstruction is required), then gradual mobilization. Intravenous antibiotics are administered while in hospital, followed by 10 days of oral antibiotics, and twice-daily saline irrigations using a high-volume high-pressure squeeze bottle is started on discharge. The patient follows up in clinic at 3 weeks postoperatively for evaluation. Silastic sheets are removed at this time and the cavity is cleaned of residual absorbable packing materials.

COMPLICATIONS AND COMORBIDITIES

Clearance of a malignant tumor in an area like the PPF or ITF can often mean sacrifice of neighboring neurovascular structures. Therefore, there are some postoperative comorbidities that are routine for this type of surgery and patients should be counseled accordingly. The descending palatine nerve is often transected, with permanent ipsilateral palate numbness, which is rarely troublesome but worthwhile preparing patients for preoperatively. Similarly, the vidian nerve is resected. Although this may intuitively seem like it could lead to problematic xerophthalmia, in practice, these symptoms are rarely bothersome for patients postoperatively in the senior author's experience. However, a noticeable lack of emotional tearing on that side is expected. Transection of the eustachian tube can result in eustachian tube dysfunction, although effusion is not typical. Immediate postoperative pterygoid muscle swelling from surgical manipulation and partial resection also commonly cause temporary trismus. Other postoperative comorbidities vary based on the extent of the malignancy. However, in many cases, patients with a malignant tumor in such an anatomically critical location as the PPF or ITF have no more than unilateral palate numbness and lack of emotional tearing postoperatively, which is a testament to the benefits of an endoscopic approach.

SUMMARY

The endoscopic resection of PPF and ITF malignancies allows excellent visualization and manipulation of tissues in an anatomically complex area compared with open approaches. With less approach morbidity, endoscopic endonasal surgery allows an easier recovery and early transition to adjuvant radiotherapy. The endoscopic approach is minimal access but rarely minimally invasive. Surgeons should gain wide access to ensure comfortable maneuverability and easy visualization of both the tumor and its adjacent normal tissue with use of a 0° endoscope and straight instruments. This method maximizes the chances of complete resection and good postoperative surveillance.

REFERENCES

1. Goffart Y, Jorissen M, Daele J, et al. Minimally invasive endoscopic management of malignant sinonasal tumours. Acta Otorhinolaryngol Belg 2000;54(2):221–32.
2. Kim BJ, Kim DW, Kim SW, et al. Endoscopic versus traditional craniofacial resection for patients with sinonasal tumors involving the anterior skull base. Clin Exp Otorhinolaryngol 2008;1(3):148–53.
3. Nicolai P, Battaglia P, Bignami M, et al. Endoscopic surgery for malignant tumors of the sinonasal tract and adjacent skull base: a 10-year experience. Am J Rhinol 2008;22(3):308–16.
4. de Almeida JR, Witterick IJ, Vescan AD. Functional outcomes for endoscopic and open skull base surgery: an evidence-based review. Otolaryngol Clin North Am 2011;44(5):1185–200.
5. McIntyre JB, Perez C, Penta M, et al. Patterns of dural involvement in sinonasal tumors: prospective correlation of magnetic resonance imaging and histopathologic findings. Int Forum Allergy Rhinol 2012;2(4):336–41.
6. Harvey RJ, Gallagher RM, Sacks R. Extended endoscopic techniques for sinonasal resections. Otolaryngol Clin North Am 2010;43(3):613–38, x.
7. Harvey RJ, Sheehan PO, Debnath NI, et al. Transseptal approach for extended endoscopic resections of the maxilla and infratemporal fossa. Am J Rhinol Allergy 2009;23(4):426–32.
8. Prosser JD, Figueroa R, Carrau RI, et al. Quantitative analysis of endoscopic endonasal approaches to the infratemporal fossa. Laryngoscope 2011;121(8): 1601–5.
9. Simmen DB, Raghavan U, Briner HR, et al. The anatomy of the sphenopalatine artery for the endoscopic sinus surgeon. Am J Rhinol 2006;20(5):502–5.
10. Labib MA, Prevedello DM, Carrau R, et al. A road map to the internal carotid artery in expanded endoscopic endonasal approaches to the ventral cranial base. Neurosurgery 2014;10(Suppl 3):448–71 [discussion: 471].
11. Ziyal IM, Ozgen T, Sekhar LN, et al. Proposed classification of segments of the internal carotid artery: anatomical study with angiographical interpretation. Neurol Med Chir (Tokyo) 2005;45(4):184–90 [discussion: 190–1].

12. Falcon RT, Rivera-Serrano CM, Miranda JF, et al. Endoscopic endonasal dissection of the infratemporal fossa: anatomic relationships and importance of eustachian tube in the endoscopic skull base surgery. Laryngoscope 2011;121(1): 31–41.
13. Liu J, Pinheiro-Neto CD, Fernandez-Miranda JC, et al. Eustachian tube and internal carotid artery in skull base surgery: an anatomical study. Laryngoscope 2014; 124(12):2655–64.
14. Liu J, Sun X, Liu Q, et al. Eustachian tube as a landmark to the internal carotid artery in endoscopic skull base surgery. Otolaryngol Head Neck Surg 2016; 154(2):377–82.
15. Ozturk K, Snyderman CH, Gardner PA, et al. The anatomical relationship between the eustachian tube and petrous internal carotid artery. Laryngoscope 2012; 122(12):2658–62.
16. Rivera-Serrano CM, Terre-Falcon R, Fernandez-Miranda J, et al. Endoscopic endonasal dissection of the pterygopalatine fossa, infratemporal fossa, and poststyloid compartment. Anatomical relationships and importance of eustachian tube in the endoscopic skull base surgery. Laryngoscope 2010;120(Suppl 4): S244.
17. Kassam AB, Vescan AD, Carrau RL, et al. Expanded endonasal approach: vidian canal as a landmark to the petrous internal carotid artery. J Neurosurg 2008; 108(1):177–83.
18. Ho B, Jang DW, Van Rompaey J, et al. Landmarks for endoscopic approach to the parapharyngeal internal carotid artery: a radiographic and cadaveric study. Laryngoscope 2014;124(9):1995–2001.
19. Harvey RJ, Smith JE, Wise SK, et al. Intracranial complications before and after endoscopic skull base reconstruction. Am J Rhinol 2008;22(5):516–21.
20. Harvey RJ, Nogueira JF, Schlosser RJ, et al. Closure of large skull base defects after endoscopic transnasal craniotomy. Clinical article. J Neurosurg 2009; 111(2):371–9.
21. Harvey RJ, Parmar P, Sacks R, et al. Endoscopic skull base reconstruction of large dural defects: a systematic review of published evidence. Laryngoscope 2012;122(2):452–9.
22. Harvey RJ, Sheahan PO, Schlosser RJ. Inferior turbinate pedicle flap for endoscopic skull base defect repair. Am J Rhinol Allergy 2009;23(5):522–6.

Endoscopic Resection of Clival Malignancies

Adam J. Folbe, MD[a,b], Peter F. Svider, MD[a,*], James K. Liu, MD[c,d], Jean Anderson Eloy, MD[c,d,e,f]

KEYWORDS

- Clivus • Clival tumor • Clival lesion • Clival chordoma • Chordoma
- Chondrosarcoma • Endoscopic endonasal approach • Skull base surgery

KEY POINTS

- Managing clival lesions using a minimally invasive approach presents numerous therapeutic challenges because of the close proximity of surrounding critical structures, including the basilar artery, brain stem structures, and cranial nerves.
- In leading skull base centers, the surgical management of clival lesions has evolved considerably from aggressive external approaches to endoscopic endonasal approaches in select cases.
- Although chordomas and chondrosarcomas are the most common clival lesions, a broad differential diagnosis should be considered during evaluation of clival lesions.
- Identification of the vidian nerve intraoperatively is of paramount importance, because finding this structure helps keep the surgeon below the internal carotid artery.

INTRODUCTION

When the tumors appeared at the base of the skull, death usually followed a history of cranial nerve disturbances with pressure symptoms.
— Dr Ernest M. Daland, 1919[1]

Disclosures: None.
Conflicts of Interest: None.
[a] Department of Otolaryngology–Head and Neck Surgery, Wayne State University School of Medicine, 4201 St. Antoine, 5E-UHC, Detroit, MI 48201, USA; [b] Department of Neurosurgery, Wayne State University School of Medicine, 4201 St. Antoine, 5E-UHC, Detroit, MI 48201, USA; [c] Department of Otolaryngology–Head and Neck Surgery, Rutgers New Jersey Medical School, 90 Bergen Street, Suite 8100, Newark, NJ 07103, USA; [d] Department of Neurological Surgery, Center for Skull Base and Pituitary Surgery, Neurological Institute of New Jersey, Rutgers New Jersey Medical School, 90 Bergen Street, Suite 8100, Newark, NJ 07103, USA; [e] Endoscopic Skull Base Surgery Program, Rhinology and Sinus Surgery, Otolaryngology Research, Department of Otolaryngology–Head and Neck Surgery, Rutgers New Jersey Medical School, 90 Bergen Street, Suite 8100, Newark, NJ 07103, USA; [f] Department of Ophthalmology and Visual Science, Rutgers New Jersey Medical School, 90 Bergen Street, Suite 8100, Newark, NJ 07103, USA
* Corresponding author.
E-mail address: psvider@gmail.com

http://dx.doi.org/10.1016/j.otc.2016.12.008
oto.theclinics.com

Managing clival lesions using a minimally invasive approach presents numerous therapeutic challenges because of the close proximity of surrounding critical structures, including the basilar artery, internal carotid artery, brain stem structures, and the cranial nerves. Discussing his operative technique in *Curetting Tumor at Base of Skull*, Dr C.A. Porter detailed surgical steps in the management of a patient with a chordoma in the early twentieth century:

> Incision [was] made over [the] growth and colloid like material curetted out with free hemorrhage. [The] curette [was] passed upwards and inwards and large masses of material obtained. The greater part of the base of the skull was denuded and the base bone felt everywhere. Bleeding gradually ceased.[1]

Surgical management of clival lesions has evolved considerably since then, as endoscopic endonasal approaches now represent the standard of care for many lesions at leading skull base centers.[2–5] Nonetheless, the significant potential for serious neurologic consequences makes an understanding of the complex anatomic relationships encountered exceedingly important. Principles of preoperative workup, surgical preparation, intraoperative management, and postsurgical care are discussed in this article, with illustrative examples of diagnostic imaging and endoscopic anatomy. In addition, the various disorders presenting as clival lesions are discussed.

DIFFERENTIAL DIAGNOSIS OF CLIVAL LESIONS

Although chordomas are the most common clival lesions, they are not the only disorder identified. A differential diagnosis can have implications in terms of patient counseling and prognosis. Surgical resection is the mainstay of treatment of most lesions, and radiation therapy can be considered either as primary therapy among poor surgical candidates or as adjuvant therapy for aggressive or recurrent disease.

Radiologic Characteristics of Clival Lesions

Differentiating factors affecting imaging interpretation are detailed in **Table 1**. Importantly, chordomas usually originate at the midline (**Fig. 1**) whereas chondrosarcomas are more commonly paramedian (**Figs. 2** and **3**). Depending on the primary tumor, metastasis to the clivus usually has lower signal on T2-weighted magnetic resonance (MR), compared with greater signaling from chordomas and chondrosarcomas.[6] Lesions originating from the clivus as well as the nasopharynx tend to elevate the pituitary gland, in contrast with invasive pituitary macroadenoma involving the clivus, which surrounds the pituitary and makes discrete identification of the pituitary difficult.[6]

Chordoma

Developing from cells thought to be remnants of the embryonic notochord, clival chordomas can commonly present with nonspecific symptoms such as pain and headaches. Furthermore, patients may present with abducens nerve (cranial nerve VI) deficits caused by the close proximity of Dorello's canal, trigeminal nerve (cranial nerve V) involvement, and in some cases lower cranial nerve deficits. In more advanced disease, there can also be cerebellopontine angle extension (**Fig. 4**). Analysis of population-based resources such as the Surveillance, Epidemiology, and End Results (SEER) database reveals that chordomas occur predominantly among men more than 40 years of age, and have an incidence of 0.08 per 100,000 people.[7] Younger patients are more likely to have intracranial and clival lesions, and the overall 5-year survival rate has been reported to be 65% to 67.6%,[7] which is significantly

Table 1
Radiologic characteristics of clival lesions

Lesion	Characteristics
Chordoma	CT: originates midline, bone destruction
	Tumor margin is sharp
	MR: T1, hypointense, isointense (may have cystic components with protein bright on T1)
	MR: T2, hyperintense
	Decreasing intensity with increasing grade
	Heterogeneous enhancement
Chondrosarcoma	CT: originates off midline
	Stippled foci of calcification
	More calcification with low grade
	MR: T1, low/intermediate signal
	MR: T2, hyperintense
Plasmacytoma	Plain radiograph: lytic lesions, clear margins
	CT: invasive outline
	MR: T1, isointense
	MR: T2, hyperintense
	MR: homogenous uptake with gadolinium
Metastasis	MR: T2, depends on origin, but may be hypointense
Pituitary adenoma	Epicenter is in sella
	Does not narrow cavernous carotids (in contrast with meningioma)
NPC	Increases pituitary gland (in contrast with pituitary macroadenoma)

Abbreviations: CT, computed tomography; MR, magnetic resonance; NPC, nasopharyngeal carcinoma.
Data from Refs.[6,41,50–56]

worse than patients with ventral skull base chondrosarcoma. Although chordomas are technically considered a low-grade neoplasm and metastasis is exceedingly uncommon, they are usually locally aggressive, with significant clinical sequelae caused by the close proximity of surrounding structures.[8,9]

Chondrosarcoma

Arising from endochondral cartilage found within the base of the skull, chondrosarcomas most commonly originate spontaneously, although an association has been suggested in patients with Paget disease and osteochondromas.[10–13] These lesions comprise as much as 6% of ventral skull base tumors, with a recent review of the literature encompassing 560 intracranial chondrosarcomas noting a plurality (32%) of tumors being associated with the clivus.[10] Hence, diplopia, headaches, and other sequelae related to brainstem compression are the most common presenting complaints.[14] The 5-year survival is nearly 90%, with a median survival of 2 years.[15] It has also been noted that there are differences in recurrence rate depending on single modality (surgical) management versus surgery and adjuvant radiotherapy (44% vs 9%). Chondrosarcomas are graded from I to III based on the level of dedifferentiation, with the mesenchymal and conventional subtypes being the histologic variants found intracranially.[10,15] No statistical difference in recurrence was noted on evaluation of tumors by histologic grading, although mesenchymal subtype tumors have a markedly increased recurrence rate (63%) relative to conventional tumors (16%).[10] A significant proportion of studies comprising these aforementioned percentages contained patients operated on before the recent development and popularization of endoscopic endonasal resections for these lesions.[4,14]

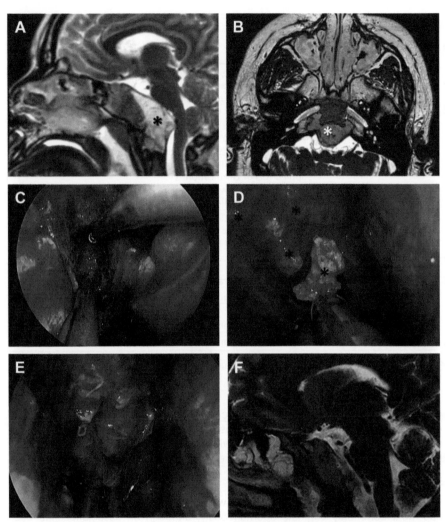

Fig. 1. Preoperative sagittal (*A*) and axial (*B*) T2-weighted magnetic resonance (MR) imaging of a young female patient with a clival chordoma with significant brainstem compression. Intraoperative endoscopic images of the patient during the endoscopic endonasal approach (*C*), resection (*D*), and final brainstem decompression (*E*). (*F*) Postoperative sagittal T2-weighted MR imaging of the patient showing adequate brainstem decompression. The asterisks mark the lesion.

Plasmacytoma

Although exceedingly uncommon,[16,17] plasmacytomas of the clivus have been reported in the literature and may be a challenging diagnosis. These lesions have ambiguous presentations, and may be difficult to discern radiologically (**Fig. 5**). They may present with many of the same cranial neuropathies and related sequelae characteristic of other clival lesions. Formed by monoclonal proliferation of plasmocytes, these represent an underappreciated consideration in the differential diagnosis of clival lesions, and present as solitary lesions in contrast with multiple myeloma, which is a

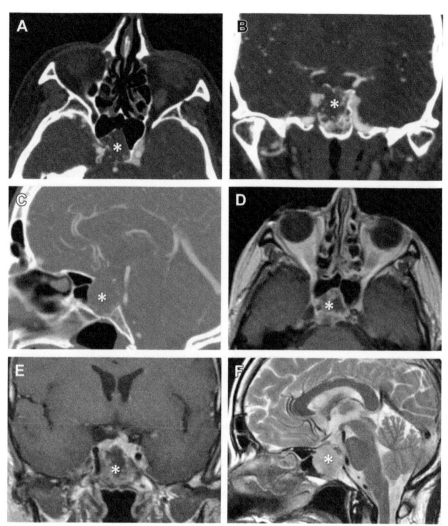

Fig. 2. Preoperative axial (*A*), coronal (*B*), and sagittal (*C*) CT angiography scan of a patient with a large right paramedian clival chondrosarcoma. Axial (*D*) and coronal (*E*) T1-weighted gadolinium-enhanced MR imaging of the patient showing significant heterogeneity in the lesion. (*F*) Sagittal T2-weighted MR imaging of the same patient showing mild brainstem compression. The asterisks mark the lesion.

multifocal/disseminated entity; however, they do harbor a risk of progression to multiple myeloma.[16] Intracranial plasmacytomas progress to multiple myeloma in less than a third of cases, whereas solitary lesions elsewhere in the body have progression rates exceeding 50%.[18–21] One case series revealed that patients had preoperative imaging indicating clival destruction on computed tomography (CT) that was strongly enhancing on MRI; lesions were isointense on T1 MRI and ranged from isointense to hyperintense on T2 MRIs.[22] These lesions are frequently misdiagnosed as other conditions, such as pituitary adenomas or chordomas (see **Fig. 5**). Note that, because of their high level of radiosensitivity in other locations, radiation therapy is the optimal

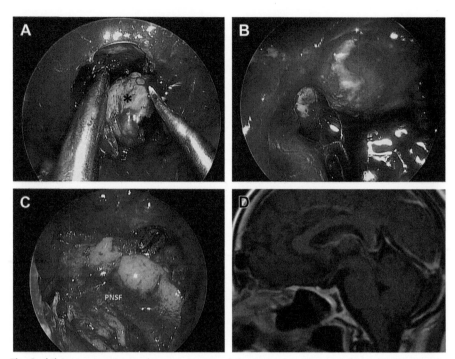

Fig. 3. (A) Intraoperative endoscopic image of the patient in **Fig. 2** while undergoing endo-scopic endonasal resection of the chondrosarcoma. The asterisk marks the lesion. (B) Endo-scopic view of the resection bed after gross total resection of the lesion. (C) Endoscopic view of the repair of the created ventral skull base defect using a vascularized pedicled naso-septal flap (PNSF). (D) Postoperative sagittal T1-weighted gadolinium-enhanced MR imaging of the patient showing adequate brainstem decompression and no gross residual disease.

treatment. Nonetheless, these represent diagnostic challenges and may often be operated on as a result.[16,22] On histology, immunohistochemical staining is positive for CD138 and CD38, and in many cases CD56.[22,23] Importantly, proliferation is restricted to immunoglobulin light chains, supporting a clonal cause.[16,22,24,25]

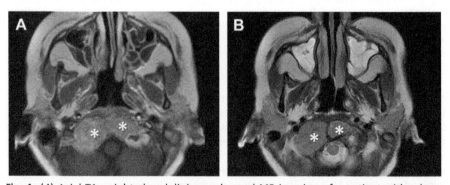

Fig. 4. (A) Axial T1-weighted gadolinium-enhanced MR imaging of a patient with a large chordoma involving the lower clivus and both occipital condyles and hypoglossal canals. (B) Axial T2-weighted MR imaging of the same patient. The asterisks mark the lesion.

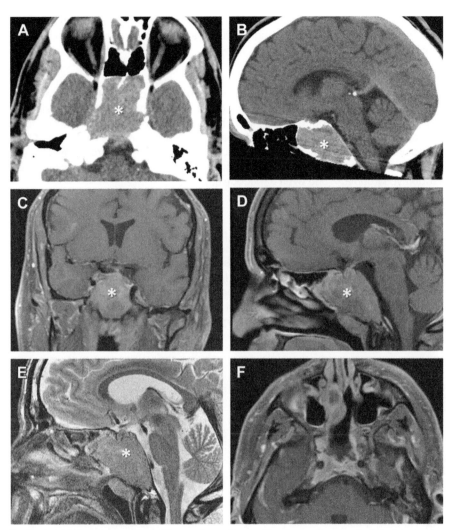

Fig. 5. Axial (*A*) and sagittal (*B*) CT scan of a patient with a large clival/ventral skull base plasmacytoma. Coronal (*C*) and sagittal (*D*) T1-weighted gadolinium-enhanced MR imaging of the patient showing significant enhancement of the lesion. (*E*) Sagittal T2-weighted MR imaging of the same patient. (*F*) Axial T1-weighted gadolinium-enhanced MR imaging of the patient after endoscopic endonasal biopsy of the lesion, and subsequent management with radiotherapy and chemotherapy. The asterisks mark the lesion.

Metastasis

Metastasis to the clivus represents another uncommon but underappreciated consideration. Although this should be low on the differential diagnosis, there have been cases reported in the literature. In one review of 47 cases involving metastatic disease to the clivus, this was often the initial presentation of a malignancy elsewhere.[26] Abducens nerve palsy was noted to be the most common specific presenting symptom (61.9%). The most common causes identified were prostate cancer, hepatocellular carcinoma, and thyroid follicular carcinoma.[26,27] Hence, completing a review of symptoms may be essential to raise suspicion for a primary lesion elsewhere. Further-more, this diagnosis should be strongly considered in patients with a personal history of malignancy (**Fig. 6**).

Other Lesions

There are numerous other lesions that have been reported in the literature and can potentially involve the clivus. Direct spread from surrounding structures should be kept in mind and ruled out on imaging. For example, an invasive pituitary adenoma or a nasopharyngeal carcinoma can have direct extension into the clivus.[28–30] Other entities in the differential diagnosis include lymphoma,[31,32] fibrous dysplasia,[33] keloid/scarring,[34] meningioma,[35,36] craniopharyngioma,[37] a sphenoid sinus mass, rhabdomyosarcoma,[38] and even a mucocele.[6]

PREOPERATIVE CONSIDERATIONS

As in any other interventions, preoperative planning and appropriate patient selection are paramount for maximizing surgical success in the management of clival lesions, and this takes on special importance because of the close proximity of neurovascular structures within a tight anatomic space. Much as the endoscopic transsphenoidal technique has largely replaced open approaches for pituitary lesions,[39] this minimally invasive approach is gaining favor for clival lesions among leading skull base centers in recent years. Because surgery plays the primary role in the treatment of most clival lesions, patients obviously need to be cleared for administration of general anesthesia.

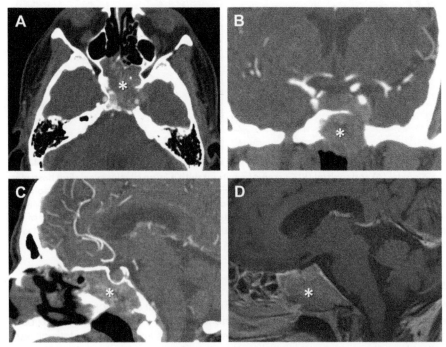

Fig. 6. Axial (*A*), coronal (*B*), and sagittal (*C*) CT angiography scan of a patient with a large clival/ventral skull base metastatic renal cell carcinoma. (*D*) Sagittal T1-weighted gadolin-ium-enhanced MR imaging of the same patient showing enhancement of the lesion. The asterisks mark the lesion.

When nonsurgical entities, such as metastasis, myeloma, or lymphoma, are suspected, there should be consideration of less extensive alternatives, such as a biopsy, particularly in patients possessing a greater number of risk factors. In patients who are not surgical candidates because of medical comorbidities, other modalities, such as radiation therapy and/or chemotherapy, may play a role, depending on the specific cause.

A history and physical examination, with special focus on the cranial nerve, neurologic, and ophthalmologic evaluation may offer important clues to the extent and clinical impact of the lesion. Furthermore, nasal endoscopy is essential in any attempt to characterize endoscopic anatomy, because this can affect accessibility and surgical approach. Importantly, nasal septal deviations may need to be corrected intraoperatively, and this potentially affects skull base reconstruction depending on the techniques considered.

Obtaining imaging from several modalities may enhance surgical planning. In addition to relaying extent of tumor extension, preoperative CT may offer clues about specific disorders (see **Table 1**). CT can also provide valuable information about the presence of anatomic variations, including posterior ethmoid cells (Onodi cells), skull base integrity, clival thickness, and the presence or absence of sphenoid sinus disease. Furthermore, it can help identify whether lesions have arisen from the clivus or represent direct extension from surrounding structures. MR can further characterize lesion involvement of surrounding structures, because it offers better differentiation of soft tissue structures. MR enhancement patterns of several more common lesions are listed in **Table 1**. Furthermore, MRI can also offer detail about cranial nerve anatomy.[9,40] An additional reason for imaging relates to the potential for clival lesions to represent metastasis from another site. In any patient with a known history of cancer, this should be further explored.

In addition to conventional CT and MR, preoperative evaluation with angiography facilitates appropriate surgical planning. The authors favor CT angiography rather than conventional angiography for preoperative planning in appropriate ventral skull base lesions, because it is less invasive; however, conventional angiography may be helpful if any major vessels are suspected to have extensive tumor involvement, particularly for evaluating the integrity of collateral circulation.[5,9,41] The authors also use CT angiography as our imaging of choice for intraoperative navigation and stereotactic image guidance because this allows localization of the course of the paraclival carotid arteries in relation to the bony involvement of the clival tumor.

In recent years, microscopic approaches have given way to endoscopic endonasal approaches for a variety of disorders of the ventral skull base.[9,39] Although lesions lacking lateral involvement are typically amenable to the endoscopic endonasal technique, planning for adjunct approaches may be necessary for lesions deviating significantly from the midline.

ANATOMIC OVERVIEW

Although this is not an exhaustive review of sphenoid sinus anatomy, several key points of surgical anatomy relevant to the clivus must be appreciated. On preoperative review of imaging, it is important to look for sphenoid sinus anatomic variants, such as Onodi cells, and deviation of the intersinus septum, as well as to be familiar with whether there is bony dehiscence over the internal carotid artery and/or the optic nerve.[42]

Representing the bony division between the nasopharynx and posterior fossa, clival anatomy can be organized into 3 portions. The upper third is posterior to the sphenoid sinus and sellar floor, whereas the middle third is behind the posterior sphenoid body and the basiocciput, between the sellar floor and the floor of the sphenoid sinus.[5] The inferior portion of the clivus is the caudal basiocciput portion below the floor of the sphenoid sinus. Incision of the dura at the junction of the middle and lower clivus reveals the basilar venous plexus, as well as the abducens nerves bilaterally; the distance of these cranial nerves from each other is approximately 2 cm.[43] Incising the dura reveals a view of the basilar and vertebral arteries, cranial nerves III to VI, and the pons.[5] Superiorly, the pituitary gland and optic chiasm can be appreciated.

INTRAOPERATIVE APPROACH FOR THE ENDOSCOPIC ENDONASAL TECHNIQUE

Many basic principles applicable to successful endoscopic sinus surgery can play an important role in the endoscopic endonasal approach for clival lesions. Note that many of the nuances the authors use in these procedures are discussed later, and some of these steps may vary depending on surgeon preference. The importance of appropriate preparation, patient positioning, and hemostasis cannot be overemphasized. Although the focus of our training is on understanding surgical anatomy, neuronavigation is helpful to evaluate the proximity of critical structures throughout the clivus. The patient is positioned supine with the head slightly rotated to the right side. The authors ensure appropriate nasal decongestion with oxymetazoline-soaked pledgets and meticulous injection of the tail of the middle turbinate (lidocaine with 1:100,000 epinephrine). After allowing appropriate time for decongestion and injections to take effect, we occasionally resect the inferior third of the middle turbinate on 1 side. After this, the posterior nasal septum is used to identify the tail of the middle turbinate as well as the superior turbinate. We then excise the inferior portion of the superior turbinate, identify the anterior face of the sphenoid sinus by going up the posterior wall of the nasal cavity, then enlarge the sphenoid sinus os on the side we are working medially and inferiorly with careful attention to protecting the pedicle of the nasoseptal flap. After this, we further enlarge the os laterally, whereat this stage, detailed preoperative review of imaging can come into play, because operating surgeons should be familiar with any anatomic variants, such as Onodi cells, dehiscence over the carotid or optic nerves, and the presence of the intersinus septum (vs the presence of other septations).[42]

After completing our sphenoidotomy on both sides in a similar fashion, we then design our nasoseptal flaps. Typically, we make a Killian incision, elevate a subperichondrial/subperiosteal flap all the way posteriorly toward the sphenoid sinus, and use a Cottle elevator to cross over to the other side, elevating a similar flap on the other side to the level of the sphenoid sinus. We then remove the rostrum of the sphenoid sinus using Kerrison rongeurs or a high-speed drill, after which we design a pedicled nasoseptal flap in anticipation of our ventral skull base defect.

Discussed in further detail later, along with variations, the authors advise the use of pedicled nasoseptal flaps when feasible. After this, we divide the inferior portion of the flap along the maxillary crest bilaterally and the superior portion so that it rides along the inferior third of the inferior middle turbinate superiorly from the sphenoid rostrum anteriorly. Exposed flaps are then removed and tucked into the nasopharynx, and we gently strip overlying mucosa off the clivus and posterior sphenoid wall. Removing bone from the sella allows for elevation of the pituitary gland to be able to address lesions involving the posterior clinoid processes.[44] After this point, we recommend using a 3-mm or 4-mm cutting burr, drilling down the clivus, bringing this along the vidian nerve bilaterally inferior to the second genu of the carotid arteries. The importance of identifying the vidian nerve cannot be overemphasized, because finding this structure helps keep the surgeon below the internal carotid artery.[4] If the sphenoid sinus is not well pneumatized, the vidian nerve can typically be identified superior to the medial pterygoid plate. Care is taken to avoid injury to the vertical paraclival carotid arteries located laterally. Use of image guidance, micro-Doppler, and careful eggshelling of bone with a diamond burr and copious irrigation can be useful in avoiding carotid injury. Skeletonization and exposure of the paraclival carotid arteries is performed judiciously on a select basis, because this can increase the risk of vascular injury. Drilling is continued posteriorly along the clivus until the dura is exposed. In cases in which opening the dura is necessary, incision is initiated medially in order to protect the abducens nerves. Alternately, the dura can be identified superiorly along the floor of the sella, and surgeons can continue dissecting in that plane posteriorly and inferiorly until the posterior clival dura is addressed.

The surgeon can further progress inferiorly depending on the extent of the mass; on reaching the nasopharyngeal portion of the clivus, a vertical cut in the roof of the nasopharynx is made, and mucosa and fascia are increased, with continued drilling. The eustachian tubes are the lateral borders of this. It is of paramount importance to drill out the entire rostrum and face of the sphenoid sinus inferiorly, from sphenopalatine foramen to sphenopalatine foramen anteriorly. Once all dimensions of the mass are exposed, the lesion can be debulked and removed as appropriate with suction, curettes, or other instruments of choice. Depending on the extent of intracranial involvement, it is important to be meticulous and deliberate in removing mucosa from a mass. In addition, any adherent attachments to bony areas may need to be further drilled out.

RECONSTRUCTION

Repair of clival skull base dural defects may present unique challenges because of a potential for significant cerebrospinal fluid (CSF) drainage, and is often optimized by multilayer closure. Furthermore, defects from these lesions may be considerably larger than those noted in the surgical management of ventral skull base lesions in other locations.

Multilayer Repair

One of the challenging aspects of multilayer repair in endoscopic clival surgery is the inability to exert forceful pressure posteriorly, because this can compress the basilar artery, brainstem, and other critical structures. For larger ventral skull base defects involving dural penetration, the authors generally use a collagen allograft or acellular dermal allograft as an inlay followed by an autologous fascia lata graft as an onlay.[3] A single layer of Surgicel is placed over the fascia lata in order to minimize graft movement. Next, an autologous fat graft is placed over the fascial graft to fill the clival bony dead space. This graft can help prevent pontine herniation through the clivus defect.[45] In addition we rotate a vascularized pedicled nasoseptal flap over our multilayered repair. Before application of the vascularized flap, there should be no gross appearance of CSF leakage.

Mucosa-sparing Techniques

The posterior bony and mucosal septectomy often performed with approaches to the clivus have a significant potential to compromise the vascular supply of the pedicled nasoseptal flap. Note that the nasoseptal flaps are not necessary in cases in which there is no CSF leak. After elevating bilateral nasoseptal flaps with incisions in offsetting locations, the flaps are freed from the septum both superiorly and inferiorly.[46] Each flap, in which the anterior border of the incision establishes the length, is inserted into the middle meatus to prevent damage, and the exposed posterior bony portion of the septum is removed to optimize exposure. After resection of the lesion, 1 of the nasoseptal flaps (occasionally both) is draped over the defect and reinforced with packing materials.[2,46] The mucoperichondrial surface should be the side contacting the defect.[3] There may be several different approaches for designing these flaps depending on the extent and location of the anticipated defect. One variation preserves the superior and inferolateral nasoseptal flap attachments; although this limits the versatility of the flap, it allows simpler closure and maximizes preservation of sinonasal architecture.[2] Another approach also using nasoseptal flap elevation bilaterally involves inferolateral release, optimized by making the inferior incisions extend under the inferior turbinates. This variation does not involve releasing the superior attachment to the septum. These flaps are then displaced superiorly and inserted into the middle meatus on each side, which allows for wider lateral exposure after subsequent posterior septectomy.[2] Regardless of which variation is used, we typically apply cottonoids followed by Gelfoam onto the nasoseptal flap, then deploy Merocel packing, which is then inflated. In addition to using bacitracin on the Merocel pack, we place patients on third-generation cephalosporin antibiotics and remove packing at 10 to 14 days postoperatively.

Postoperative Care

As detailed earlier, patients should be on antibiotic prophylaxis with either a third-generation cephalosporin or a β-lactamase–containing penicillin while packing is in place. We reinforce the importance of nasal precautions with all of our patients, including avoidance of Valsalva maneuvers, nose blowing, and drinking with straws. Although we avoid using lumbar drains in transcribriform and transsellar defects, and in our early experience did not use diversion for clival dural defects, currently we typically use lumbar drainage at 5 to 10 mL/h for 3 to 4 days for these defects.[47–49] For patients who develop postoperative CSF leakage, endoscopic exploration in the operating room should be performed. The same nasoseptal flap can be used as long as it is viable.[3]

SUMMARY

Surgical management of clival lesions presents numerous therapeutic challenges because of the close proximity of surrounding critical structures. With a detailed understanding of the endoscopic endonasal approach and relevant considerations, appropriate lesions can be removed in a safe and minimally invasive manner. Use of this technique as a primary approach represents the standard of care for many lesions at leading skull base centers, although adjunct techniques may be necessary in extensive lesions and those with significant lateral extension.

REFERENCES

1. Daland EM. Chordoma. Boston Med Surg J 1919;21:571–6. CLXXX.
2. Eloy JA, Vazquez A, Marchiano E, et al. Variations of mucosal-sparing septectomy for endonasal approach to the craniocervical junction. Laryngoscope 2016;126:2220–5.
3. Liu JK, Schmidt RF, Choudhry OJ, et al. Surgical nuances for nasoseptal flap reconstruction of cranial base defects with high-flow cerebrospinal fluid leaks after endoscopic skull base surgery. Neurosurg Focus 2012;32:E7.

4. Moussazadeh N, Kulwin C, Anand VK, et al. Endoscopic endonasal resection of skull base chondrosarcomas: technique and early results. J Neurosurg 2015;122: 735–42.
5. Stamm AC, Pignatari SS, Vellutini E. Transnasal endoscopic surgical approaches to the clivus. Otolaryngol Clin North Am 2006;39:639–56, xi.
6. Neelakantan A, Rana AK. Benign and malignant diseases of the clivus. Clin Radiol 2014;69:1295–303.
7. McMaster ML, Goldstein AM, Bromley CM, et al. Chordoma: incidence and survival patterns in the United States, 1973-1995. Cancer Causes Control 2001;12: 1–11.
8. Jones PS, Aghi MK, Muzikansky A, et al. Outcomes and patterns of care in adult skull base chordomas from the Surveillance, Epidemiology, and End Results (SEER) database. J Clin Neurosci 2014;21:1490–6.
9. Mangussi-Gomes J, Beer-Furlan A, Balsalobre L, et al. Endoscopic endonasal management of skull base chordomas: surgical technique, nuances, and pitfalls. Otolaryngol Clin North Am 2016;49:167–82.
10. Bloch OG, Jian BJ, Yang I, et al. Cranial chondrosarcoma and recurrence. Skull Base 2010;20:149–56.
11. Brandolini F, Bacchini P, Moscato M, et al. Chondrosarcoma as a complicating factor in Paget's disease of bone. Skeletal Radiol 1997;26:497–500.
12. Ibanez R, Gutierrez R, Fito C, et al. Chondrosarcoma in Paget's disease of bone. Clin Exp Rheumatol 2005;23:275.
13. Watanabe M, Funayama M, Soeda K. Paget's disease complicated by chondrosarcoma. A case report. Fukushima J Med Sci 1965;12:121–9.
14. Ditzel Filho LF, Prevedello DM, Dolci RL, et al. The endoscopic endonasal approach for removal of petroclival chondrosarcomas. Neurosurg Clin N Am 2015;26:453–62.
15. Bloch OG, Jian BJ, Yang I, et al. A systematic review of intracranial chondrosarcoma and survival. J Clin Neurosci 2009;16:1547–51.
16. Kalwani N, Remenschneider AK, Faquin W, et al. Plasmacytoma of the clivus presenting as bilateral sixth nerve palsy. J Neurol Surg Rep 2015;76:e156–9.
17. Patel TD, Vazquez A, Choudhary MM, et al. Sinonasal extramedullary plasmacytoma: a population-based incidence and survival analysis. Int Forum Allergy Rhinol 2015;5:862–9.
18. Liu ZY, Qi XQ, Wu XJ, et al. Solitary intracranial plasmacytoma located in the spheno-clival region mimicking chordoma: a case report. J Int Med Res 2010; 38:1868–75.
19. Soutar R, Lucraft H, Jackson G, et al. Guidelines on the diagnosis and management of solitary plasmacytoma of bone and solitary extramedullary plasmacytoma. Br J Haematol 2004;124:717–26.
20. Soutar R, Lucraft H, Jackson G, et al. Guidelines on the diagnosis and management of solitary plasmacytoma of bone and solitary extramedullary plasmacytoma. Clin Oncol 2004;16:405–13.
21. Tanaka M, Shibui S, Nomura K, et al. Solitary plasmacytoma of the skull: a case report. Jpn J Clin Oncol 1998;28:626–30.
22. Gagliardi F, Losa M, Boari N, et al. Solitary clival plasmocytomas: misleading clinical and radiological features of a rare pathology with a specific biological behaviour. Acta Neurochir (Wien) 2013;155:1849–56.
23. Gagliardi F, Boari N, Mortini P. Solitary nonchordomatous lesions of the clival bone: differential diagnosis and current therapeutic strategies. Neurosurg Rev 2013;36:513–22 [discussion: 522].

24. Ustuner Z, Basaran M, Kiris T, et al. Skull base plasmacytoma in a patient with light chain myeloma. Skull base 2003;13:167–71.
25. Yamaguchi S, Terasaka S, Ando S, et al. Neoadjuvant therapy in a patient with clival plasmacytoma associated with multiple myeloma: a case report. Surg Neurol 2008;70:403–7.
26. Deconde AS, Sanaiha Y, Suh JD, et al. Metastatic disease to the clivus mimicking clival chordomas. J Neurol Surg B Skull Base 2013;74:292–9.
27. Pallini R, Sabatino G, Doglietto F, et al. Clivus metastases: report of seven patients and literature review. Acta Neurochir (Wien) 2009;151:291–6 [discussion: 296].
28. Chong VF, Fan YF. Skull base erosion in nasopharyngeal carcinoma: detection by CT and MRI. Clin Radiol 1996;51:625–31.
29. Karras CL, Abecassis IJ, Abecassis ZA, et al. Clival ectopic pituitary adenoma mimicking a chordoma: case report and review of the literature. Case Rep Neurol Med 2016;2016:8371697.
30. Wong K, Raisanen J, Taylor SL, et al. Pituitary adenoma as an unsuspected clival tumor. Am J Surg Pathol 1995;19:900–3.
31. Aronson PL, Reilly A, Paessler M, et al. Burkitt lymphoma involving the clivus. J Pediatr Hematol Oncol 2008;30:320–1.
32. Grau S, Schueller U, Weiss C, et al. Primary meningeal T-cell lymphoma at the clivus mimicking a meningioma. World Neurosurg 2010;74:513–6.
33. Heman-Ackah SE, Boyer H, Odland R. Clival fibrous dysplasia: case series and review of the literature. Ear Nose Throat J 2014;93:E4–9.
34. Kanumuri VV, Raikundalia MD, Khan MN, et al. Clival keloid after nasopharyngeal radium irradiation masquerading as skull base malignancy. Laryngoscope 2014; 124:1767–70.
35. Sekhar LN, Jannetta PJ, Burkhart LE, et al. Meningiomas involving the clivus: a six-year experience with 41 patients. Neurosurgery 1990;27:764–81 [discussion: 781].
36. Steno J, Bizik I, Krajina A, et al. Meningioma of the clivus. Bratisl Lek Listy 2000; 101:200–5 [in Slovak].
37. Ragel BT, Bishop FS, Couldwell WT. Recurrent infrasellar clival craniopharyngioma. Acta Neurochir (Wien) 2007;149:729–30 [discussion: 730].
38. Seiz M, Radek M, Buslei R, et al. Alveolar rhabdomyosarcoma of the clivus with intrasellar expansion: case report. Zentralbl Neurochir 2006;67:219–22.
39. Svider PF, Keeley BR, Husain Q, et al. Regional disparities and practice patterns in surgical approaches to pituitary tumors in the United States. Int Forum Allergy Rhinol 2013;3:1007–12.
40. Mikami T, Minamida Y, Yamaki T, et al. Cranial nerve assessment in posterior fossa tumors with fast imaging employing steady-state acquisition (FIESTA). Neurosurg Rev 2005;28:261–6.
41. Erdem E, Angtuaco EC, Van Hemert R, et al. Comprehensive review of intracranial chordoma. Radiographics 2003;23:995–1009.
42. Svider PF, Baredes S, Eloy JA. Pitfalls in sinus surgery: an overview of complications. Otolaryngol Clin North Am 2015;48:725–37.
43. Puxeddu R, Lui MW, Chandrasekar K, et al. Endoscopic-assisted transcolumellar approach to the clivus: an anatomical study. Laryngoscope 2002;112:1072–8.
44. Fraser JF, Nyquist GG, Moore N, et al. Endoscopic endonasal transclival resection of chordomas: operative technique, clinical outcome, and review of the literature. J Neurosurg 2010;112:1061–9.

45. Koutourousiou M, Filho FV, Costacou T, et al. Pontine encephalocele and abnormalities of the posterior fossa following transclival endoscopic endonasal surgery. J Neurosurg 2014;121:359–66.
46. Eloy JA, Vazquez A, Mady LJ, et al. Mucosal-sparing posterior septectomy for endoscopic endonasal approach to the craniocervical junction. Am J Otolaryngol 2015;36:342–6.
47. Eloy JA, Kuperan AB, Choudhry OJ, et al. Efficacy of the pedicled nasoseptal flap without cerebrospinal fluid (CSF) diversion for repair of skull base defects: incidence of postoperative CSF leaks. Int Forum Allergy Rhinol 2012;2:397–401.
48. Eloy JA, Choudhry OJ, Shukla PA, et al. Nasoseptal flap repair after endoscopic transsellar versus expanded endonasal approaches: is there an increased risk of postoperative cerebrospinal fluid leak? Laryngoscope 2012;122:1219–25.
49. Eloy JA, Choudhry OJ, Friedel ME, et al. Endoscopic nasoseptal flap repair of skull base defects: is addition of a dural sealant necessary? Otolaryngol Head Neck Surg 2012;147:161–6.
50. Brackmann DE, Teufert KB. Chondrosarcoma of the skull base: long-term follow-up. Otol Neurotol 2006;27:981–91.
51. Cho YH, Kim JH, Khang SK, et al. Chordomas and chondrosarcomas of the skull base: comparative analysis of clinical results in 30 patients. Neurosurg Rev 2008; 31:35–43 [discussion: 43].
52. Firooznia H, Pinto RS, Lin JP, et al. Chordoma: radiologic evaluation of 20 cases. AJR Am J Roentgenol 1976;127:797–805.
53. Meyers SP, Hirsch WL Jr, Curtin HD, et al. Chordomas of the skull base: MR features. AJNR Am J Neuroradiol 1992;13:1627–36.
54. Oot RF, Melville GE, New PF, et al. The role of MR and CT in evaluating clival chordomas and chondrosarcomas. AJR Am J Roentgenol 1988;151:567–75.
55. Weber AL, Liebsch NJ, Sanchez R, et al. Chordomas of the skull base. Radiologic and clinical evaluation. Neuroimaging Clin N Am 1994;4:515–27.
56. Yeom KW, Lober RM, Mobley BC, et al. Diffusion-weighted MRI: distinction of skull base chordoma from chondrosarcoma. AJNR Am J Neuroradiol 2013;34: 1056–61. S1051.

Combined Endoscopic and Open Approaches in the Management of Sinonasal and Ventral Skull Base Malignancies

CrossMark

James K. Liu, MD[a,b,*], Anni Wong, MS[c,d],
Jean Anderson Eloy, MD[e,f,g,h]

KEYWORDS

- Skull base malignancy • Skull base defect • Skull base surgery
- Sinonasal malignancy • Endoscopic endonasal surgery • Craniotomy • Transbasal
- Nasoseptal flap

KEY POINTS

- The use of combined transcranial and endoscopic endonasal approaches or so-called cranionasal approaches to the anterior ventral skull base and paranasal sinuses remain an important option in the surgical treatment of sinonasal and ventral skull base malignancies.
- The modified 1-piece extended transbasal approach provides wide panoramic exposure to tumor that invades the frontal lobes, orbital roofs, and cribriform plate without using a transfacial incision or orbital bar removal.

Continued

Financial Disclosures: None.
Conflicts of Interest: None.
[a] Department of Neurological Surgery, Center for Skull Base and Pituitary Surgery, Neurological Institute of New Jersey, Rutgers New Jersey Medical School, 90 Bergen Street, Suite 8100, Newark, NJ 07103, USA; [b] Department of Otolaryngology – Head and Neck Surgery, Rutgers New Jersey Medical School, Newark, NJ, USA; [c] Department of Neurological Surgery, Neurological Institute of New Jersey, Rutgers New Jersey Medical School, 90 Bergen Street, Suite 8100, Newark, NJ 07103, USA; [d] Department of Otolaryngology – Head and Neck Surgery, Neurological Institute of New Jersey, Rutgers New Jersey Medical School, 90 Bergen Street, Suite 8100, Newark, NJ 07103, USA; [e] Department of Neurological Surgery, Rutgers New Jersey Medical School, Newark, NJ, USA; [f] Rhinology and Sinus Surgery, Otolaryngology Research, Endoscopic Skull Base Surgery Program, Department of Otolaryngology – Head and Neck Surgery, Neurological Institute of New Jersey, Rutgers New Jersey Medical School, 90 Bergen Street, Suite 8100, Newark, NJ 07103, USA; [g] Center for Skull Base and Pituitary Surgery, Neurological Institute of New Jersey, Rutgers New Jersey Medical School, Newark, NJ, USA; [h] Department of Ophthalmology and Visual Science, Rutgers New Jersey Medical School, Newark, NJ, USA
* Corresponding author: Department of Neurological Surgery, Center for Skull Base and Pituitary Surgery, Neurological Institute of New Jersey, Rutgers New Jersey Medical School, 90 Bergen Street, Suite 8100, Newark, NJ 07103.
E-mail address: liuj10@njms.rutgers.edu

Continued

- The endoscopic endonasal approach can be combined with the transbasal approach for secondary inspection from below after tumor removal from the transcranial exposure, further resection of tumor within the sinonasal cavity, and reconstruction with a vascularized pedicled nasoseptal flap, if needed.
- Skull base reconstruction can be performed using a simultaneous pericranial flap from above and a nasoseptal flap from below (double flap), especially when postoperative adjuvant radiation therapy is anticipated.

Abbreviations
CTA Computed tomography angiography
EEA Endoscopic endonasal approach
CSF Cerebrospinal fluid

INTRODUCTION

Since the conception of the bifrontal craniotomy by Frazier in 1913,[1] Derome[2] and Tessier and colleagues[3] popularized the transbasal approach to the anterior ventral skull base. Numerous modifications of the transbasal approach have been developed, each adding varying degrees of bone removal of the supraorbital bar, orbital roof and wall, lateral orbital rims, nasal bones, and paranasal sinuses (frontal, ethmoid, and sphenoid sinuses). In 1988, Raveh and Vuillemin,[4,5] described the subcranial approach for the removal of fronto-orbital and anteroposterior skull base tumors, which entailed nasal and orbital osteotomies and minimal frontal lobe retraction. In 1991, Kawakami and colleagues,[6] presented the extensive transbasal approach, performing en bloc bilateral orbital roof and frontal sinus osteotomy. This allowed for access to tumors extending laterally into the anterior cranial fossa. Sekhar and colleagues[7] discussed the extended frontal approach in 1992, which added an orbitofrontal or orbitofrontoethmoidal osteotomy. These transbasal modifications have allowed for increased posterior and inferior surgical view toward the clivus with less frontal lobe retraction. These midline subfrontal approaches to the anterior ventral skull base and paranasal sinuses remain critical in the treatment of anterior ventral skull base and sinonasal malignancies.

In the past decade the role of the pure endoscopic endonasal approach (EEA) has gained increasing popularity, driven by continuous advances in endoscopic instrumentation, intraoperative image guidance, and surgical technique. Resections with negative margins via a purely EEA have been successfully performed for tumors confined to the nasal cavity and paranasal sinuses with radiologic evidence of normal cribriform plate and upper ethmoid sinuses.[8]

However, limitations of the pure EEA arise when there is significant intracranial extension or considerable extension beyond the lamina papyracea.[8,9] For instance, when en bloc resection of the tumor including the cribriform plate is necessary, it may be best accomplished with an anterior craniotomy.[8,10] Thus, open approaches remain an integral component in our surgical armamentarium. In the bifrontal transbasal approach, one can access the cribriform plate and perform a total ethmoidectomy, sphenoidotomy, and midline clivectomy down to the craniovertebral junction. Traditionally, the transbasal approach was often combined with a transfacial approach (combined craniofacial approaches) to treat a vast majority of sinonasal skull base malignancies. This combined approach allowed for access to tumors residing beneath the orbit in the superolateral aspect of the maxillary sinus, where the bifrontal approach alone was restricted from.[11] Although the transfacial approach provides ample exposure for complete tumor removal, it often involved rather invasive techniques, including extensive facial incisions, facial disassembly, lateral rhinotomy, midfacial degloving, and/or facial osteotomies, leaving displeasing cosmetic results.[11,12] Infectious complications or inadequate healing may lead to malunion of bones or loss of grafts, resulting in unsightly scars and disfigurement.[12] Additionally, compared with craniofacial resection, transnasal endoscopic resection of anterior ventral skull base tumors has been demonstrated to be associated with decreased hospital and intensive care unit (ICU) stay, decreased estimated blood loss, and faster recovery.[13–15] Subsequently, the EEA has become a more favorable adjunct (endoscopic-assisted craniofacial approaches or cranionasal approaches) due to its superior panoramic visualization, illumination, and avoidance of transfacial skin incisions.[11] In this article, we discuss the role of combined transcranial and EEA approaches (combined cranionasal approach) in the surgical management of ventral skull base malignancies (**Figs. 1–3**).

COMBINED TRANSBASAL AND ENDOSCOPIC ENDONASAL APPROACH

With the advent of skull base endoscopy, the EEA and its extended variations have changed the paradigm by which ventral skull base lesions are treated. In recent years, the surgical landscape of endoscopic skull base surgery has evolved as this anatomic territory became better understood. By taking advantage of the natural anatomic corridors, such as the transnasal, transsphenoidal, transethmoidal, and transmaxillary corridors, structures from the clivus to the Meckel cave to the pterygopalatine fossa

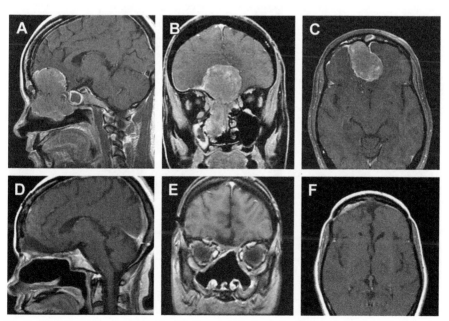

Fig. 1. (A–C) Preoperative MRI of esthesioneuroblastoma in sinonasal cavity with extension through anterior skull base and significant intracranial invasion. A combined cranionasal approach was performed to achieve complete resection. Reconstruction of the skull base defect was performed using the double-flap technique. (D–F) Postoperative MRI at 4 years shows no evidence of tumor recurrence.

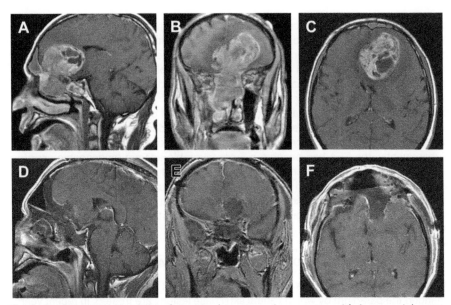

Fig. 2. (A–C) Preoperative MRI of sinonasal teratocarcinosarcoma with intracranial extension through the anterior skull base and significant brain invasion. A combined cranionasal approach was performed to achieve complete resection. Reconstruction of the skull base defect was performed using the double-flap technique. (D–F) Immediate postoperative MRI shows no evidence of residual tumor.

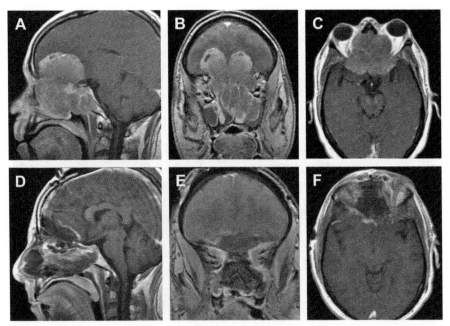

Fig. 3. (A–C) Preoperative MRI of sinonasal undifferentiated carcinoma with significant brain invasion and lateral extension. A combined cranionasal approach was performed to achieve near total resection. Reconstruction of the skull base defect was performed using the double-flap technique. (D–F) Immediate postoperative MRI shows tumor adherent to the orbital apex bilaterally.

are now accessible without external incisions.[11,16–18] The versatility of EEA has increased minimally invasive surgical access to the ventral skull base dramatically. In our practice, most sinonasal and anterior ventral skull base malignancies are treated with a purely endoscopic endonasal transcribriform approach. However, if one is to choose a transbasal approach from above, this can be used in conjunction with a complementary EEA from below to treat large lesions involving multiple anatomic compartments (see **Figs. 1–3**). The transbasal approach provides exposure from the third ventricle to the base of the clivus with relatively limited frontal lobe retraction.[19] In the past, such lesions were traditionally treated with extended transbasal approaches combined with open transfacial approaches involving facial skin incisions and facial osteotomies. Because the extended EEAs provide wide panoramic access and visualization to the ventral skull base in the sagittal and coronal planes, the traditional transfacial approaches have gradually fallen out of favor and use. From a transcranial approach, the anterior nasal cavity and superolateral regions of the maxillary sinus are difficult to visualize (blind spots). However, the EEA allows excellent visualization and access to the entire paranasal sinuses, including these blind spots, particularly with angled endoscopy. Through this synergistic combined approach, the surgeon can work from above to control and remove intracranial tumor, and also from "below" to control tumor in the sinonasal cavity. A combined approach also can be used from a reconstruction strategy because the EEA can provide an additional vascularized pedicled nasoseptal flap, if needed. This may be useful in cases in which the pericranial flap is compromised from prior craniotomies, or needs to be supplemented from below. Alternatively, the pericranial flap can serve as the primary source of vascularized reconstruction if the nasoseptal flap is compromised or invaded by a sinonasal malignancy.

SURGICAL CONSIDERATIONS: APPROACH SELECTION

Several considerations go into deciding on an appropriate operative approach for sinonasal skull base malignancies, such as anatomic location, degree of tumor extension in the sagittal and coronal plane, degree of intracranial involvement, vascular or cranial nerve encasement, brainstem compression, tumor consistency, history of prior surgical approach, surgeon's preference, and level of experience. When selecting the optimal approach based on anatomic location, consideration should be taken to choose an approach that not only has the most direct route to the tumor, but also optimizes exposure and visualization of the tumor interface with critical structures so as to avoid neurologic damage and surrounding vital structures, such as the orbit, optic nerves, carotid arteries, cavernous sinus, and frontal lobes.

History of prior surgery is important and may affect the surgical approach selected. Postoperative changes, such as altered anatomy, loss of landmarks, edema, and fibrosis may make definitive surgical resection and accurate evaluation of the extent of disease more challenging.[20] Individual surgeons may have different thresholds as to when an open approach should be warranted or added to their endoscopic resection. Hanna and colleagues[20] held a low threshold for adding a craniotomy to the EEA (combined cranionasal approach) if there was dural involvement or transdural spread and/or invasion of the skull base, whereas Nicolai and colleagues[21] continued EEA for selected patients with skull base invasion and focal dural infiltration. The surgeon must also be aware that some cases with significant tumor extension into multiple compartments may require a combination of more than 1 approach to adequately remove the tumor. Typically, the use of EEA exclusively is contraindicated when there is involvement of skin and subcutaneous tissue, nasolacrimal sac, anterior table of frontal sinus, carotid artery, and extensive dural and brain parenchymal involvement. In these instances, the addition of a transfacial or transcranial approach is warranted for optimal resection of the malignancy.[18,21] Thus, it is important to maintain the open approaches in the surgical repertoire for various indications.

PREOPERATIVE CONSIDERATIONS

Preoperative MRI is essential to assess the tumor and to check for intracranial extension. Computed tomography angiography (CTA) is useful to assess the anatomy of the anterior and posterior arterial circulation relative to the tumor, to rule out any vascular encasement, and to study the neighboring venous anatomy, including the cavernous sinus, petrosal sinuses, and any large draining veins. CTA is preferred over magnetic resonance angiography, as it also shows the bony anatomy of the skull base in high resolution. Digital subtraction angiography is reserved for complicated vascular anatomy not adequately assessed on CTA or for balloon test occlusion in cases of significant arterial encasement. In patients with sellar and suprasellar tumor involvement, baseline pituitary function should be assessed with appropriate endocrine testing. It is important to obtain formal baseline neuro-ophthalmological testing for patients who present with visual disturbances due to optic nerve and/or orbital involvement.

SURGICAL TECHNIQUE
Patient Positioning

After general endotracheal anesthesia and appropriate arterial and venous access is obtained, the patient is positioned supine and the head placed in 3-pin fixation (**Fig. 4**). The bed is flexed 10 to 15° to facilitate venous drainage. The neck is slightly extended to promote frontal lobe relaxation away from the anterior ventral skull base and to reduce the need for brain retraction.

Neuronavigation can be useful and can be used to plan the craniotomy and verify anatomic landmarks. Neurophysiologic monitoring of somatosensory and motor evoked potentials are performed. Additional neurophysiologic monitoring modalities can be used as needed depending on the location of the tumor. Antibiotics, mannitol, decadron, and antiepileptics are administered before skin incision.

Skin Incision

A preauricular bicoronal skin incision is planned behind the patient's hairline that extends from one zygoma to the other, no more than 1 cm anterior to the tragus (see **Fig. 4**). The nose and nares are also prepped, in case endoscopic endonasal

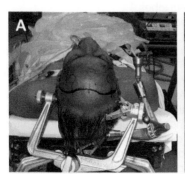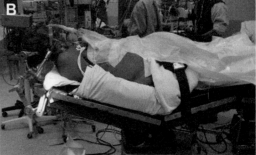

Fig. 4. (*A, B*) For a combined cranionasal approach, the patient is positioned supine with the head in 3-pin fixation. A standard bicoronal incision is used.

exploration is required to remove additional tumor from the sinuses or to harvest a vascularized pedicled nasoseptal flap to aid in anterior ventral skull base reconstruction. The face can be prepped in case an additional open transfacial is required. Abdominal and thigh incisions also can be prepared for fat and fascia lata graft harvesting, if needed.

A bicoronal skin incision is made and the scalp is elevated in a 2-layer fashion. A galeocutaneous flap is elevated anteriorly, leaving the pericranium and temporalis fascia and muscle attached to the skull. Interfascial dissection of the temporalis fascia is performed so that the superficial fat pad is elevated with the scalp to protect the frontotemporal branch of the facial nerve. When dissecting around the orbital rims, care is taken to preserve the supraorbital and supratrochlear neurovascular bundles, which provide the blood supply to the pericranium. The galeocutaneous flap is undermined posteriorly to the incision by several centimeters to allow for a longer pericranial flap harvest. The pericranium is then incised posteriorly behind the skin incision and laterally just above the superior temporal line, and elevated as a separate vascularized flap that is pedicled anteriorly (**Fig. 5**A, B).

Subperiosteal elevation of the scalp and pericranial flap exposes the orbital rims anteriorly, with care to preserve the supraorbital nerve at the supraorbital notch. In cases in which the supraorbital notch is closed by a fibrous ring, the nerve can be displaced inferiorly away from the orbital roof subperiosteally. However, in cases in which the supraorbital nerve exits from a closed osseous ring, an osteotome may be used to release the nerve from the orbital rim. The frontonasal suture is also exposed in the midline to obtain a low-lying bifrontal osteotomy at the nasion. The lateral orbital rims also can be exposed subperiosteally down to the frontozygomatic suture after performing interfascial dissection of the temporalis fascia. The superior aspect of temporalis muscle and fascia is reflected inferiorly to expose the frontal keyhole just below the superior temporal line, behind the orbital rim.

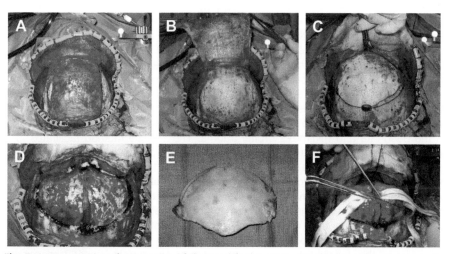

Fig. 5. Intraoperative photographs of the modified 1-piece extended transbasal approach. (*A, B*) Harvest of vascularized pedicled pericranial flap. (*C–E*) Bifrontal craniotomy incorporates the anterior wall of the frontal sinus down to the nasion and along the roofs of the orbit. This allows the lowest basal trajectory to the skull base without having to remove the supraorbital bar. (*F*) The superior sagittal sinus is ligated at the level of the crista galli and the falx cerebri is incised to the free edge.

Modified 1-Piece Extended Transbasal Approach

The standard transbasal approach is simply a bifrontal craniotomy without removal of the supraorbital bar. Access to the cribriform region and paranasal sinuses can be limited without significant frontal lobe retraction due to obstruction of line of sight by the overhang of the supraorbital bar. On the other hand, the extended transbasal approach, which typically involves a standard bifrontal craniotomy followed by a supraorbital bar osteotomy that is performed in a 2-piece fashion, provides a low basal trajectory into the anterior skull base without significant brain retraction.[19] Cosmetic reconstruction of the frontal bone and supraorbital bar in the traditional 2-piece approach can be a bit more cumbersome, as small gaps between the bone flaps can be apparent and titanium plates used in the forehead area can be more sensitive in some patients. We previously described a modified 1-piece extended transbasal approach that incorporates the bifrontal bone flap with the anterior table of the frontal sinus without requiring removal of the supraorbital bar (see **Fig. 5C–E**).[22,23] A low-lying osteotomy is made through the outer table of the frontal sinus that follows the contour of the floor of the anterior cranial fossa to provide a low basal exposure to the anterior fossa without any obstruction of line of sight.

A burr hole is made directly over the superior sagittal sinus superiorly with exposure of dura on each side of the sinus. Another set of bur holes is made in the keyhole region behind the orbital rim and below the superior temporal line to expose the frontal lobe dura. A craniotome is used to connect the midline burr hole to both frontal keyholes. The craniotome is then used to make a cut from the frontal burr hole across the lateral aspect of the supraorbital rim in a lateral-to-medial fashion. Inferiorly, an osteotomy is made through the outer table of the frontal sinus at the nasofrontal suture using a C-1 drill bit (Medtronic, Minneapolis, MN). The osteotomy is carried laterally on both sides, and follows the contour of the anterior cranial fossa and orbital rims. The intersinus septum of the frontal sinus anchors the bifrontal bone flap to the skull base and needs to be disconnected to allow elevation of the flap. This osteotomy is made by using an osteotome at the nasofrontal suture, and tapping it with a mallet. It is important to visualize incremental advancement of the osteotome while tapping with gentle force. The bone over the supraorbital rim tends to be thick as well, and may need an osteotome to release the bone flap. Once the bone flap is loose and mobile, a curved dissector is used lift the bone flap from the frontal dura and a periosteal elevator is used to fracture the posterior table of the frontal sinus to release the bone flap.

This technique provides a low basal exposure of the cribriform plate and orbital rims. In essence, it provides the same midline exposure as an extended transbasal approach without having to remove the supraorbital bar and thus avoids dissection of the periorbita and minimizes orbital trauma. The 1-piece method facilitates fast and easy cosmetic reconstruction and avoids titanium plates in the supraorbital region. Although others have described variations of a 1-piece transbasal approach with removal with the supraorbital bar,[24] our technique eliminates the need for supraorbital removal by taking advantage of the frontal sinus anatomy. After removal of the bone flap, the frontal sinus is exenterated and cranialized by removing the sinus mucosa and the posterior table of the frontal sinus. The nasofrontal ducts are packed with betadine-soaked Gelfoam before opening the dura.

To expose the intradural component of the tumor, the dura is opened transversely along the frontal base and the superior sagittal sinus is ligated as anteriorly as possible, near the crista galli (see **Fig. 5F**). The sinus is then divided sharply and the incision is carried along the falx cerebri toward the free edge.[25] With bilateral frontal lobes exposed, dissection can be carried out using either a subfrontal or interhemispheric corridor. Care is taken to avoid compromise of any bridging veins so as to avoid a venous infarct. The intradural portion of the tumor is removed with care to create a plane to separate the frontal lobes from the tumor capsule (**Fig. 6**A–C). Solid and firm tumors can be debulked with an ultrasonic aspirator, whereas hemorrhagic and friable tumor may need to be removed in a piecemeal fashion suctions and bipolar cautery. After tumor removal, the frontal lobes are inspected and frozen sections are sent for margins.

Before entering the sinonasal cavity via the cribriform plate, the dura can be closed in a watertight fashion with a dural patch graft (**Fig. 6**D). The remainder of the extradural tumor can be removed and access to the clivus can be achieved through the transcribriform corridor microsurgically (**Fig. 6**E, F). The cribriform plate and crista galli are drilled off to expose the anterior and posterior ethmoid sinuses and lamina papyracea. The anterior and posterior ethmoidal arteries and coagulated and divided sharply. Care is taken to avoid retraction of an incompletely coagulated ethmoidal artery back into the globe to avoid an orbital hematoma. Removal of the planum sphenoidale posteriorly provides exposure of the sphenoid sinus. Both optic canals are identified posterolaterally within the sphenoid sinus. Bilateral bony prominences formed by the cavernous segment of the internal carotid arteries are identified on either side of the sella. The sphenoid sinus can be widened, and the sellar floor can be removed if access to the clivus is needed. Exposure of both maxillary sinuses can also be achieved. However, visualization to the anterior nasal cavity and superolateral aspect of the maxillary sinus is limited from above (blind spots).[11] Thus, further inspection for remaining tumor from below via an EEA is performed. Endoscopic debulking of the intranasal portion of the lesion also can be performed if necessary.[21] It is important to preserve the nasal septum and mucosa during the tumor removal, in case a nasoseptal flap is needed for reconstruction (see later in this article).

Reconstruction

The large skull base defects and communication with the nasal sinuses present a unique challenge in reconstruction. Although endonasal repair of smaller skull base

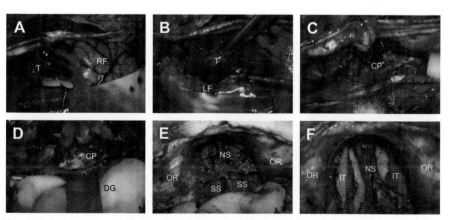

Fig. 6. Intraoperative photographs of patient in **Fig. 2**. (*A, B*) Intracranial tumor (T) is removed and dissected away from the right frontal lobe (RF) and left frontal lobe (LF). (*C*) The cribriform plate (CP) is exposed after removal of the intracranial portion of the tumor. (*D*) The intracranial cavity is closed in a watertight fashion by suturing a dural graft (DG) to secure the brain contents from the sinonasal cavity. (*E, F*) The CP is entered and the tumor is removed from the sinonasal cavity through the transcranial approach. IT, inferior turbinate; NS, nasal septum; OR, orbital roof; SS, sphenoid sinus.

defects with fascial or mucosal grafts in conjunction with tissue sealants have been successful in preventing cerebrospinal fluid (CSF) leaks, its adequacy for endonasal reconstruction of major skull base and dural defects is of debate.[13,20,26] Vascularized tissue is optimal for reconstruction with goals of separation of the intracranial compartment from the sinonasal cavity and prevention of postoperative CSF leakage. Additionally, vascularized flaps promote rapid and complete healing.[26–28] Pericranium is a commonly used vascularized tissue flap that is readily available with a bicoronal incision. Undermining beneath the incision posteriorly provides several additional centimeters of pericranium for increased surface area of coverage. It is important to attempt watertight closure of durotomies and dural defects, if possible, before placement of the pericranial flap. We typically suture a dural patch using acellular dermal allograft at the cribriform dural defect of the anterior ventral skull base. Endoscopic endonasal inspection of the skull base reconstruction from below can be very useful in ensuring an adequate pericranial flap reconstruction to prevent CSF leakage. This strategy can allow an endoscopic-assisted repair with direct visualization of the anterior ventral skull base repair and optimal positioning of the pericranial flap.

If postoperative radiation therapy is anticipated, particularly for sinonasal skull base malignancies, one can consider using a "double-flap" technique in which a pericranial flap is simultaneously used with a nasoseptal flap (**Figs. 7** and **8**).[29] The 2 flaps can complement each other at their respective areas of weakness. The pericranial flap is strongest anteriorly at the region of the frontal sinus and cribriform plate, whereas the nasoseptal flap is strongest at the area of the clivus defect. When used together, these 2 vascularized tissue flaps can provide optimal skull base reconstruction in select cases that are at high risk of postoperative CSF leakage.

In some instances, a vascularized pedicled nasoseptal flap may be used as a salvage strategy if the pericranial flap is unavailable due to prior usage in revision craniotomies.[27] This durable yet pliable flap is robustly vascularized by the posterior nasoseptal arteries arising from the sphenopalatine artery. Its large surface area and superior rotational arc allow for flexibility in flap design, contributing to its high

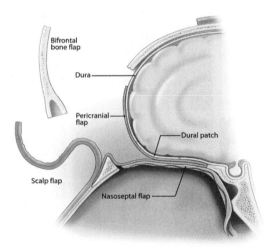

Fig. 7. Illustration demonstrating the double-flap reconstruction technique used in combined cranionasal approach. Simultaneous pericranial flap from above and nasoseptal flap from below are used for reconstruction of the extensive anterior skull base defect. (*Courtesy of* Chris Gralaap, MA, CMI, Fairfax, CA.)

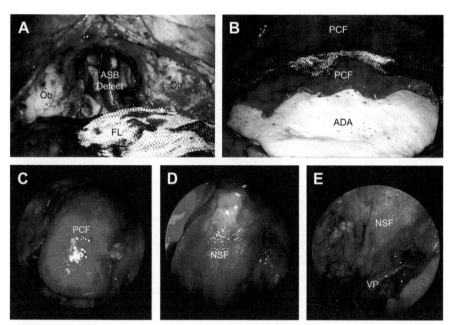

Fig. 8. Intraoperative photographs of a simultaneous double-flap reconstruction after combined cranionasal removal of an anterior skull base malignancy. (*A*) Anterior skull base (ASB) defect is visualized anterior and inferior to the frontal lobes (FL) and between the orbits (Ob). (*B*) The vascularized pericranial flap (PCF) is rotated over the ASB defect. The distal redundant portion is used to cover the frontal lobe dural closure. Here, an additional acellular dermal allograft (ADA) was placed as an onlay graft over the dural closure. (*C*) Endonasal endoscopic view of the PCF. (*D, E*) A vascularized pedicled nasoseptal flap (NSF) is rotated over the PCF to provide double-flap reconstruction. The vascular pedicle (VP) is preserved.

rate of success in ventral skull base reconstruction.[26,27] It is paramount to inspect the nasal septal mucosa to ensure that it is free of tumor invasion before considering it for reconstruction. The surface area and dimensions of the nasoseptal flap available for use is limited by tumor involvement of the nasal septum. In cases of tumor involvement of the superior nasal septum, tissue from the nasal floor mucosa, lateral wall of the nasal cavity, and lower septum can be harvested to create an extended nasoseptal flap.[18,30] However, if there is significant bilateral septal involvement, the nasoseptal flap may not be a viable option, and thus one has to rely solely on pericranial flap reconstruction. In cases of revision surgery in which the pericranial and nasoseptal flap are both unavailable, other vascularized reconstructive alternatives, such as the temporoparietal fascial, galeopericranial, and palatal flaps can be considered.[18,26] Free tissue transfer with microvascular anastomosis (free flap) is another feasible option.[26,31]

The flap reconstruction is bolstered with Surgicel, followed by gentamicin-soaked Gelfoam pledgets, and finally buttressed with several inflatable Merocel (Medtronic Xomed, Jacksonville, FL) nasal tampons. The packing is left in the nasal cavity for approximately 10 to 12 days to promote adherence of the flap to the ventral skull base. The patient is maintained on oral antibiotics until the nasal packing is removed endoscopically as an outpatient. The bone flap is replaced and fixed with titanium plates. Care is taken not to compress or strangulate the pericranial flap to avoid ischemic compromise to the reconstruction. Meticulous multilayered wound closure is then performed. We generally avoid lumbar drains for transcribriform defects[32] so as to avoid complications of intracranial hypotension, tension pneumocephalus, and thromboembolic complications associated with prolonged bedrest.

POSTOPERATIVE MANAGEMENT

Postoperatively, the patient is monitored in the neurosurgical ICU. Hourly neurologic examinations in the ICU should be performed for the first 24 to 48 hours, including assessment for CSF leakage. Hemodynamic monitoring with an arterial line is used with intravenous infusion of an antihypertensive or hypertensive (pressor) agents to maintain normal blood pressures. Routine blood work is performed including complete blood count, coagulation profile, electrolytes, and arterial blood gas. Strict intake and output is monitored, especially if there is concern for diabetes insipidus in cases of parasellar involvement. We typically administer broad-spectrum intravenous antibiotics postoperatively that cover sinonasal flora with blood-brain-barrier penetration for 72 hours after surgery. This is transitioned to oral antibiotics that are continued for the duration of nasal packing.

Both intracranial hypertension and hypotension can be concerns in the immediate postoperative period and the clinical presentations can be similar. Any change of neurologic examination should warrant an immediate computed tomography scan to rule out a mass lesion such as a hematoma or tension pneumocephalus, or signs of intracranial hypotension.[33] Prophylactic lumbar drainage should be used judiciously, as it can precipitate intracranial hypotension and tension pneumocephalus. In our practice, we typically do not use postoperative lumbar drainage for cranionasal approaches so as to avoid these risks.[32]

CSF leakage can present in the immediate postoperative period or in a delayed fashion. Although very low-flow CSF leaks can sometimes be successfully treated with lumbar drainage, most significant CSF leaks require surgical exploration to directly repair the site of the fistula. A revision craniotomy can be avoided by using an EEA to inspect the site of the fistula, reinforce any persistent defects with tissue grafts (fat, fascia lata, acellular dermal allografts), reposition the pericranial flap, and/or augment the repair with a vascularized nasoseptal flap.

DISCUSSION

Traditionally, extensive malignant tumors of the paranasal sinuses and ventral skull base have been surgically managed via a transcranial-transfacial (combined craniofacial) approach and postoperative radiotherapy with satisfactory success. However, craniofacial resection is associated with significant perioperative morbidity, mortality, and complications.[8,13,34] These limitations prompted the search for safer and improved methods for the surgical management of extensive paranasal sinus and anterior ventral skull base malignancies, which would improve the patient's functionality and quality of life with satisfactory cosmetic results while preserving oncological principles. Advancing developments in endoscopic surgical technology, refinements in endoscopic techniques, and increased familiarity of the endoscopic endonasal anatomy have allowed the EEA to transcend its expected uses, where its applicability has expanded from its initial use for the treatment of inflammatory paranasal sinus disease to resection of benign sinonasal neoplasms,[9,35,36] and ultimately to resection of malignant neoplasms, including those of the ventral skull base.[21,37,38] In tumors with significant intracranial extension that is not amenable to a pure EEA, a combined transcranial/EEA (combined cranionasal approach) can be performed.[8,10,12,37,39]

In 1997, Yuen and colleagues[39] first described the combined transcranial and endoscopic transnasal approach for the resection of an esthesioneuroblastoma that infiltrated the ethmoidal cribriform plate and their subsequent experience with the implementation of the approach in a series of esthesioneuroblastomas that do not require free-flap reconstruction, demonstrating complete tumor removal with no local recurrences.[40] Carrau and colleagues,[12] demonstrated that endoscopic-assisted surgery in the treatment of juvenile angiofibromas, was a suitable complement to the traditional approaches, thus avoiding additional transfacial incisions. In the pediatric population, this was of particular importance, as it avoided additional interference with developing facial growth centers and minimized functional and cosmetic deficits. Castelnuovo and colleagues[41] also described the combined cranionasal approach for en bloc resection of malignant neoplasms with minimal disturbance to the facial skeleton. These advantages were similarly echoed by Galassi and colleagues,[42] in their report of the combined cranionasal approach for the resection of infantile myofibromatosis of the ethmoid and anterior ventral skull base. Although most studies have focused mainly on specific neoplasms, Hanna and colleagues[20] reported the use of the combined cranionasal approach to a wide range of malignant tumors of the sinonasal tract. Their study demonstrated that there was no significant difference in disease-specific or overall survival rate between groups of patients surgically treated exclusively via EEA and those treated via combined cranionasal approach. This is probably due to appropriate patient selection for each approach strategy. For example, smaller, less extensive tumors were selected for EEA, and larger tumors with significant intracranial extension were selected for a cranionasal approach.

It is important to emphasize that the combined cranionasal approach should be performed only in specialized centers with an experienced skull base team consisting of an endoscopic/skull base–trained otolaryngologist and neurosurgeon to ensure optimal success of the operation. When managing malignancies, definitive resection should, whenever possible, result in complete oncologic removal with tumor-free surgical margins regardless of the approach, as principles of surgical oncology should be upheld. Although surgery is the mainstay of treatment of most sinonasal and ventral skull base malignancies, the use of adjuvant or neoadjuvant therapy when appropriate is critical to achieving optimal oncologic outcomes.[20] Advancements in microsurgical and endoscopic skull base techniques have further added to the armamentarium of surgical management of sinonasal and ventral skull base malignancies in both the resection and reconstruction process. The EEA has made great strides in the management of anterior ventral skull base malignancies and has consistently yielded good oncologic outcomes in well-selected patients. When used in conjunction with the transcranial approach, the combined cranionasal approach is a suitable option in those with significant intracranial disease, to improve tumor resection and skull base repair.[20] The surgical treatment of sinonasal and ventral skull base malignancies has evolved to be one of integrated collaboration between the otolaryngologist and neurosurgeon, necessitating their combined advanced technical expertise and knowledge.

SUMMARY

Combined transcranial and EEA approaches remain useful in the treatment of sinonasal and ventral skull base malignancies. The modified 1-piece extended transbasal approach provides wide access to the anterior ventral skull base and paranasal sinuses. The endoscopic endonasal approach has largely replaced transfacial approaches for combined craniofacial approaches and also can provide additional vascularized tissue for skull base reconstruction, if needed, via the nasoseptal flap. Double-flap reconstruction with simultaneous vascularized pericranial and nasoseptal flaps is a useful strategy for malignant tumors that require postoperative adjuvant radiation therapy.

REFERENCES

1. Frazier CH. I. An approach to the hypophysis through the anterior cranial fossa. Ann Surg 1913;57:145–50.
2. Derome P. Spheno-ethmoidal tumors. Possibilities for exeresis and surgical repair. Neurochirurgie 1972;18(Suppl 1):1–164 [in French].
3. Tessier P, Guiot G, Rougerie J, et al. Cranio-naso-orbito-facial osteotomies. Hypertelorism. Ann Chir Plast 1967;12:103–18 [in French].
4. Raveh J, Vuillemin T. Advantages of an additional subcranial approach in the correction of craniofacial deformities. J Craniomaxillofac Surg 1988;16:350–8.
5. Raveh J, Vuillemin T. Subcranial-supraorbital and temporal approach for tumor resection. J Craniofac Surg 1990;1:53–9.
6. Kawakami K, Yamanouchi Y, Kubota C, et al. An extensive transbasal approach to frontal skull-base tumors. Technical note. J Neurosurg 1991;74:1011–3.
7. Sekhar LN, Nanda A, Sen CN, et al. The extended frontal approach to tumors of the anterior, middle, and posterior skull base. J Neurosurg 1992;76:198–206.
8. Komotar RJ, Starke RM, Raper DM, et al. Endoscopic endonasal compared with anterior craniofacial and combined cranionasal resection of esthesioneuroblastomas. World Neurosurg 2013;80:148–59.
9. Liu JK, Husain Q, Kanumuri V, et al. Endoscopic graduated multiangle, multicorridor resection of juvenile nasopharyngeal angiofibroma: an individualized, tailored, multicorridor skull base approach. J Neurosurg 2016;124:1328–38.
10. Devaiah AK, Larsen C, Tawfik O, et al. Esthesioneuroblastoma: endoscopic nasal and anterior craniotomy resection. Laryngoscope 2003;113:2086–90.
11. Liu JK, Decker D, Schaefer SD, et al. Zones of approach for craniofacial resection: minimizing facial incisions for resection of anterior cranial base and paranasal sinus tumors. Neurosurgery 2003;53:1126–35 [discussion: 1135–7].
12. Carrau RL, Snyderman CH, Kassam AB, et al. Endoscopic and endoscopic-assisted surgery for juvenile angiofibroma. Laryngoscope 2001;111:483–7.
13. Eloy JA, Vivero RJ, Hoang K, et al. Comparison of transnasal endoscopic and open craniofacial resection for malignant tumors of the anterior skull base. Laryngoscope 2009;119:834–40.
14. Belli E, Rendine G, Mazzone N. Malignant ethmoidal neoplasms: a cranionasal endoscopy approach. J Craniofac Surg 2009;20:1240–4.
15. Wood JW, Eloy JA, Vivero RJ, et al. Efficacy of transnasal endoscopic resection for malignant anterior skull-base tumors. Int Forum Allergy Rhinol 2012;2:487–95.
16. Hosemann W, Schroeder HW. Comprehensive review on rhino-neurosurgery. GMS Curr Top Otorhinolaryngol head Neck Surg 2015;14:Doc01.
17. Zacharia BE, Romero FR, Rapoport SK, et al. Endoscopic endonasal management of metastatic lesions of the anterior skull base: case series and literature review. World Neurosurg 2015;84:1267–77.
18. Su SY, Kupferman ME, DeMonte F, et al. Endoscopic resection of sinonasal cancers. Curr Oncol Rep 2014;16:369.
19. Terasaka S, Day JD, Fukushima T. Extended transbasal approach: anatomy, technique, and indications. Skull Base Surg 1999;9:177–84.

20. Hanna E, DeMonte F, Ibrahim S, et al. Endoscopic resection of sinonasal cancers with and without craniotomy: oncologic results. Arch Otolaryngol Head Neck Surg 2009;135:1219–24.
21. Nicolai P, Battaglia P, Bignami M, et al. Endoscopic surgery for malignant tumors of the sinonasal tract and adjacent skull base: a 10-year experience. Am J Rhinol 2008;22:308–16.
22. Liu JK. Modified one-piece extended transbasal approach for translamina terminalis resection of retrochiasmatic third ventricular craniopharyngioma. Neurosurg Focus 2013;34. Video 1.
23. Liu JK, Eloy JA. Modified one-piece extended transbasal approach for resection of giant anterior skull base sinonasal teratocarcinosarcoma. J Neurosurg 2012; 32(Suppl):E4.
24. Effendi ST, Rao VY, Momin EN, et al. The 1-piece transbasal approach: operative technique and anatomical study. J Neurosurg 2014;121:1446–52.
25. Liu JK, Christiano LD, Gupta G, et al. Surgical nuances for removal of retrochiasmatic craniopharyngiomas via the transbasal subfrontal translamina terminalis approach. Neurosurg Focus 2010;28:E6.
26. Kassam AB, Thomas A, Carrau RL, et al. Endoscopic reconstruction of the cranial base using a pedicled nasoseptal flap. Neurosurgery 2008;63:ONS44–52 [discussion: ONS52–3].
27. Eloy JA, Kalyoussef E, Choudhry OJ, et al. Salvage endoscopic nasoseptal flap repair of persistent cerebrospinal fluid leak after open skull base surgery. Am J Otolaryngol 2012;33:735–40.
28. Liu JK, Schmidt RF, Choudhry OJ, et al. Surgical nuances for nasoseptal flap reconstruction of cranial base defects with high-flow cerebrospinal fluid leaks after endoscopic skull base surgery. Neurosurg Focus 2012;32:E7.
29. Eloy JA, Choudhry OJ, Christiano LD, et al. Double flap technique for reconstruction of anterior skull base defects after craniofacial tumor resection: technical note. Int Forum Allergy rhinology 2013;3:425–30.
30. Pinheiro-Neto CD, Fernandez-Miranda JC, Wang EW, et al. Anatomical correlates of endonasal surgery for sinonasal malignancies. Clin Anat 2012;25:129–34.
31. Zweig JL, Carrau RL, Celin SE, et al. Endoscopic repair of cerebrospinal fluid leaks to the sinonasal tract: predictors of success. Otolaryngol Head Neck Surg 2000;123:195–201.
32. Eloy JA, Kuperan AB, Choudhry OJ, et al. Efficacy of the pedicled nasoseptal flap without cerebrospinal fluid (CSF) diversion for repair of skull base defects: incidence of postoperative CSF leaks. Int Forum Allergy Rhinology 2012;2:397–401.
33. Diaz L, Mady LJ, Mendelson ZS, et al. Endoscopic ventral skull base surgery: is early postoperative imaging warranted for detecting complications? Laryngoscope 2015;125:1072–6.
34. Krischek B, Carvalho FG, Godoy BL, et al. From craniofacial resection to endonasal endoscopic removal of malignant tumors of the anterior skull base. World Neurosurg 2014;82:S59–65.
35. Kopec T, Borucki L, Szyfter W. Fully endoscopic resection of juvenile nasopharyngeal angiofibroma: own experience and clinical outcomes. Int J Pediatr Otorhinolaryngol 2014;78:1015–8.
36. Kennedy DW, Keogh B, Senior B, et al. Endoscopic approach to tumors of the anterior skull base and orbit. Oper Tech Otolaryngol Head Neck Surg 1996;7:257–63.
37. Liu JK, O'Neill B, Orlandi RR, et al. Endoscopic-assisted craniofacial resection of esthesioneuroblastoma: minimizing facial incisions–technical note and report of 3 cases. Minim Invasive Neurosurg 2003;46:310–5.

38. Casiano RR, Numa WA, Falquez AM. Endoscopic resection of esthesioneuroblastoma. Am J Rhinol 2001;15:271–9.

39. Yuen AP, Fung CF, Hung KN. Endoscopic cranionasal resection of anterior skull base tumor. Am J Otolaryngol 1997;18:431–3.

40. Yuen AP, Fan YW, Fung CF, et al. Endoscopic-assisted cranionasal resection of olfactory neuroblastoma. Head Neck 2005;27:488–93.

41. Castelnuovo P, Battaglia P, Locatelli D, et al. Endonasal micro-endoscopic treatment of malignant tumors of the paranasal sinuses and anterior skull base. Oper Tech Otolayngol Head Neck Surg 2006;17:152–67.

42. Galassi E, Pasquini E, Frank G, et al. Combined endoscopy-assisted cranionasal approach for resection of infantile myofibromatosis of the ethmoid and anterior skull base. Case report. J Neurosurg Pediatr 2008;2:58–62.

Management of Orbital Involvement in Sinonasal and Ventral Skull Base Malignancies

Gregory S. Neel, MD[a], Thomas H. Nagel, MD[a],
Joseph M. Hoxworth, MD[b], Devyani Lal, MD[c],*

KEYWORDS

- Sinonasal malignancy • Orbit • Orbital invasion • Orbital exenteration
- Orbital clearance • Orbital sacrifice • Orbit preservation • Endoscopic resection

KEY POINTS

- Multimodality therapy with surgery and radiation therapy is usually necessary to manage the orbit infiltrated with sinonasal or ventral skull base malignancy.
- Surgical resection with negative margins is the cornerstone of management.
- In carefully selected situations, orbital preservation does not adversely affect survival.
- Imaging and frozen section histopathology are critical in assessing candidacy for orbital preservation.
- Appropriate reconstruction of surgical defects is essential to minimize complications and optimize functional and aesthetic outcomes.

 Video content accompanies this article at http://www.oto.theclinics.com.

INTRODUCTION: ORBITAL INVOLVEMENT IN SINONASAL AND VENTRAL SKULL BASE MALIGNANCIES

Malignancies of the sinonasal cavity and skull base involve the orbit in in 50% to 80% of cases.[1–4] The incidence of orbital involvement depends on primary tumor site and histopathology, being reported in 62% to 82% of ethmoid tumors and 46% of nasal cavity tumors.[2,5] Orbital invasion bodes poorer prognosis for overall and

Disclosure Statement: No relevant disclosures or Conflicts of Interest.
[a] Department of Otolaryngology-Head & Neck Surgery, Mayo Clinic, 5777 East Mayo Bouelvard, Phoenix, AZ 85054, USA; [b] Section of Neuroradiology, Department of Radiology, Mayo Clinic, 5777 East Mayo Bouelvard, Phoenix, AZ 85054, USA; [c] Department of Otolaryngology-Head & Neck Surgery, Mayo Clinic College of Medicine, Mayo Clinic, 5777 East Mayo Bouelvard, Phoenix, AZ 85054, USA
* Corresponding author.
E-mail address: Lal.Devyani@mayo.edu

Otolaryngol Clin N Am 50 (2017) 347–364
http://dx.doi.org/10.1016/j.otc.2016.12.010
oto.theclinics.com

Table 1
Staging of orbital invasion

Primary tumor (T)	
Maxillary sinus, nasal cavity and ethmoid sinus	
T3	Tumor invades floor or medial wall of the orbit
T4a	Moderately advanced local disease: tumor invades the anterior orbital contents
T4b	Very advanced local disease: tumor invades orbital apex

From Edge SB, Byrd DR, Compton CC, et al, editors. AJCC cancer staging manual. 7th edition. New York: Springer; 2010.

disease-free survival[2,5,6] and is associated with poorer outcome from salvage surgery.[7] Involvement of the orbit therefore upgrades local tumor stage to at least T3, with invasion of the orbital apex and beyond (T4b) having the gravest prognosis (**Table 1**).[8]

DIAGNOSIS

The proximity of the orbit to the sinonasal and ventral skull base facilitates tumor infiltration into the eye through many pathways (**Table 2**). Although diplopia, epiphora, chemosis, visual changes, and proptosis may be present in approximately 50% of cases,[3,5] the absence of these findings does not rule out tumor invasion. Symptoms can result from orbital compression, nasolacrimal duct obstruction, and true invasion. The periorbita is a robust barrier against invasion. However, once the tumor invades through the periorbita, there are no further barriers to diffuse orbital infiltration. Computerized tomography (CT) of the paranasal sinuses is useful in studying loss of orbital bone and enlargement of fissures and foramina. MRI is superior for delineating orbital soft tissue

Table 2
Pathways for orbital invasion by sinonasal and ventral skull base tumors

Route of Extension	Orbital Involvement
Direct invasion through bone	• Lamina papyracea, orbital floor and orbital roof → orbital periosteum, extraconal fat, extraocular muscles, intraconal fat, globe, orbital apex • Nasal bone, frontal process of maxilla (nasal tumor) → skin of medial canthal area, eyelids • Lateral sphenoidal wall → optic canal, orbital apex, cavernous sinus, cranial fossa
Direct extension through preformed pathways	• Sphenopalatine foramen → pterygopalatine fossa → inferior oblique fissure → orbit • Inferior orbital fissure • Superior orbital fissure • Anterior and posterior ethmoidal foramina
Perineural extension	• Infraorbital nerve • Supraorbital and supratrochlear nerves
Subperiosteal or intraperiosteal extension	• Orbital apex, cavernous sinus, cranial fossa
Nasolacrimal duct	• Lacrimal sac, medial and inferior orbit, upper and lower eyelids
Blood borne	• Metastatic tumors (eg, renal cell carcinoma)

involvement, and distinguishing retained secretions (eg, in the lacrimal sac) from tumor.[9–11] However, imaging may not be able to distinguish true periorbital and extraocular muscle invasion from other changes. Peritumoral edema can lead to muscle enhancement, which may be mistaken for muscle invasion.[9–11] The final determination of orbital involvement is often made intraoperatively on frozen section pathology.[10]

STAGING OF ORBITAL INVOLVEMENT AND SURGICAL IMPLICATIONS

Different systems have been proposed for staging orbital involvement by sinonasal tumors (**Tables 3–5**).[1,10] These staging systems attempt to stratify patients along a spectrum of invasiveness. **Table 5** proposes a contemporary grading system that can be used for treatment planning. The most minimal form of orbital involvement is rarefaction or focal erosion of the lamina papyracea without transgression of the periorbita (**Fig. 1**). As tumors progressively invade the orbit, periorbita can become focally or extensively involved with tumor, eventually infiltrating orbital fat (**Fig. 2**). Ultimately, extraocular muscles can become involved either by focal tumor contact or frank invasion/encasement (**Fig. 3**). In terms of vision preservation and the need for reconstruction, tumor extension into the nasolacrimal duct/sac and eyelids is particularly relevant (**Fig. 4**). Adjacency to or invasion of a nerve must be noted preoperatively to counsel patients regarding potential postoperative neurologic deficits and to map out neurotropic cancer spread with MRI (**Fig. 5**). Invasion of the orbital apex, cavernous sinus, and other intracranial structures will significantly impact resectability and patient outcome (**Fig. 6**).

PROGNOSIS

An international collaborative analysis of 334 patients with ethmoid malignancies undergoing craniofacial resection found orbital involvement reduced 5-year disease-specific survival from 78.0% to 44.4%.[2] Although survival may not be adversely affected if orbital invasion is limited to the orbital periosteum, orbital apex involvement significantly decreases survival.[2] Tumor histology may affect survival. Nishino and colleagues[12] reported a statistically superior 5-year overall survival rate of 74% for squamous cell carcinoma versus 40% for other sinonasal malignancy invading the orbit.

MANAGEMENT OF ORBITAL INVASION

A combination of surgery and radiation therapy is used for advanced sinonasal and ventral skull base malignancies with invasion of the orbit.[1–6,12–15] Induction and postoperative chemotherapy also may have a role.[1–6,12–15] Surgery to address orbital disease may require orbital exenteration (complete removal of orbital contents,

Table 3	
Grades of orbital involvement	
Grade	**Criteria**
I	Erosion or destruction of medial orbital wall
II	Extraconal invasion of periorbital fat
II	Invasion of medial rectus muscle, optic nerve, ocular bulb, or skin overlying the eyelid

Adapted from Iannetti G, Valentini V, Rinna C, et al. Ethmoido-orbital tumors: our experience. J Craniofac Surg 2005;16(6):1087.

Table 4
Grades of orbital involvement

Grade	Criteria
A	Tumor adjacent the orbit, without infiltration of the orbital wall, which appears thinner
B	Tumor eroding the orbital wall without ocular bulb displacement
C	Tumor eroding and infiltrating the orbital wall, displacing the orbital wall, without periorbital involvement
D	Tumor invading the orbit with periorbital invasion

Adapted from McCary WS, Levine PA, Cantrell RW. Preservation of the eye in the treatment of sinonasal malignant neoplasms with orbital involvement. A confirmation of the original treatise. Arch Otolaryngol Head Neck Surg 1996;122(6):659.

Table 5
Authors' staging of orbital invasion for surgical management

Grade	Criteria	Surgical Approach
1	Tumor adjacent to orbital wall, which may be thinned, bowed, or eroded without periorbital involvement	Orbital preservation is undertaken (Video 1)
2	Tumor eroding orbital wall, with resectable periorbital involvement	Orbital preservation is attempted; periorbita is resected and preservation is likely feasible (Video 2)
3	Tumor with extraocular muscle, intraconal fat, globe, or orbital apex invasion	Orbital clearance is performed
4	Tumor invading the nasolacrimal system, eyelids duct and/or sac	Orbital preservation may be feasible; reconstruction performed for functional eye
5	Tumor with cavernous sinus, optic canal or massive intracranial invasion	Unresectable tumor

Table 6
Options for orbital floor reconstruction

Option	Material	Advantages and Limitations
Nonvascularized grafts	• Titanium or synthetic mesh • Bone grafts (rib, calvarial or iliac crest bone)	In a previous or soon to be irradiated bed, nonvascular grafts are subject to infection, resorption in the case of bone and cartilage grafts, or exposure
Vascularized local flap	The coronoid-temporalis sling procedure	Is a readily available local vascularized option in which the temporalis muscle is transferred medially with the coronoid process across the orbital floor and affixed
Combined avascular- vascular option	Synthetic mesh or bone graft with vascularized soft tissue flap	Reduces graft complications and optimizes tolerance of radiotherapy

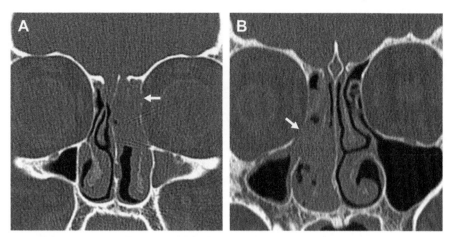

Fig. 1. (*A*) Coronal noncontrast CT from a 36-year-old woman with esthesioneuroblastoma. The left lamina papyracea demonstrates subtle rarefaction and irregularity (*arrow*) without frank tumor entering the orbit. (*B*) Coronal noncontrast CT from a 72-year-old woman with melanoma. The tumor causes focal erosion of the inferior aspect of the right lamina papyracea (*arrow*).

including the eyelids) or orbital clearance (complete removal of orbital contents with preservation of the lid and palpebral conjunctiva). For the purposes of this article, we use the term "orbital sacrifice" to refer to either.

RADIATION THERAPY

Radiation may be used before or after surgery, based on tumor stage and histology. Preoperative radiotherapy can be used to reduce tumor bulk and eliminate peripheral

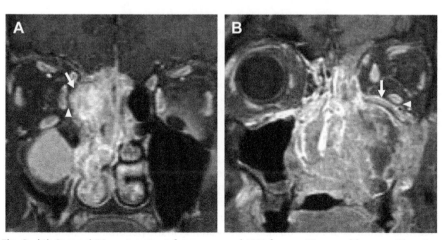

Fig. 2. (*A*) Coronal T1 postcontrast fat-suppressed MRI from a 44-year-old man with esthesioneuroblastoma. Tumor invades the medial right orbital fat (*arrow*), but a fat plane (*arrowhead*) still separates it from the medial rectus muscle. (*B*) Coronal T1 postcontrast fat-suppressed MRI from a 64-year-old man with squamous cell carcinoma. Tumor infiltrates the left inferior orbital fat (*arrow*), though a fat plane (*arrowhead*) between the mass and left inferior rectus muscle is preserved.

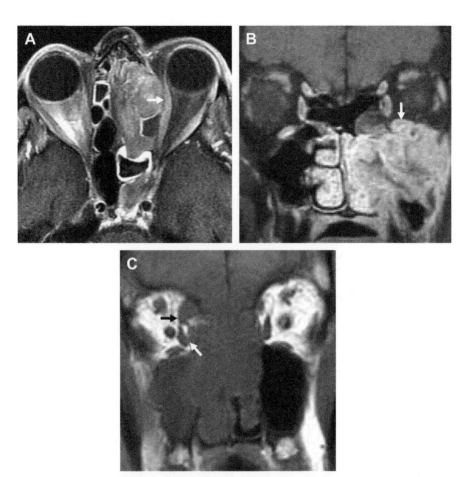

Fig. 3. (A) Axial T1 postcontrast fat-suppressed MRI from a 69-year-old woman with mela-noma. Tumor extends through the left lamina papyracea to directly contact the left medial rectus muscle (*arrow*). (B) Coronal T1 postcontrast fat-suppressed MRI from a 52-year-old man with squamous cell carcinoma. The left inferior rectus muscle (*arrow*) is partially en-cased by tumor infiltrating the inferior left orbit. (C) Coronal noncontrast T1 MRI from a 34-year-old man with esthesioneuroblastoma. The right superior oblique muscle (*black arrow*) is inseparable from tumor, whereas there is only minimal contact between the mass and medial rectus muscle (*white arrow*).

tumor microfoci in an effort to perform orbit-sparing surgery, or to facilitate resectability of disease.[13,16] Conversely, postoperative radiotherapy following orbit-preserving surgery also has been used.[12,15,17] Intensity modulated radiation therapy (IMRT) may minimize ocular toxicity, while preserving disease control and survival rates.[18] Re-irradiation with hypofractionated IMRT also has been reported to be feasible for sino-nasal and ventral skull base malignancies recurring in the periorbital region.[19]

SURGICAL MANAGEMENT
Preoperative Considerations and Controversies in Surgical Management

Investigators until the 1970s advocated for orbital sacrifice in all cases with bony orbital invasion.[20,21] However, beginning with Sisson in 1970,[16] many investigators[4,13,17]

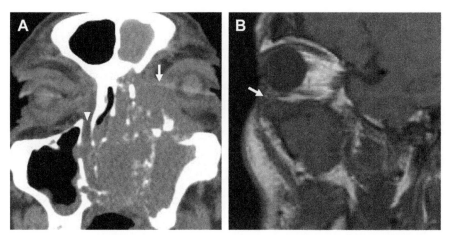

Fig. 4. A 64-year-old man with squamous cell carcinoma. (*A*) Coronal noncontrast CT shows tumor obliterating the left nasolacrimal duct and infiltrating the medial canthal region (*arrow*). The normal contralateral nasolacrimal duct is displayed for reference (*arrowhead*). (*B*) Sagittal noncontrast T1 MRI exhibits tumor invading the left inferior eyelid (*arrow*).

started reporting comparable survival with orbital preservation surgery and adjuvant radiation therapy. However, other investigators eschew such approaches as oncologically unsound.[22] In the absence of consensus, contemporary surgeons must consider oncologic soundness as well as functional outcome in preserved eyes.

SURGICAL APPROACH

Surgery for sinonasal and ventral skull base tumors can be undertaken by appropriately selected external or expanded endoscopic endonasal approaches,[1–6,12–15,23–25] The authors reserve orbital sacrifice for invasion of extraocular muscles, intraconal fat, globe, or orbital apex (see **Table 5**). Frozen sections are routinely used. Tumors deemed unresectable are those with internal carotid artery encasement, cavernous sinus invasion, or massive intracranial invasion, in which negative margins may not be possible. For low-grade ventral skull base tumors (eg, meningioma), orbital preservation is used with adjuvant radiation depending on the grade of resection (**Fig. 7**). In addition to oncologic soundness, residual eye function and cosmesis are considered when proceeding with orbital preservation.

SURGICAL TECHNIQUE

Please see Thomas J. Willson and colleagues' article, "Anatomic Considerations for Sinonasal and Ventral Skull Base Malignancy," in this issue and the reader is also referred to the review of orbital anatomy by Turvey and Golden.[26] Disease abutting the orbital wall without bony erosion is addressed by drilling and resection of the involved bone. The underlying periosteum is sampled by frozen sections. When the disease penetrates through the orbital wall, a wide resection of involved bone with or without limited resection of the underlying periorbita is performed. Gross periorbital invasion where the tumor cannot be dissected off the periorbita is managed by wide resection of periorbita and a cuff of underlying extraconal orbital fat. Gross invasion into extraocular muscles, intraconal orbital fat, globe, or orbital apex is managed by orbital clearance. If the eyelids are also invaded, then orbital exenteration may be

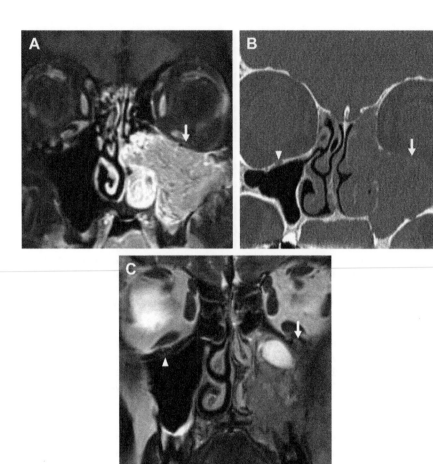

Fig. 5. (*A*) Coronal T1 postcontrast fat-suppressed MRI from a 57-year-old man with squamous cell carcinoma. Although there is extensive contact between the left maxillary sinus tumor and the orbital floor, the left infraorbital nerve appears normal (*arrow*). (*B*) Coronal noncontrast CT from an 80-year-old woman with melanoma. Left maxillary sinus tumor has extensively eroded the left orbital floor such that a normal infraorbital canal is no longer apparent (*arrow*). The normal contralateral infraorbital canal is displayed for reference (*arrowhead*). (*C*) Coronal T2 MRI from a 34-year-old man with squamous cell carcinoma. Left maxillary sinus tumor has invaded the left infraorbital nerve, which appears expanded and edematous (*arrow*). The normal contralateral infraorbital nerve is displayed for reference (*arrowhead*).

undertaken. Careful presurgical planning is undertaken (**Box 1**). The patient is then prepped and positioned (**Box 2**). Steps in surgical management of the involved orbit are outlined in **Box 3** (orbital preservation) and **Box 4** (orbital sacrifice). **Box 5** outlines postprocedure care.

RECONSTRUCTION OF ORBITAL DEFECTS

The orbit and its contents sit adjacent to the air-filled cavities of the maxillary, ethmoid, and frontal sinuses. Reconstructive goals include appropriate support and positioning

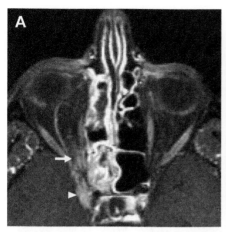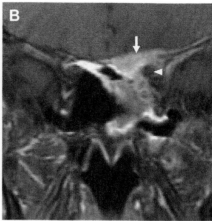

Fig. 6. (*A*) Axial T1 postcontrast fat-suppressed MRI from a 54-year-old woman with squamous cell carcinoma. Tumor in the right sphenoid sinus invades the right orbital apex (*arrow*) and cavernous sinus (*arrowhead*). (*B*) Coronal T1 postcontrast fat-suppressed MRI from a 61-year-old man with squamous cell carcinoma. Tumor infiltrates the skull base (*arrow*) surrounding the optic canal resulting in encasement of the left optic nerve (*arrowhead*).

of preserved orbital contents, dural and skull base repair, and aesthetic reconstitution of bony and soft tissue defects.[27]

Techniques and options for repairing orbital defects depend on the extent of resection (**Tables 6** and **7**). Reconstructive options range from no reconstruction to simple grafts, to free tissue transfer (see **Table 7**).[28–32] The best aesthetic results are achieved with immediate reconstruction, as this helps mitigate soft tissue contraction, especially if radiation therapy has, or will be used. Limited lamina papyracea defects or limited floor defects do not require rigid reconstruction. No reconstruction, or simple fascial grafts (temporalis or fascia lata), may suffice for lamina papyracea and adjacent periorbital defects. Commercially available products, such as porcine submucosal intestinal graft, acellular dermis, titanium, or porous polyethylene implants also can be used.[27] Larger defects involving the orbital floor must undergo rigid reconstruction to minimize enophthalmos, globe malpositioning, ptosis, diplopia, and ectropion.[17,28] Larger tumor resections involving total maxillectomy, ventral skull base resection, orbital exenteration, and facial soft tissue sacrifice require both structural and aesthetic form (**Figs. 8** and **9**). These may necessitate utilization of regional flaps or distant free tissue transfer (see **Table 7**). Complementary strategies, such as prosthetics, can be exceedingly helpful in restoring form (**Fig. 10**).

CLINICAL RESULTS IN THE LITERATURE
Oncologic Outcomes

The literature supports surgery as the cornerstone in management of orbital invasion from sinonasal and ventral skull base malignancies. Carrillo and colleagues[33] reported 5-year survival to be superior in their patients with maxillary and nasal cavity cancers who underwent surgery versus those who did not undergo surgery (50% vs 20%; $P = .0003$). Lisan and colleagues[14] reported statistically significant benefit from surgery in patients with orbital invasion from sinonasal malignancy. Local control was 48% for the group treated without surgery and 72% for the group treated with surgery

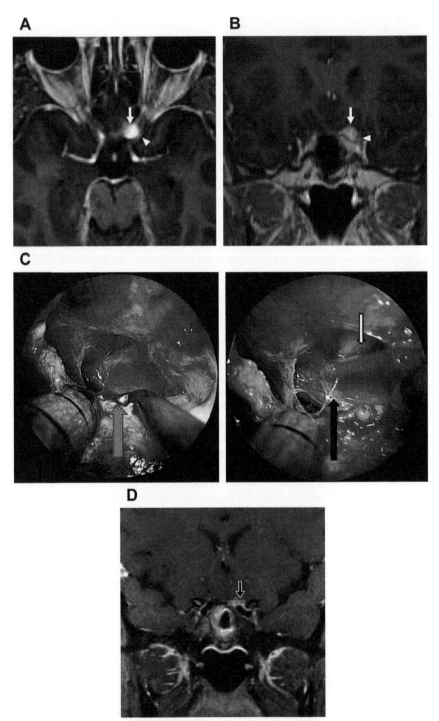

Fig. 7. Axial (*A*) and coronal (*B*) contrast-enhanced T1-weighted images demonstrate para-clinoidal meningioma (*white arrow*) causing lateral displacement of the left optic nerve

Box 1
Preoperative planning

1. Careful clinical and radiographic examination to judge surgical candidacy and approach.

2. Weigh endoscopic versus open techniques. Indications for open approach may be
   a. Soft tissue involvement of eyelids and facial skin
   b. Extensive involvement of orbital rim (floor, roof, lateral wall), nasal bone, frontal bone, and maxillary bone
   c. Tumor involvement far laterally over orbital roof

2. Anticipate equipment (instruments, image guidance), blood products, and reconstructive needs required at time of surgery

3. Optimization of general medical condition

Box 2
Preparation and patient positioning

1. The patient is laid supine.

2. General anesthesia is induced.

3. The field is prepped in a sterile fashion.

4. The eyes are draped into the field. If endoscopic techniques are used, a transparent tape is used to tape the eyes shut. If an external approach is used, a temporary tarsorrhaphy or corneal shield is placed.

5. Additional sites for reconstructive grafts and flap harvest also are prepped and draped.

Box 3
Procedural approach

1. Incision: Appropriate incisions are made for external approaches (eg, lateral rhinotomy, midfacial degloving, Lynch approach). If an endonasal approach is used, the tumor is visualized endoscopically and the tumor is carefully debulked piecemeal to find the site of attachment (Video 1). Adjunctive approaches, such as the sublabial, frontal trephination, or Lynch incisions, may be combined with the endoscopic endonasal approach (Video 2).

2. The site of attachment is resected with margin clearance as outlined in **Table 5**.

3. If needed, endoscopic dacryocystorhinostomy or lacrimal stenting may also preemptively be used to prevent nasolacrimal duct stenosis

4. Reconstruction is performed as necessary

(white arrowhead). (C) Endoscopic transsphenoidal resection of meningioma. Blue arrow shows tumor being resected; black solid arrow points to decompressed optic nerve and white arrow shows olfactory tract. (D) Coronal contrast-enhanced T1-weighted fat-suppressed image with minimal postoperative enhancement at the site of the meningioma resection (black arrow).

Box 4
Steps in orbital clearance and orbital exenteration

1. Incision: In orbital clearance, the lids are preserved. Incisions are made several millimeters away from the lash line, parallel to the lid margin, leaving the lash on the orbital specimen. If exenteration is performed, the involved lid and periorbital skin is resected with an adequate margin and then subperiosteal dissection conducted to the orbital rims. Surgery then proceeds in a similar fashion to orbital clearance.

2. The skin and subcutaneous tissue are dissected off the underlying tarsal plate down to the orbital rims.

3. A circumferential incision is made through the periosteum to the bone of the underlying orbital socket.

4. Subperiosteal dissection is conducted to free the orbital contents from the bony orbit.

5. The attachments of the medial and lateral canthal tendon are sharply detached.

6. The zygomaticofacial and zygomaticotemporal vessels are cauterized in the lateral wall, the anterior and posterior ethmoidal vessels in the medial wall, and the supratrochlear and supraorbital vessels in the roof of the orbit. Bipolar cautery is preferred in the posterior orbit and the orbital roof.

7. Medially the lacrimal sac is lifted off and sharply divided at the junction with the nasolacrimal duct, and laterally, the lacrimal gland is dissected.

8. The origin of the extraocular muscles is divided. Care is taken not to breach through the inferior and superior oblique fissures, dividing sharply through their contents.

9. The stump of the orbit close to the orbital apex is circumferentially freed. The stump is clamped and a stay suture placed before cutting the stump with curved Mayo scissors. Care must be taken when cutting through this stump. There may be brisk bleeding from the ophthalmic artery. If the stump is cut too close to the apex without adequate control of the ophthalmic artery, the artery may retract intracranially, causing potentially catastrophic complications. Bradycardia may occur during transection of the optic nerve.

10. After resection, the stay suture helps in ligation of the ophthalmic artery and prevention of cerebrospinal fluid leak through the optic nerve sheath.

11. The orbit is then packed with saline gauze for 5 to 10 minutes.

12. Reconstruction is performed.

Box 5
Immediate postprocedural care

1. If preserved, the eye is carefully examined postoperatively to judge vision, and monitored in the postoperative period.

2. Diplopia, exposure keratitis, etc are anticipated and managed.

3. Postoperative care acuity is judged individually and an appropriate monitored setting provided to patient.

4. Ancillary monitoring and care provided as necessary. Perioperative antibiotics are used per standard guidelines.

5. Free flaps are monitored per standard guidelines and may require intensive care in the early postoperative period.

Table 7
Options for reconstruction after orbital clearance and exenteration

Option	Source	Advantages and Limitations
Regional flaps	• Temporalis muscle flap • Temporoparietal fascial flap	Compared to free tissue transfer, they minimize operative time. Disadvantages: • Provide less tissue bulk for volume repletion • Have less mobility to adapt to 3-dimensional defects • Require traversing an intact lateral orbital wall to reach defect • Can result in a secondary temporal contour depression at donor site
Soft tissue free flaps	• Radial forearm flap • Rectus abdominis flap • Parascapular flap • Anterolateral thigh flap	• For larger and more complex defects, free tissue transfer has become the gold standard • The choice of flap depends on the amount of tissue volume required and defect variables • The cutaneous components replace nasal, oral, or external lining, whereas the fascial or muscular components can be used to support dural repair and create cranio-nasal separation
Bony free flap	• Scapular or scapular tip flap • Iliac crest • Fibular free flap	• Can replace the midface facial buttresses • Can reestablish malar projection and prevent soft tissue contraction into the maxillary sinus
Orbital prosthetics	• Osseointegrated • Spectacle-held • Customized	• Complementary adjunct to flap for restoring form • Secondary procedures may be required to soft tissue reconstructions to provide adequate foundation to which prosthetics can be applied • Osseointegrated implants can be placed into bony reconstructions to aid in supporting a prosthetic

(P<.05). Patients treated without surgery had a 3-year survival rate of 19% versus 65% for patients treated with surgery. The 5-year survival rates were 10% and 58%, respectively. These results reflect a selection bias, as patients treated without surgery are more likely to have advanced disease.

Although Sisson[16] proposed that the eye could be spared when tumor invasion was limited to the bony orbit, later investigators recommended orbital preservation even if the orbital periosteum was breached.[5,13,28,34] Howard and colleagues[3] reported similar survival whether the patient had orbital clearance or orbital preservation using this strategy. Imola and Schramm[17] reported on 66 tumors abutting or invading into the orbit, of which 54 were treated with orbital preservation. Local recurrence at the original site of orbital involvement was seen in only 7.8% of cases. They found no statistically significant differences in oncologic outcomes in patients with squamous cell carcinoma, adenomatous carcinomas, and undifferentiated carcinoma when managed by orbital preservation or sacrifice. Lisan and colleagues[14]

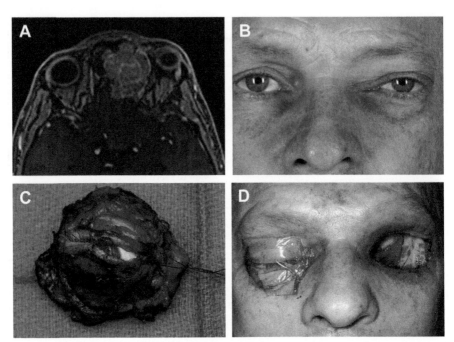

Fig. 8. (*A*) Axial contrast-enhanced T1-weighted images demonstrate extensive invasion of poorly differentiated sinonasal carcinoma into left eye (extraocular muscle, intraconal fat, and medial canthus soft tissue). (*B*) Left-sided proptosis is evident on examination. (*C*) Orbital exenteration specimen. (*D*) Defect following orbital exenteration.

reported 58 patients with sinonasal malignancy invading the orbit who underwent surgery. Orbital preservation was feasible in 66%. Orbital clearance was performed for invasion of extraocular muscles, ocular globe, or orbital apex. Mean follow-up was 45 months. Local control was similar in those treated with orbital clearance (70%) or orbital preservation (74%), as were 5-year survival and 5-year relapse-free survival.

Some recent studies report even more aggressive preservation strategies.[12,15] Itami and colleagues[15] reported 5-year local recurrence-free survival of 59% in patients who underwent piecemeal debulking followed by conventional fractionated radiation therapy. Orbital exenteration had to be performed in only 1 patient. Nishino and colleagues[12] examined oncologic and functional outcomes in patients with advanced malignant maxillary sinus tumors with orbital invasion. Patients were treated with conservative surgery through a sublabial approach, radiotherapy, and regional chemotherapy. The 5-year overall survival and local control rates were 68% and 66%, respectively. However, other investigators have cautioned that such approaches may be oncologically flawed.[4,22] Dulguerov and colleagues[22] reported on retrospectively collected data from 220 patients. The investigators reported local control rate of 79% with orbital sacrifice and 14% with orbital preservation in patients with orbital invasion.

FUNCTIONAL OUTCOMES FOR ORBITAL PRESERVATION

Enophthalmos, diplopia, lid ectropion, epiphora from lid malposition, canthal dystopia, exposure keratitis, and loss of visual acuity may become problematic in preserved

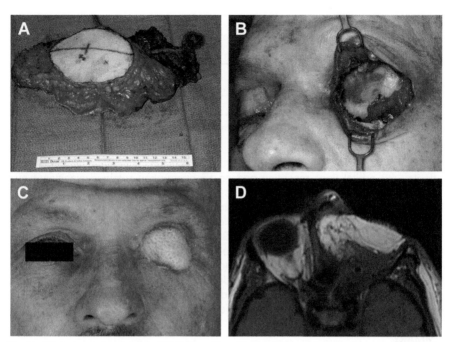

Fig. 9. (*A*) Anterolateral thigh (ALT) flap. The skin paddle will be used to reconstruct the cutaneous exenteration defect. The muscle and fascia will reconstruct the skull base and support the dural repair. (*B*) Intraoperative view of orbital soft tissue reconstruction with the ALT flap. (*C*) Postoperative view of orbital reconstruction at 1 year following flap refining. (*D*) Postoperative axial T1-weighted MRI at 1 year demonstrating fat and muscle from the flap reconstruction.

orbits.[17] Imola and Schramm[17] assessed and graded postoperative function in the preserved orbit (**Table 8**). Eye function was reported as functional without impairment in 54%, functional with impairment in 37%, and nonfunctional in 9%. The most common problem was globe malposition (63%) due to lack of adequate rigid reconstruction of the orbital floor, or multisegmental orbital defects. Enophthalmos was clinically inconsequential in most, but diplopia was persistent in 9% of patients. Ocular sequelae occurred in 41% of functional eyes, being more frequent in those treated with radiation. Radiation increased the risk of optic atrophy, cataract formation, excessive dryness, and ectropion. Stern and colleagues[28] reported that only 17% of

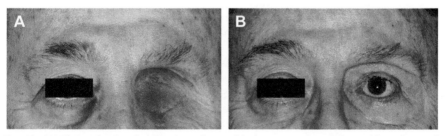

Fig. 10. (*A*, *B*) Prosthetic rehabilitation of an orbital exenteration defect with mature soft tissue reconstruction.

Table 8
Classification of postoperative functional outcomes from orbital preservation

Grade of Function	Orbital Function
I	Functional eye without impairment
II	Functional eye with some impairment
III	Nonfunctional eye

Adapted from Imola MJ, Schramm VL. Orbital preservation in surgical management of sinonasal malignancy. Laryngoscope 2002;112(8 Pt 1):1358.

patients with orbital floor resection and no reconstruction retained significant eye function. Patients with adequate floor support or orbit-sparing radiation fields had minimal problems. Recently, Rajapurkar and colleagues[35] reported functional outcomes in 19 patients with orbital preservation. Sixteen patients remained recurrence free and were reported to have Grade I or Grade II function even after adjuvant radiotherapy (mean dosage 6000 cGy). Two developed decreased visual acuity, one due to radiation-induced retinopathy. Epiphora can result from stenosis of the nasolacrimal duct system, lid malposition, or dry eye. Andersen and colleagues[36] reported epiphora in 36%, whereas Imola and Schramm[17] reported a decreased epiphora rate of 13% with preemptive silastic stenting of the nasolacrimal system.

SUMMARY

Orbital involvement with sinonasal and ventral skull base malignancy is not infrequent, and should be carefully assessed for. Invasion into orbital soft tissue and the apex adversely affects oncological outcomes. Multimodality therapy is usually attempted to optimize local control and overall survival. Contemporary studies show that in carefully selected cases of orbital invasion, orbital preservation can be attempted, without adversely impacting survival. Reconstructive needs should be anticipated and addressed at the time of surgery so as to optimize orbital function and aesthetic outcomes.

SUPPLEMENTARY DATA

Supplementary data related to this article can be found at http://dx.doi.org/10.1016/j. otc.2016.12.010.

REFERENCES

1. Iannetti G, Valentini V, Rinna C, et al. Ethmoido-orbital tumors: our experience. J Craniofac Surg 2005;16(6):1085–91.
2. Ganly I, Patel SG, Singh B, et al. Craniofacial resection for malignant paranasal sinus tumors: report of an International Collaborative Study. Head Neck 2005; 27:575–84.
3. Howard DJ, Lund VJ, Wei WI. Craniofacial resection for tumors of the nasal cavity and paranasal sinuses: a 25-year experience. Head Neck 2006;28(10):867–73.
4. Carrau RL, Segas J, Nuss DW, et al. Squamous cell carcinoma of the sinonasal tract invading the orbit. Laryngoscope 1999;109(2 Pt 1):230–5.
5. Lund VJ, Howard DJ, Wei WI, et al. Craniofacial resection for tumors of the nasal cavity and paranasal sinuses–a 17-year experience. Head Neck 1998;20(2): 97–105.

6. Suarez C, Llorente JL, Fernandez De Leon R, et al. Prognostic factors in sinonasal tumors involving the anterior skull base. Head Neck 2004;26:136–44.
7. Kaplan DJ, Kim JH, Wang E, et al. Prognostic indicators for salvage surgery of recurrent sinonasal malignancy. Otolaryngol Head Neck Surg 2016;154(1):104–12.
8. Edge SB, Byrd DR, Compton CC, et al, editors. AJCC cancer staging manual. 7th edition. New York: Springer; 2010.
9. Eisen MD, Yousem DM, Loevner LA, et al. Preoperative imaging to predict orbital invasion by tumor. Head Neck 2000;22:456–62.
10. Loevner LA, Sonners AI. Imaging of neoplasms of the paranasal sinuses [review]. Magn Reson Imaging Clin N Am 2002;10(3):467–93.
11. Yousem DM, Gad K, Tufano RP. Resectability issues with head and neck cancer. AJNR Am J Neuroradiol 2006;27(10):2024–36.
12. Nishino H, Ichimura K, Tanaka H, et al. Results of orbital preservation for advanced malignant maxillary sinus tumors. Laryngoscope 2003;113(6):1064–9.
13. McCary WS, Levine PA, Cantrell RW. Preservation of the eye in the treatment of sinonasal malignant neoplasms with orbital involvement. A confirmation of the original treatise. Arch Otolaryngol Head Neck Surg 1996;122(6):657–9.
14. Lisan Q, Kolb F, Temam S, et al. Management of orbital invasion in sinonasal malignancies. Head Neck 2016;38(11):1650–6.
15. Itami J, Uno T, Aruga M, et al. Squamous cell carcinoma of the maxillary sinus treated with radiation therapy and conservative surgery. Cancer 1998;82:104–7.
16. Sisson GA. Symposium: paranasal sinuses. Laryngoscope 1970;80:945–53.
17. Imola MJ, Schramm VL. Orbital preservation in surgical management of sinonasal malignancy. Laryngoscope 2002;112(8 Pt 1):1357–65.
18. Duprez F, Madani I, Morbée L, et al. IMRT for sinonasal tumors minimizes severe late ocular toxicity and preserves disease control and survival. Int J Radiat Oncol Biol Phys 2012;83(1):252–9.
19. Thiagarajan A, Mechalakos J, Lee N. Feasibility of reirradiation of recurrent sinonasal carcinoma in the periorbital region using hypofractionated image-guided intensity-modulated radiation therapy. Head Neck 2011;33(9):1372–8.
20. Harrison DFN. Problems in surgical management of neoplasms arising in the paranasal sinuses. J Laryngol Otol 1976;90(1):69–74.
21. Jackson RT, Fitz-Hugh GS, Constable WC. Malignant neoplasms of the nasal cavities and paranasal sinuses: (a retrospective study). Laryngoscope 1977;87(5 Pt 1):726–36.
22. Dulguerov P, Jacobsen MS, Allal AS, et al. Nasal and paranasal sinus carcinoma: are we making progress? A series of 220 patients and a systematic review. Cancer 2001;92(12):3012–29.
23. Lund VJ, Wei WI. Endoscopic surgery for malignant sinonasal tumours: an eighteen year experience. Rhinology 2015;53:204–11.
24. Castelnuovo P, Turri-Zanoni M, Battaglia P, et al. Endoscopic endonasal management of orbital pathologies. Neurosurg Clin N Am 2015;26(3):463–72.
25. Christianson B, Perez C, Harrow B, et al. Management of the orbit during endoscopic sinonasal tumor surgery. Int Forum Allergy Rhinol 2015;5(10):967–73.
26. Turvey TA, Golden BA. Orbital anatomy for the surgeon. Oral Maxillofac Surg Clin North Am 2012;24(4):525–36.
27. Lal D, Cain RB. Updates in reconstruction of skull base defects [review]. Curr Opin Otolaryngol Head Neck Surg 2014;22(5):419–28.
28. Stern SJ, Goepfert H, Clayman G, et al. Orbital preservation in maxillectomy. Otolaryngol Head Neck Surg 1993;109(1):111–5.

29. Cordeiro PG, Santamaria E, Kraus DH, et al. Reconstruction of total maxillectomy defects with preservation of the orbital contents. Plast Reconstr Surg 1998; 102(6):1874–84 [discussion: 1885–7].
30. Yamamoto Y, Kawashima K, Sugihara T, et al. Surgical management of maxillectomy defects based on the concept of buttress reconstruction. Head Neck 2004; 26(3):247–56.
31. Dediol E, Uglešić V, Zubčić V, et al. Brown class III maxillectomy defects reconstruction with prefabricated titanium mesh and soft tissue free flap. Ann Plast Surg 2013;71(1):63–7.
32. Heffelfinger R, Murchison AP, Parkes W, et al. Microvascular free flap reconstruction of orbitocraniofacial defects. Orbit 2013;32(2):95–101.
33. Carrillo JF, Guemes A, Ramırez-Ortega MC, et al. Prognostic factors in maxillary sinus and nasal cavity carcinoma. Eur J Surg Oncol 2005;31:1206–12.
34. Suárez C, Ferlito A, Lund VJ, et al. Management of the orbit in malignant sinonasal tumors. Head Neck 2008;30(2):242–50.
35. Rajapurkar M, Thankappan K, Sampathirao LM, et al. Oncologic and functional outcome of the preserved eye in malignant sinonasal tumors. Head Neck 2013; 35(10):1379–84.
36. Andersen PE, Kraus DH, Arbit D, et al. Management of the orbit during anterior fossa craniofacial resection. Arch Otolaryngol Head Neck Surg 1996;122:1305–7.

Management of Cavernous Sinus Involvement in Sinonasal and Ventral Skull Base Malignancies

CrossMark

Amol Raheja, MBBS, MCH, William T. Couldwell, MD, PhD*

KEYWORDS

- Cavernous sinus • Skull base tumor • Sinonasal and ventral skull base malignancy
- Surgical approach • Technical nuances • Cerebral revascularization

KEY POINTS

- For a malignant tumor involving the cavernous sinus, the approach must be individualized to optimize the treatment strategy. Often a combination of surgical approaches is necessary for optimal resection of aggressive ventral skull base malignancies with cavernous sinus involvement, including frequent collaboration between the disciplines of otorhinolaryngology and neurosurgery.
- To confirm the diagnosis in cases of inconclusive radiological impressions or suspicious-looking lesions, use of minimally invasive approaches aided with stereotactic neuronavigation is helpful.
- Once the diagnosis is confirmed, and if the patient is healthy and has no metastatic disease, aggressive surgical resection may be indicated, especially if the removal of the cavernous sinus lesion may result in total tumor resection.
- For patients with more advanced and recurrent malignant disease, whereby carotid preservation would prevent a meaningful resection, en bloc resection of the tumor and cavernous sinus with cerebrovascular revascularization may be justified.
- Frequently, en bloc resection will require cavernous sinus exenteration, including sacrifice of the cavernous internal carotid artery, possible high-flow extracranial-to-intracranial bypass, and placement of a vascularized pedicled flap for ventral skull base reconstruction along with adjuvant chemotherapy and radiotherapy to effectively eradicate the microscopic tumor remnants.

 Video content accompanies this article at http://www.oto.theclinics.com.

Department of Neurosurgery, Clinical Neurosciences Center, University of Utah, 175 North Medical Drive East, Salt Lake City, UT 84132, USA
* Corresponding author.
E-mail address: neuropub@hsc.utah.edu

Otolaryngol Clin N Am 50 (2017) 365–383
http://dx.doi.org/10.1016/j.otc.2016.12.011
0030-6665/17/© 2016 Elsevier Inc. All rights reserved.

INTRODUCTION

Sinonasal and ventral skull base malignancy refers to tumors arising from the nasal cavity, paranasal sinuses, orbit, salivary glands, and soft tissue and bone along the ventral skull base.[1,2] This broad spectrum of malignant diseases includes, but is not limited to, nasopharyngeal squamous cell carcinoma, adenoid cystic carcinoma, lymphoma, chordoma, chondrosarcoma, hemangiopericytoma, malignant meningioma, osteosarcoma, rhabdomyosarcoma, adenocarcinoma, mucoepidermoid carcinoma, acinic cell carcinoma, undifferentiated carcinoma, clear cell carcinoma, liposarcoma, and esthesioneuroblastoma.[1,2] These lesions spread to the cavernous sinus (CS) either directly (83.2%) via the superior orbital fissure, inferior orbital fissure, foramen rotundum, and foramen ovale or through metastasis (16.8%) via perineural extension or hematogenous or lymphatic spread.[3] Malignant tumors of the nasal cavity and paranasal sinuses are rare, accounting for 0.2% to 0.5% of all cancer cases and only 3.0% of malignant tumors in the head and neck region.[4] According to the Surveillance, Epidemiology, and End Results database of all reported sinonasal malignancies between 1973 and 2006, the cumulative incidence of sinonasal malignancy was 0.556 cases per 100,000 population per year; the most common sites of origin were the nasal cavity (43.9%) and the maxillary sinus (35.9%).[2] CS involvement by sinonasal and ventral skull base malignancies carries dismal prognosis overall, because it precludes radical oncological resection in many instances.[1,5,6] However, the overall and progression-free survival in a particular malignant ventral skull base tumor case with CS involvement depends on many factors besides the extent of resection, which include tumor burden, pathologic conditions, presence of metastasis, positive tumor margins, and age of patients. Aggressive surgical resection followed by adjuvant chemotherapy and radiotherapy offers the best possible chance of prolonging overall survival in most sinonasal and ventral skull base malignancies.[7,8]

Since the seminal articles by Ketcham and colleagues[9,10] in 1963 and 1966 detailing the role of surgery in intracranial involvement of head and neck malignancy, innovation of radical surgical resection procedures for the eradication of malignant ventral skull base tumors is arguably one of the most important advancements in the treatment of head and neck malignancy in the past half century. Besides the use of conventional open transcranial and transfacial approaches to achieve the surgical goal of oncologic resection, minimally invasive endoscopic approaches have been applied more recently to selected patients with reasonable outcomes.[11–13] It was not uncommon in the past that malignant skull base tumors were considered inoperable. With advancement in skull base microneurosurgery, availability of better endoscopic devices, expertise in cerebral revascularization, more effective hemostatic agents, and improved ventral skull base reconstruction techniques, the collective opinion of the neurosurgical community has changed from this conventional thinking. More aggressive groups preferred piecemeal removal of tumor, including parts extending into the CS proper[14]; however, the oncological principle of en bloc resection was still not realized until the pioneering efforts of Sekhar and Moller,[15] Saito and colleagues,[1] and others.[16,17] This review discusses the current surgical strategies, their indications, techniques, nuances, advantages, limitations, and complications of operative approaches for CS involvement of malignant ventral skull base tumors.

SURGICAL MANAGEMENT

Since the pioneering work of Parkinson[18] and others,[19–21] more refined intradural and extradural transcranial surgical approaches have been described to access CS lesions; more recently, the extended endonasal/transmaxillary endoscopic approaches have been introduced in the realm of microneurosurgery. For a malignant tumor involving the CS, the approach needs to be individualized to optimize the treatment strategy. Firstly, confirming the diagnosis is of paramount importance in cases of inconclusive radiological impressions or suspicious-looking lesions. Use of minimally invasive approaches aided with stereotactic neuronavigation helps to achieve that goal safely. Once the diagnosis is confirmed, and if the patient is healthy and has no metastatic disease, aggressive surgical resection may be indicated, especially if the removal of the CS lesion may result in total tumor resection. Some investigators think that tumor resection with carotid preservation carries the lowest risk of cerebrovascular accidents and should generally be the treatment of choice.[14] For patients with more advanced and recurrent malignant disease, whereby carotid preservation would prevent a meaningful resection, en bloc resection of the tumor and CS with cerebrovascular revascularization may be justified.[1,16]

Frequently, en bloc resection will require CS exenteration (CSE), including sacrifice of the cavernous internal carotid artery (ICA), possible high-flow extracranial-to-intracranial bypass, and placement of a vascularized pedicled flap for ventral skull base reconstruction along with adjuvant chemotherapy and radiotherapy to effectively eradicate the microscopic tumor remnants.[1,16] Often a combination of surgical approaches is necessary for optimal resection of aggressive ventral skull base malignancies with CS involvement, including frequent collaboration between the disciplines of otorhinolaryngology and neurosurgery. The surgical approach to the CS region includes the intradural and extradural transcranial and transfacial routes. When planning for a CS approach, preoperative planning is very important to prepare for any potential intraoperative events like ICA injury requiring vascular repair or cerebral revascularization or nerve damage requiring reanastomosis.

Minimally Invasive Transcavernous Biopsy of Cavernous Sinus Lesions

With the diverse radiological differentials for complex skull base lesions with CS involvement including infectious and inflammatory pathologies as well as benign and malignant tumors, whenever the radiological findings are inconclusive or suspicious for malignancy, minimally invasive tissue sampling methods should be attempted before proceeding with an aggressive surgical strategy because a precise identification of the cause of the lesion helps to optimize the treatment planning. The use of frameless stereotactic neuronavigation can be of great assistance in safely performing such blind procedures. Tissue sampling of radiologically inconclusive or suspicious CS lesions yields a positive diagnosis of malignant skull base tumor in as many as 37% to 40% of patients.[22,23] Different surgical approaches can then be optimized to target the CS lesion based on the precise anatomic location of the lesion and surgeon's preference.

Lateral orbitotomy approach

Altay and colleagues[24] originally described the minimally invasive lateral orbitotomy extradural transcavernous approach in 2012. It is a practical, reliable, and low-risk minimally invasive technique for CS biopsy.[24] The primary indication for this procedure is a lesion situated in the lateral compartment of the CS (primary position lateral to the carotid artery). Patients are positioned supine with the head stabilized on a Mayfield head holder with slight contralateral rotation ($\sim 10°$–$15°$). The LO approach to the CS involves a small 2-cm Y-shaped incision along the natural skin crease (Video 1). Next, the periosteum is dissected off the lateral orbital rim to expose the orbitozygomatic and fronto-orbital junctions. Subsequently, the temporalis muscle fibers and periorbita are carefully dissected from both sides of the lateral orbit wall. A 2-cm segment of the lateral orbital rim is cut using a fine-tip C1 drill bit to expose the inferior orbital fissure inferiorly, the orbitotemporal junction posteriorly, and up to the lower margin of sphenoid ridge superiorly (**Fig. 1**). Before the bony rim is removed, thin-profile miniplates are screwed in and corresponding holes are tentatively made on either side of the bone removed to optimize the cosmesis of bony closure at the end. The remaining lateral orbital rim and lateral sphenoid wing are drilled to expose the temporal dura mater. Drilling the lateral orbital wall and deeper sphenoid wing under neuronavigation guidance helps in precise localization of the CS lesion.

The superior orbital fissure is centered in the operative trajectory, enabling easy detachment of 2 layers of the lateral CS, which is performed using an extradural Dolenc technique.[24] Anterior clinoid process drilling can be added to augment the superior exposure of the CS and to decompress the optic nerve if desired. This drilling also aids in more posterior exposure as far back as the geniculate ganglion at a wider craniocaudal angle, besides proving an immediate vascular control of the clinoidal ICA. With further drilling superiorly along the lower aspect of sphenoid ridge and inferiorly along the remaining lateral orbital wall toward the inferior orbital fissure, the Meckel cave and the foramen rotundum are well within the operative reach. To access the more lateral aspect of the middle cranial fossa, including the mandibular division of the trigeminal nerve (V3), foramen ovale, foramen spinosum, greater superficial petrosal nerve (GSPN), and petrous ICA, an extended version of this approach that involves further drilling of the lateral aspect of greater sphenoid wing is required.[24] The advantages of this approach are the small skin incision, minimal soft tissue dissection and blood loss, sparing of the temporalis muscle insertion, and, consequently,

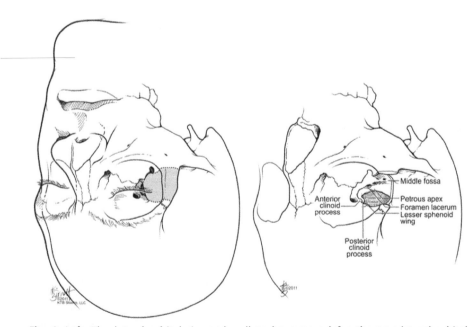

Fig. 1. Left: The lateral orbital rim and wall to be removed for the translateral orbital approach to the CS. Right: The parasellar area and middle fossa structures after removal of the lateral orbital rim and wall in the translateral orbital approach. (*From* Altay T, Patel BC, Couldwell WT. Lateral orbital wall approach to the cavernous sinus. J Neurosurg 2012;116(4):756; with permission.)

reduced risk of muscle atrophy. In addition, there is a shorter incision-to-target distance, with minimal brain retraction. These patients have a reduced hospital stay (usually 1 day). The primary limitation of this approach is the unfamiliar anatomy of the sphenocavernous region when viewed from below at a translateral orbital angle of view. Although infrequently encountered, potential complications include cerebrospinal fluid (CSF) leak, pseudomeningocele, orbital hematoma, and transient cranial neuropathy.

Percutaneous needle biopsy via the foramen ovale

Stechison and Bernstein[25] reported the first attempt of a middle fossa biopsy through the foramen ovale in 1989.[25] Lesions amenable to this approach are those involving the Meckel cave, the posterior part of the CS, and the upper part of the petroclival region. Patients are placed supine with the head under fluoroscopic control, and the procedure is performed under small-dose and short-lasting general anesthesia. After the local anesthetic is injected, the trajectory for percutaneous biopsy is made using the Hartel technique. The skin entry point is 3 cm lateral to the labial commissure. The tip of the biopsy needle is directed toward the foramen ovale, which corresponds to 3 cm anterior to the tragus on a horizontal line along the inferior border of the zygoma and pupilla.[22] Depth is continuously assessed using fluoroscopy or stereotactic neuronavigation.[22,26] Extreme care is required not to take a wrong trajectory and violate the internal jugular vein or the ICA at its entrance to the petrous canal and jugular foramen posterolaterally, the lateral segment of the ICA medially, or the optic nerve anteriorly along the orbital apex.[22] Along the correct trajectory, the needle may encounter, successively, the parotid duct, maxillary artery, or auditory tube, with corresponding potential complications of hemosialorrhea, cheek hematoma, or middle ear hemoserous otitis, respectively.[22]

The advantages of this approach include shorter operative time, short length of hospitalization, no brain retraction, and an acceptable safety profile.[22,26] The primary limitations include the technically challenging nature of the approach, which requires adequate expertise, and the blind nature of tissue sampling with a significant number of nonproductive biopsies. In a series of 50 cases with percutaneous biopsy of CS lesions via the foramen ovale, Messerer and colleagues[22] demonstrated that a productive biopsy was obtained in 86% (n = 43) of cases. Among those 43 cases, 28 patients underwent second (open) surgery and a second set of confirmatory histopathologic evaluation and resection. They demonstrated that percutaneous biopsy via foramen ovale had a sensitivity of 83% and specificity of 100%.[22] Complications included 2 cases of facial cellulitis and cheek hematoma, with no permanent sequelae. Procedure-related complications have a low incidence but may include potential injury to the optic nerve, ICA, internal jugular vein, maxillary artery, and V3 resulting in possibly visual decline, ICA pseudoaneurysm, massive blood loss, cheek hematoma, and facial pain/numbness, respectively. This procedure is associated with some degree of facial hypesthesia, dysesthesia, or paresthesia in approximately two-thirds of cases[22]; however, most of the symptoms are short lasting, with associated permanent sequelae in only a fraction of cases.[22]

Endoscopic transfacial approaches

Unlike the LO and percutaneous transforamen ovale approaches, which provide access to primarily the lateral CS compartment (lateral to carotid siphon), transfacial approaches (endonasal and transmaxillary endoscopic) provide access to the medial and lateral compartments of the CS.[27,28] The extended endoscopic endonasal transsphenoidal trans-sellar and extended endoscopic endonasal transethmoidal transsphenoidal parasellar approaches are optimal for lesions situated primarily medial to the carotid siphon, whereas an extended endoscopic transmaxillary transpterygoid approach provides an access to the lateral CS lesions.[27,28] Patients are placed supine with the head stabilized on Mayfield fixation in slight extension, lateral tilt, and ipsilateral rotation to provide a comfortable working trajectory. Use of stereotactic neuronavigation is essential in these extended approaches where surface landmarks may be erroneous at times, and the close proximity to vital neurovascular structures in the CS does not allow any margin of error in this narrow operative corridor. No incision is required for endonasal approaches while a sublabial incision is necessary for the transmaxillary approach. The endonasal approach requires a binostril, 2- or 3-handed technique to make the best use of the narrow working corridors. Lateralization of the middle turbinates, removal of distal bony nasal septum, and wide opening of the sphenoid sinus are common to both endonasal approaches to enhance exposure.[27,28]

Apart from the steps these approaches have in common, for the trans-sellar approach, the sellar floor is removed, the pituitary gland is mobilized if needed, and biopsy of the CS lesion is done under direct vision using an angled endoscope, whereas for a parasellar endonasal approach, the superior turbinate and anterior and posterior ethmoidal air cells are opened. The parasellar endonasal approach aims to enter the CS more anteriorly than the trans-sellar approach, with the steps of removing the cavernous carotid bony wall, gently mobilizing the ICA, and obtaining the biopsy of the CS lesion.[27,28] For a transmaxillary approach, the anterior and posterior walls of the maxillary sinus are opened to access the pterygopalatine fossa. Next, the pterygoid process is removed along with the ethmoid and sphenoid to expose the lateral aspect of CS, which allows for tissue sampling.[27,28] The primary advantages of these approaches are the lack of incision and ability to achieve tissue sampling under direct vision; however, certain limitations to these approaches include protracted sinonasal symptoms after surgery, a risk of CSF leak, a higher risk of meningitis because of potential contamination in crossing the nasal cavity or paranasal sinuses, and risk of cavernous ICA injury. For a transmaxillary approach, damage to the neurovascular structures along paramedian skull base, including maxillary, mandibular, and vidian neurovascular bundles, is a possible procedure-related complication.[27,28]

Aggressive Transcranial Approaches to the Cavernous Sinus

In most young, healthy patients who have been diagnosed with malignant ventral skull base tumors with CS involvement and limited metastatic disease, aggressive surgical exploration of the CS and resection of the diseased tissue remains an option as an initial modality of therapy.[14] It differs from radical en bloc resection in principle in that it allows only piecemeal removal of tumor rather than aiming at oncological resection of malignant disease. This approach has been tailored to achieve maximal safe resection of the tumor with minimum possible risk of iatrogenic neurovascular injury, aiming at a functional preservation for better quality of life. Although it may benefit patients from a functional standpoint, it may compromise on the best possible overall and progression-free survival for a given ventral skull base malignancy. Patients with multiple metastases and poor overall health status with multiple comorbidities are relative contraindications for extensive skull base surgery (both aggressive and radical en bloc resections), whereby high intraoperative blood loss is expected along with the requirement of prolonged general anesthesia.[29]

It is critical to understand the surgical anatomy of the 4 CS and 4 middle fossa triangles to grasp the concept of transcranial transcavernous surgical approaches.[30,31]

These surgically relevant triangles provide invaluable working operative corridors and help with accessing different CS tumors with middle and posterior fossa extensions. For performing a transcranial route to the CS, a frontotemporal craniotomy with or without orbitozygomatic or transzygomatic osteotomy is required.[31] There are 3 primary safe operative trajectories to enter the CS transcranially, vis-á-vis anteromedially through the roof of CS via the Hakuba (oculomotor) triangle using the Hakuba/Dolenc approach; anterolaterally through the lateral wall of the CS via various CS and middle fossa triangles using a modified Dolenc approach; and posterolaterally through the posterolateral wall of the CS using the Kawase approach.[32–35] A suitable approach (or a combination of these approaches) to the CS is chosen depending on the tumor size, location, epicenter, extent of the tumor, nature of pathology, and the preference of the operating surgeon.

There are certain common operative steps in all 3 transcranial approaches. The patient is placed supine with the head turned 30° to 60° to the contralateral side (depending on the epicenter of the lesion and suitable operative corridor) and slightly extended. Intraoperative electrophysiologic monitoring for motor evoked potential, somatosensory evoked potential, and electroencephalogram is set up. A standard curvilinear incision is made from just anterior to the tragus to the midline along the hairline, and a single myocutaneous flap is elevated to expose the frontotemporal bone, the root of the zygoma, and the Key burr-hole point. After a frontotemporal craniotomy is performed, the sphenoid ridge and lateral sphenoid wing are drilled flush to the anterior and middle cranial fossa. Once the meningo-orbital band is identified, it is coagulated and divided. To achieve adequate access in all 3 transcranial transcavernous approaches, expansion of the operative corridor can be achieved by augmenting bone removal in the form of orbitozygomatic osteotomy and transzygomatic osteotomy. Specific further primary operative steps are highlighted later in their respective sections. Closure is done in a standard fashion at the end of the procedure, and the skull base defect is reconstructed and plugged using a fat graft, free fascia lata, pedicled nasoseptal flap from below, pedicled pericranial flap, temporalis muscle graft, or a combination of these depending on the size of the dural defect and the surgeon's preference.

The primary advantages of the microscopic transcranial approach over the endoscopic transfacial approach include the wide operative corridor between various cranial nerves located in the lateral wall of the CS, better vascular control in case of inadvertent ICA injury, and a lower risk of CSF leak and associated complications. There is no limitation in the size and extent of the intracranial disease process beyond the CS involvement. Limitations include large scalp incisions with higher wound-related postoperative morbidity, a higher risk of iatrogenic cranial neuropathy, and possible brain retraction–related complications. In addition, extracranial sinus disease is less amenable to resection via a transcranial approach. Extensive skull base malignancies with CS involvement often warrant combined otorhinolaryngology and neurosurgery surgical procedures, with simultaneous transcranial and transfacial approaches for the best possible outcome (Video 2). Overall, the possible complications for transcranial approaches include wound complications, infection, CSF leak, pseudomeningocele, cranial neuropathy, vascular injury, retraction hematoma/contusions, seizures, and neurologic deficits.

Anteromedial transcavernous approach

For entry into the CS roof, a combined intradural and extradural approach is required including drilling of the anterior clinoid process either intradurally or extradurally.[31,34] Once the anterior clinoid process is drilled, it exposes the clinoidal ICA, carotid-oculomotor membrane, optic strut, superior orbital fissure, and optic canal.[31,34] Adequate irrigation must be used while drilling the anterior clinoid process to prevent optic nerve damage from thermal injury. Additionally, a thin rim of bone along the optic nerve and ICA should be left after the drilling; it is safer to remove this thin shell of bone with microdissectors to avoid any inadvertent damage to the optic nerve and clinoidal ICA while drilling. Careful preoperative assessment of the bony anatomy of the skull base should be used to rule out physiologic variations like an osseous bridge between the anterior clinoid process and middle clinoid process, forming a caroticoclinoid foramen. Care should be taken to seal off any air spaces, which might open inadvertently while drilling.

Besides anterior clinoid process drilling, adequate CS roof exposure requires wide splitting of the sylvian fissure. In addition, the temporal lobe should be freed from arachnoid adhesions along its medial and basal surface to allow gentle retraction to access the roof of CS. After the distal dural ring is opened, the supraclinoidal and clinoidal ICA can be mobilized to increase the access to the CS roof. Vertical entry into the CS roof via the oculomotor (Hakuba) triangle is then achieved by carefully dividing the dural membrane along the anterosuperior aspect of the oculomotor nerve entry into CS roof, until the nerve becomes incorporated into the lateral wall of the CS. The next step is to open the carotid-oculomotor membrane in the clinoidal (Dolenc) triangle medial to the oculomotor nerve to widen the intracavernous operative corridor. Any venous bleeding can be controlled using absorbable hemostatic agents.

Anterolateral transcavernous approach

Umansky and Nathan[21] described the 2-layer composition of the lateral wall of the CS, which allows safe peeling of the outer layer of dura mater away from the inner layer along the middle cranial fossa to provide adequate extradural access to the lateral wall of the CS and its contents through the various CS and middle fossa triangles. Dolenc[32,33] also pioneered this technique of the interdural transcavernous approach, followed by piecemeal removal of tumor via the narrow operative corridors between the nerves in the lateral wall of the CS. The dissection starts at the greater sphenoid wing and proceeds posteromedially toward the superior orbital fissure, where the intracranial periosteum is continuous with the periorbita. A shallow cut is made, which allows gentle separation of the dura mater from the lateral wall of the CS and middle cranial fossa floor. This outer (meningeal) layer is peeled away from the inner (endosteal) layer to expose cranial nerves III, IV, V1, V2, V3 and gasserian ganglion, along with the CS and middle fossa triangles. The appropriate operative corridor is chosen to access the tumor filling the CS (**Fig. 2**).[36]

Posterolateral transcavernous approach

In contrast to the anteromedial and anterolateral approaches, this approach requires reflection of the middle fossa dura mater in a posterior-to-anterior direction to prevent undue stress and avulsion of the GSPN and consequent facial paresis. The middle meningeal artery is identified, coagulated, and divided to allow smooth retraction of the basal dura mater. Using this extradural approach and sharp dissection between the two layers of the CS lateral wall, V3 is delineated to the gasserian ganglion and Meckel cave posteromedially. Using the GSPN, V3, and Meckel cave as surgical landmarks, the surgeon delineates the Kawase triangle and drills to expose 180° to 270° of the internal acoustic canal posterolaterally, inferior petrosal sinus inferiorly, Dorello canal medially, and petrous ICA anterolaterally.[31,35] Care is taken not to violate the bony labyrinth and cochlea situated just anterolaterally to the internal auditory canal in the premeatal triangle and the superior semicircular canal located laterally to the internal auditory canal in the postmeatal triangle. The dura mater is opened at the porus trige-minus above the superior petrosal sinus and extended laterally to the arcuate eminence to reveal the tentorium. A parallel dural incision is made below the superior petrosal sinus, which is subsequently ligated and divided.[31,35] With gravity-assisted temporal lobe retraction, the posterior CS is exposed along with the abducens nerve in the Dorello canal, and the tumor is debulked.

Extended Endoscopic Transfacial Approaches to the Cavernous Sinus

The transsphenoidal approach to the CS was first performed in 1979 to treat bilateral carotid-cavernous fistula.[37] Later, various modifications of this technique to tackle CS lesions have been developed, especially with the advent of high-resolution endos-copy.[27,28] The CS proper is divided into its medial and lateral compartments by the cavernous carotid siphon. All the cranial nerves are present in the lateral compartment of the CS. Limitation of transcranial surgical approaches to reach this medial aspect of cavernous ICA without transgressing the cranial nerves in the lateral aspect of CS led to the innovation of minimally invasive endonasal and transmaxillary endoscopic ap-proaches.[27,28,38] These approaches are essentially extensions of a standard endo-nasal endoscopic transsphenoidal sellar approach that offer better access to the parasellar region.[27,28] As mentioned earlier, lesions situated medial to the carotid siphon are ideal candidates for resection via the extended endoscopic endonasal transsphenoidal trans-sellar and extended endoscopic endonasal transethmoidal transsphenoidal parasellar approaches, whereas the lateral CS lesions are accessed via the extended endoscopic transmaxillary transpterygoid approach. The operative technique mentioned earlier is essentially the same as for the purposes of tissue sam-pling, but a few key aspects of each approach are mentioned separately later.

The advantages of these endoscopic approaches over transcranial approaches to the CS are their minimally invasive nature, lack of brain retraction and associated com-plications, shorter hospitalization, lower risk of iatrogenic cranial neuropathy, and bet-ter cosmesis. However, to achieve oncologic resections, they are considered inferior for large malignant tumors with extensive ventral skull base involvement and also carry a higher risk of iatrogenic cavernous ICA injury. Another limitation of extended endo-nasal endoscopic approaches is a higher incidence of CSF leak and associated com-plications, as high as 15.9% overall (19.4% for extrasellar groups) as reported by Kassam and colleagues[39] in a large series of 800 patients. However, using either the single (Hadad)[40] or double (Janus, for larger skull base defects)[41] vascularized pedicled nasoseptal flap to cover the ventral skull base defect helped to reduce the CSF leak rate substantially to 5.4% overall. Similarly, Thorp and colleagues[42] observed an acceptable CSF leak rate of 3.3% in a series of 144 nasoseptal flaps after extended endonasal endoscopic approaches. In a systematic review of 38 studies (609 patients) with large dural defects after extended endonasal endoscopic proced-ures, Harvey and colleagues[43] observed statistically lower CSF leak rates in the flap group (6.7%) compared with the group that had free fat reconstruction (15.6%) of the skull base defect. Additionally, the use of perioperative lumbar drainage, use of intraoperative fluorescein dye to assess the CSF leak sites precisely along with cus-tomization of reconstruction technique appropriately, multilayer Gasket-seal closure of skull base defects using autologous fascia lata, allograft, free mucosal flap and pedicled nasoseptal flap, and a countersunk rigid buttress (like stents) further helps reduce the CSF leak rate.[44,45] Overall, the possible complications for endoscopic transfacial approaches include CSF leak, meningitis, cranial neuropathy, and vascular injury.

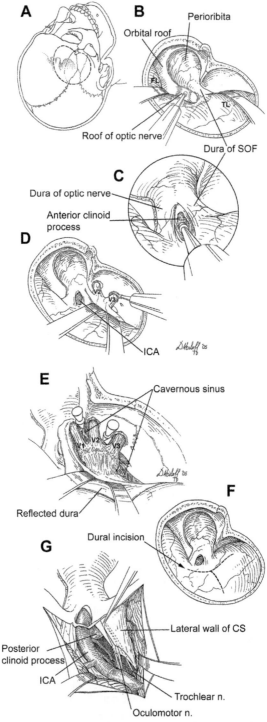

Fig. 2. The CS meningioma resection-decompression technique. A frontotemporal crani-otomy is performed (*A*), with extradural dissection of the lateral and superior orbit. The

Extended endoscopic endonasal transsphenoidal trans-sellar approach

This approach provides adequate access to the posteromedial aspect of the CS via an inferior operative trajectory.[27,28] Use of an angled endoscope is essential to have adequate visualization of lesions in the medial aspect of the CS. Pituitary transposition in the sella may be required depending on the pathological condition encountered and extent of the tumor.

Extended endoscopic endonasal transethmoidal transsphenoidal parasellar approach

This approach provides adequate access to the anteromedial aspect of the CS via an inferior operative trajectory. Anterior and posterior ethmoidectomy is done along with superior turbinate resection to reach the anteromedial aspect of the CS.[27,28] It is particularly suitable for lesions infiltrating the superior orbital fissure. The contralateral nostril is used to access the CS lesion to obtain a better viewing angle and operative trajectory.

Extended endoscopic transmaxillary transpterygoid approach

This approach provides adequate access to the lateral aspect of the CS via an inferior operative trajectory. Its advantage over a conventional transcranial approach is that the cranial nerves are encountered last, after the CS tumor is resected. Therefore, theoretically, the risk of postsurgical cranial neuropathy is lower with inferolateral transmaxillary approaches. To obtain appropriate far-lateral access to the CS lesion, removal of the pterygoid process, ethmoidectomy, transethmoidal sphenoidotomy, and maxillary antrostomy are performed.[27,28] This approach helps in addressing tumors involving the pterygopalatine fossa, lateral sphenoid sinus, Meckel cave, and infratemporal fossa. It is a more extensive surgical approach than endonasal approaches, with resultant exposure of pterygopalatine ganglion besides vidian,

---

bone of the posterior orbit is drilled, and the superior orbital fissure is exposed (*B*). The anterior clinoid process is removed and the optic canal roof is drilled to decompress the optic nerve (*C*). Any tumor within the anteromedial triangle of the CS is removed. The foramina rotundum and ovale are enlarged to provide mobilization of the second and third divisions of the trigeminal nerve (*D*). The lateral dural wall of the CS is then dissected and elevated free from the trigeminal ganglion and its branches (*E*). This technique provides decompression of the lateral aspect of the CS. Portions of tumor in the inferior CS, located between the first and second divisions (anteromedial triangle) and between the second and third divisions (anterolateral triangle), are removed to provide further decompression. More of the tumor is removed medial to the carotid artery in the petrous bone (medial to the Glasscock triangle) and in the region of the Kawase triangle. Care must be taken to avoid injury to the petrous carotid artery, located just posterior to the foramen ovale. Following the extradural procedure, the dura mater is opened in a T-shaped fashion, along the frontotemporal skull base with an arm opening to the carotid artery at the base just lateral to the optic nerve (*F*). The final decompression is achieved by opening the oculomotor foramen anteriorly to the orbit along the course of the oculomotor nerve (*G*). Care is taken to avoid injury to the trochlear nerve as it crosses the oculomotor nerve at the superior orbital fissure. At the completion of the dissection, the portion of the tumor between the oculomotor nerve and the optic nerve has been removed to reduce the volume of tumor adjacent to the optic nerve. The CS has been decompressed from the inferior, lateral, and superior directions. FL, frontal lobe; n, nerve; SOF, superior orbital fissure; TL, temporal lobe; V1, V2, V3, divisions of the fifth cranial nerve. (*From* Couldwell WT, Kan P, Liu JK, et al. Decompression of cavernous sinus meningioma for preservation and improvement of cranial nerve function. Technical note. J Neurosurg 2006;105(1):149; with permission.)

maxillary, and mandibular neurovascular bundles; thus, the risk of potential damage to the aforementioned structures may be increased.[27,28]

Radical En bloc Oncological Resection

Although en bloc resection of malignant ventral skull base tumors is an established oncological principle, the structural complexities of the skull base make en bloc resection technically challenging.[14,46,47] CS involvement represents one of the primary issues when attempting en bloc oncological resection of the sinonasal and ventral skull malignancies.[1,47,48] Different anatomic, biological, and patient-related factors govern the safety of radical en bloc surgical resection in extensive skull base malignancy with CS involvement.[29] Radical surgery is relatively contraindicated in patients with bilateral involvement of CS or distant metastasis (especially if multiple and at different anatomic sites), those in the elderly age group, and those with multiple comorbidities precluding high-risk surgery and prolonged anesthesia.[29] In 1999, Saito and colleagues[1] standardized en bloc resection techniques involving the CS and described 3 types of surgical procedures to achieve en bloc resection of the tumor, depending on the level of CS infiltration and the extent of CS resected along with the malignant skull base tumor. In their series of 25 patients with malignant skull base tumor, 15 patients had CS involvement. Among these 15 cases, they performed type I, II, and III procedures in 7, 5, and 3 patients, respectively. As expected, they demonstrated poor 2- and 5-year overall survival rates in patients with CS involvement (62% and 31%, respectively) as compared with patients whose tumors had only extracavernous involvement (88% and 88%, respectively).[1] Further dissecting their survival rates based on type of procedure performed, they observed 2-year overall survival rates of 54%, 100%, and 33% for type I, II, and III resection, respectively.[1] Common operative steps for all 3 types of en bloc resections mirror those described earlier for aggressive transcranial approaches. Specific and key operative steps and nuances of different types of radical en bloc CS resection are described separately later. Because carotid sacrifice without revascularization seems to be the treatment option with the least favorable results, cerebral revascularization is performed before most CSE or type III procedures.[1,16]

The primary advantage of such radical en bloc oncological resection of malignant ventral skull base tumor is that it theoretically helps eradicate the tumor and presumably increases the overall and progression-free survival in patients with CS involvement by reducing tumor burden and increasing the efficacy of adjuvant therapies.[1,16] However, controversy pertaining to justification of such en bloc resections for extensive malignant ventral skull base tumors with CS involvement includes the fact that once the tumor has invaded the CS, it may have already disseminated hematogenously and aggressive resection may hardly affect the overall or progression-free survival in such cases. Bumpous and colleagues[49] reported 2 out of 3 necropsies of patients with CS involvement had evidence of subclinical pulmonary metastasis. Similarly, Brisman and colleagues[14] also reported 2 deaths from distal metastasis out of 8 patients with malignant ventral skull base tumor and CS involvement. Currently, there is no strong evidence in the literature to support either claim. Optimizing the expectations of survival benefit against procedure-related complications in an individualized manner is probably a more balanced way to approach such aggressive and extensive tumors. Potential complications from such extensive skull base approaches include ophthalmic pseudoaneurysm; cerebral ischemia following poor collateral flow, failed bypass, or massive intraoperative blood loss with hypotension and hypovolemia; CSF leak; meningitis; and mortality.[1,14–17] The risk of cerebrovascular complications is much higher in patients undergoing type III procedures than in those undergoing type I/II procedures.[1] Type III procedures also have a higher associated risk of inadvertent tumor spread both locally and distally because of disruption of natural barriers to the tumor spread.[1] The ventral skull base reconstruction technique aims to plug the iatrogenic bony defect in the skull base after en bloc resections. Autologous fat/free fascial/muscle packing is usually sufficient for skull base defects smaller than 3 to 4 cm, whereas pedicled temporalis muscle, pedicled pericranial graft, or free flap muscle transfer (eg, latissimus dorsi) with vascular anastomosis to facial artery and vein is often required to address defects larger than 3 to 4 cm in maximum dimension.[1,16]

Type I Saito procedure

This procedure is indicated primarily for malignant skull base tumors with pseudoinvasion of the CS, where the tumor can be freed from the walls of CS easily and intracavernous exploration is not required at all. It essentially involves extradural dissection of the CS to reflect it posteriorly. The optic nerve, superior orbital fissure, V2, and V3 are incised after unroofing each structure in juxta-cavernous locations. All the bony cuts/osteotomies spare the CS portion and the body of sphenoid. Procedure-related morbidity is minimal using this strategy.[1]

Type II Saito procedure

This procedure is an intradural procedure indicated for tumors involving the anterolateral portion of the CS proper with ICA sparing. The optic nerve, ophthalmic artery, and sylvian veins draining into the sphenoparietal sinus are sacrificed. Intradural anterior clinoid process drilling is done along with release of both proximal and distal dural rings to mobilize the cavernous ICA posteriorly. Then the CS is transected along the lateral aspect of cavernous ICA, and osteotomies are extended along sphenoid bone and middle cranial fossa to achieve en bloc resection of the tumor.[1]

Type III Saito procedure/cavernous sinus exenteration

In addition to Saito and colleagues,[1] both Brisman and colleagues[14] and Couldwell and colleagues[16] helped to popularize this procedure for oncologic resection of malignant tumors with limited extracranial disease. It is particularly relevant for patients with recurrent/progressive benign tumors despite reasonable medical/radiation treatment and ipsilateral complete loss of vision and extraocular movements or when contralateral function is threatened by progressively growing tumor.[1,16] A combined otorhinolaryngology and neurosurgery approach may be required depending on the nature and extent of the lesion. Sacrificing the ICA without cerebral revascularization is associated with a 17% to 66% risk of cerebral infarction.[14,48,50–54] Therefore, many reports advise the use of bypass procedures to augment the blood flow to the ipsilateral brain when the ICA is sacrificed.[14,48,51,55] Yet, this still caries a risk of cerebrovascular accidents in surgery for head and neck malignant tumors with extensive skull base involvement.[14,51,54–56] The senior author prefers a selective approach and chooses to perform a balloon test occlusion before surgery (high-flow interpositional carotid artery bypass) (see later discussion). After the completion of the common surgical steps of frontotemporal craniotomy and skull base exposure mentioned previously, the neck is exposed at the level of common carotid bifurcation for proximal ICA control and the donor external carotid artery (ECA) vessel is delineated for proximal bypass anastomosis (end to end or end to side). Next, the dura mater is opened, the sylvian fissure is dissected, and a suitable M2–middle cerebral artery (MCA) division is identified as a recipient vessel for distal anastomosis as part of the cerebral revascularization procedure. Once the bypass is performed and its patency is confirmed using intraoperative indocyanine green angiogram or micro-Doppler,[16] the supraclinoid ICA is ligated distally and divided proximal to the posterior communicating artery and the ICA is ligated proximally at either the cervical ICA or the petrous ICA segment. Care should be taken to ligate the cervical ICA stump in such a way that there is no residual blind pouch, which can potentially be a source of distal thromboembolism through the ECA and interpositional graft.[16]

Subsequently, drill cuts along the skull base are planned to completely isolate the lesion and involved CS (**Fig. 3**).[16] The initial cut is made across the orbital roof, well anterior to the extent of lesion. The posterior orbital contents are divided, and the ophthalmic artery is ligated and divided. Laterally, the orbital wall anterolateral to the superior orbital fissure is disconnected with extension to the middle cranial fossa along the lateral sphenoid wing. The nerves distal to the superior orbital fissure (oculomotor, trochlear, ophthalmic division of trigeminal and abducens nerves) are divided well in front of the disease process. Similarly, the V2 and V3 nerves are divided along the foramen rotundum and foramen ovale, respectively. Posterolaterally, the petrous bone is drilled as necessary and the petrous ICA is ligated and divided.[16] A posterior cut is made across the tentorium, petrous apex, and upper clivus; the trochlear nerve is divided along the free margin of the tentorium. Both the superior and inferior petrosal sinuses are also sacrificed. Proximally, both the oculomotor and trigeminal nerves are divided close to their root entry zones in the cisternal segments. Care has to be taken to cut the optic nerve a few millimeters away from the chiasm, so as not to damage the Von Willebrand knee fibers arising from the contralateral eye.[16] If the tumor has not invaded the sphenoid sinus and the nasal cavity inferiorly and medially, the lesion along with the involved CS can be lifted away from the lateral wall of sphenoid sinus. If involved, the pituitary gland is mobilized in entirety or in part from the sella turcica depending on the extent of the lesion; the medial cut is made along the body of the sphenoid, which is connected anteriorly to the orbital cut and posteriorly to the

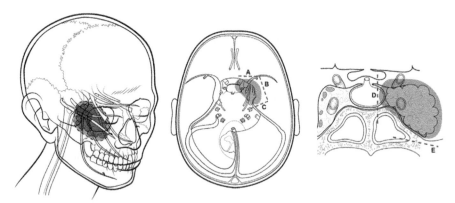

Fig. 3. The region of resection (*left*) and skull base drill cuts (*dashed lines*) (*center* and *right*) designed to incorporate the CS and involved tumor. (*A*) The initial cut is made across the orbital roof well anterior to the extent of the tumor. (*B*) Laterally, the cuts are made in the lateral orbital wall anterior to the superior orbital fissure, with extension to the middle fossa to ensure normal margins around the tumor. (*C*) The posterior cut must come across the petrous apex and tentorium. (*D*) If the tumor has not invaded the sphenoid sinus medially, it will be dissected off of the medial bony wall (lateral sphenoid sinus wall) and removed. (*E*) The inferior cut below the CS is made into the sphenoid or nasopharynx as demanded by the extent of resection. (*From* Couldwell WT, MacDonald JD, Taussky P. Complete resection of the cavernous sinus-indications and technique. World Neurosurg 2014;82(6):1266; with permission.)

petroclival cut.[16] The final inferior cut is made into the sphenoidal bone or naso-pharynx as needed. At this point, the lesion is circumferentially dissected and free of adjoining structures and can be removed en bloc as planned. The iatrogenic skull base defect is plugged as described earlier. Postoperative placement of a lumbar drain helps to divert the CSF for a few days to augment the skull base reconstruction and reduce the risk of CSF leak.[16]

Cerebral Revascularization

Cerebral revascularization is reserved for patients with extensive CS involvement and reasonably long life expectancy who have inadequate vascular reserve. Although balloon occlusion test and computed tomography perfusion imaging with acetazol-amide challenge are standard for assessing vascular reserve,[16,57,58] these methods have a false-negative rate of 3% to 8% in preoperative assessment.[57–59] Thus, the in-dications for bypass procedures may be broadened and include acute vascular injury during surgery along with preoperative evidence of intolerance of sacrifice of the same vessel; cerebrovascular reserve in a younger patient with low tumor burden and longer life expectancy; invasion of major arteries by malignant, aggressive, and recurrent dis-ease, rendering sacrifice of vessel pivotal for achieving radical tumor resection;

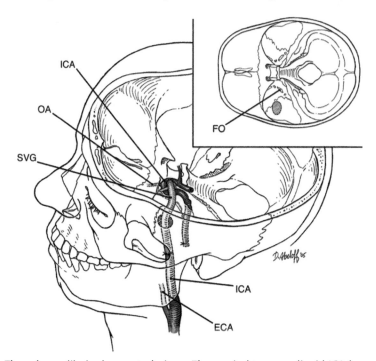

Fig. 4. The submandibular bypass technique. The cervical-to-supraclinoid ICA bypass using an interpositional saphenous vein graft. The graft is tunneled through the submandibular-infratemporal route via a middle fossa craniectomy (*shaded region*, see inset) that is located lateral to the foramen ovale. In this example, the graft is anastomosed to the supraclinoid ICA in an end-to-side fashion. An aneurysm clip is placed just proximal to the ophthalmic artery takeoff. FO, foramen ovale; OA, ophthalmic artery; SVG, saphenous vein graft. (*From* Couldwell WT, Liu JK, Amini A, et al. Submandibular-infratemporal inter-positional carotid artery bypass for cranial base tumors and giant aneurysms. Neurosurgery 2006;59(4 Suppl 2):ONS353–359 [discussion: ONS354]; with permission.)

preoperative poor vascular reserve with symptoms of preoperative ischemia; and high risk of intraoperative vessel injury because of tumor encasement or invasion, especially with prior history of surgical or radiation treatments.[57,58]

Cerebral revascularization is often performed before the CSE/type III Saito procedure. For this purpose, the neck is exposed at the level of the common carotid artery bifurcation to obtain proximal ICA control and to define the donor ECA vessel, often distal to the superior thyroid branch. ECA is preferred over ICA as a donor vessel because it reduces the chances of cerebral ischemia due to prolonged temporary clipping time on the proximal cervical ICA. End-to-end or end-to-side ECA-to–interpositional graft proximal anastomosis and end-to-side interpositional graft–to–M2-MCA distal anastomosis is done using interrupted 7-0 and 10-0 nylon monofilament suturing technique, respectively.[57,58,60] Either saphenous vein or radial artery can be used as a vascular conduit depending on the surgeon's preference and the availability of a suitable graft. The primary advantages of saphenous vein graft over radial artery graft are that it provides a higher volume of blood flow and the size matches quite nicely to both the donor and recipient sites.[57,60] A graft of an appropriate caliber can be chosen based on the preoperative Doppler ultrasonography. Saphenous vein harvest can be done using a minimally invasive endoscopic technique to prevent the morbidity associated with large skin incisions. Whether to perform the proximal or the distal anastomosis first is essentially the surgeon's preference. The graft is passed along the submandibular route (using a chest tube) through a 15-mm hole created along the middle cranial fossa, just lateral to the foramen ovale and anterolateral to the foramen spinosum (**Fig. 4**).[57,60,61] Use of a submandibular route of graft passage is optimal because it allows for the shortest possible graft length and prevents any kinking of the interpositional graft with the head movements over the neck, which the preauricular and postauricular routes do not.[57,60] To prevent ischemic damage during temporary clipping, burst suppression is performed to reduce the cerebral metabolic rate and reduce the oxygen demand to the brain.

SUMMARY

The current literature is sparse and divided on a standard management protocol for sinonasal and ventral skull base malignancies with CS involvement. Individualized case-by-case basis treatment planning provides a reasonable format for optimizing the outcome specifically tailored to a patient's need. Minimally invasive approaches for tissue sampling in cases suspicious for malignancy can help optimize management strategy. If possible and justified based on the risk-benefit ratio, oncological resection of skull base malignancy should be considered to target eradication of disease with the goal of increasing overall and progression-free survival. Interdisciplinary collaboration between multiple specialties is ideal for such extensive and aggressive ventral skull base malignancies with CS and intracranial involvement.

ACKNOWLEDGMENTS

The authors thank Kristin Kraus, MSc, their medical editor, for her contribution to article editing and Vance Mortimer, their video editor, for his contribution to editing the operative videos.

SUPPLEMENTARY DATA

Supplementary data related to this article can be found at http://dx.doi.org/10.1016/j.otc.2016.12.011.

REFERENCES

1. Saito K, Fukuta K, Takahashi M, et al. Management of the cavernous sinus in en bloc resections of malignant skull base tumors. Head Neck 1999;21(8):734–42.
2. Turner JH, Reh DD. Incidence and survival in patients with sinonasal cancer: a historical analysis of population-based data. Head Neck 2012;34(6):877–85.
3. Han J, Zhang Q, Kong F, et al. The incidence of invasion and metastasis of nasopharyngeal carcinoma at different anatomic sites in the skull base. Anat Rec (Hoboken) 2012;295(8):1252–9.
4. Grant RN. The incidence of and mortality from cancer in the United States. Prog Clin Cancer 1970;4:34–47.
5. Michel J, Fakhry N, Mancini J, et al. Sinonasal squamous cell carcinomas: clinical outcomes and predictive factors. Int J Oral Maxillofac Surg 2014;43(1):1–6.
6. Nishio N, Fujimoto Y, Fujii M, et al. Craniofacial resection for T4 maxillary sinus carcinoma: managing cases with involvement of the skull base. Otolaryngol Head Neck Surg 2015;153(2):231–8.
7. Dulguerov P, Jacobsen MS, Allal AS, et al. Nasal and paranasal sinus carcinoma: are we making progress? A series of 220 patients and a systematic review. Cancer 2001;92(12):3012–29.
8. Katz TS, Mendenhall WM, Morris CG, et al. Malignant tumors of the nasal cavity and paranasal sinuses. Head Neck 2002;24(9):821–9.
9. Ketcham AS, Hoye RC, Van Buren JM, et al. Complications of intracranial facial resection for tumors of the paranasal sinuses. Am J Surg 1966;112(4):591–6.
10. Ketcham AS, Wilkins RH, Vanburen JM, et al. A combined intracranial facial approach to the paranasal sinuses. Am J Surg 1963;106:698–703.
11. Castelnuovo P, Dallan I, Battaglia P, et al. Endoscopic endonasal skull base surgery: past, present and future. Eur Arch Otorhinolaryngol 2010;267(5):649–63.
12. Harvey RJ, Gallagher RM, Sacks R. Extended endoscopic techniques for sinonasal resections. Otolaryngol Clin North Am 2010;43(3):613–38, x.
13. Roxbury CR, Ishii M, Gallia GL, et al. Endoscopic management of esthesioneuroblastoma. Otolaryngol Clin North Am 2016;49(1):153–65.
14. Brisman MH, Sen C, Catalano P. Results of surgery for head and neck tumors that involve the carotid artery at the skull base. J Neurosurg 1997;86(5):787–92.
15. Sekhar LN, Moller AR. Operative management of tumors involving the cavernous sinus. J Neurosurg 1986;64(6):879–89.
16. Couldwell WT, MacDonald JD, Taussky P. Complete resection of the cavernous sinus-indications and technique. World Neurosurg 2014;82(6):1264–70.
17. Spetzler RF, Fukushima T, Martin N, et al. Petrous carotid-to-intradural carotid saphenous vein graft for intracavernous giant aneurysm, tumor, and occlusive cerebrovascular disease. J Neurosurg 1990;73(4):496–501.
18. Parkinson D. A surgical approach to the cavernous portion of the carotid artery. Anatomical studies and case report. J Neurosurg 1965;23(5):474–83.
19. Dolenc V. Direct microsurgical repair of intracavernous vascular lesions. J Neurosurg 1983;58(6):824–31.
20. Taptas JN. The so-called cavernous sinus: a review of the controversy and its implications for neurosurgeons. Neurosurgery 1982;11(5):712–7.
21. Umansky F, Nathan H. The lateral wall of the cavernous sinus. With special reference to the nerves related to it. J Neurosurg 1982;56(2):228–34.
22. Messerer M, Dubourg J, Saint-Pierre G, et al. Percutaneous biopsy of lesions in the cavernous sinus region through the foramen ovale: diagnostic accuracy and limits in 50 patients. J Neurosurg 2012;116(2):390–8.

23. Sekhar LN, Pomeranz S, Sen CN. Management of tumours involving the cavernous sinus. Acta Neurochir Suppl (Wien) 1991;53:101–12.
24. Altay T, Patel BC, Couldwell WT. Lateral orbital wall approach to the cavernous sinus. J Neurosurg 2012;116(4):755–63.
25. Stechison MT, Bernstein M. Percutaneous transfacial needle biopsy of a middle cranial fossa mass: case report and technical note. Neurosurgery 1989;25(6):996–9.
26. Frighetto L, De Salles AA, Behnke E, et al. Image-guided frameless stereotactic biopsy sampling of parasellar lesions. Technical note. J Neurosurg 2003;98(4):920–5.
27. Raithatha R, McCoul ED, Woodworth GF, et al. Endoscopic endonasal approaches to the cavernous sinus. Int Forum Allergy Rhinol 2012;2(1):9–15.
28. Schwartz TH, Fraser JF, Brown S, et al. Endoscopic cranial base surgery: classification of operative approaches. Neurosurgery 2008;62(5):991–1002 [discussion: 1002–5].
29. Donald PJ. Skull base surgery for malignancy: when not to operate. Eur Arch Otorhinolaryngol 2007;264(7):713–7.
30. Rhoton AL Jr. The cavernous sinus, the cavernous venous plexus, and the carotid collar. Neurosurgery 2002;51(4 Suppl):S375–410.
31. Yasuda A, Campero A, Martins C, et al. Microsurgical anatomy and approaches to the cavernous sinus. Neurosurgery 2005;56(1 Suppl):4–27 [discussion: 24–7].
32. Dolenc VV. A combined epi- and subdural direct approach to carotid-ophthalmic artery aneurysms. J Neurosurg 1985;62(5):667–72.
33. Dolenc VV. Frontotemporal epidural approach to trigeminal neurinomas. Acta Neurochir (Wien) 1994;130(1–4):55–65.
34. Hakuba A, Tanaka K, Suzuki T, et al. A combined orbitozygomatic infratemporal epidural and subdural approach for lesions involving the entire cavernous sinus. J Neurosurg 1989;71(5 Pt 1):699–704.
35. Kawase T, Shiobara R, Toya S. Anterior transpetrosal-transtentorial approach for sphenopetroclival meningiomas: surgical method and results in 10 patients. Neurosurgery 1991;28(6):869–75 [discussion: 875–6].
36. Couldwell WT, Kan P, Liu JK, et al. Decompression of cavernous sinus meningioma for preservation and improvement of cranial nerve function. Technical note. J Neurosurg 2006;105(1):148–52.
37. Laws ER Jr, Onofrio BM, Pearson BW, et al. Successful management of bilateral carotid-cavernous fistulae with a trans-sphenoidal approach. Neurosurgery 1979;4(2):162–7.
38. Couldwell WT, Sabit I, Weiss MH, et al. Transmaxillary approach to the anterior cavernous sinus: a microanatomic study. Neurosurgery 1997;40(6):1307–11.
39. Kassam AB, Prevedello DM, Carrau RL, et al. Endoscopic endonasal skull base surgery: analysis of complications in the authors' initial 800 patients. J Neurosurg 2011;114(6):1544–68.
40. Hadad G, Bassagasteguy L, Carrau RL, et al. A novel reconstructive technique after endoscopic expanded endonasal approaches: vascular pedicle nasoseptal flap. Laryngoscope 2006;116(10):1882–6.
41. Nyquist GG, Anand VK, Singh A, et al. Janus flap: bilateral nasoseptal flaps for anterior skull base reconstruction. Otolaryngol Head Neck Surg 2010;142(3):327–31.
42. Thorp BD, Sreenath SB, Ebert CS, et al. Endoscopic skull base reconstruction: a review and clinical case series of 152 vascularized flaps used for surgical skull

base defects in the setting of intraoperative cerebrospinal fluid leak. Neurosurg Focus 2014;37(4):E4.

43. Harvey RJ, Parmar P, Sacks R, et al. Endoscopic skull base reconstruction of large dural defects: a systematic review of published evidence. Laryngoscope 2012;122(2):452–9.

44. Leng LZ, Brown S, Anand VK, et al. "Gasket-seal" watertight closure in minimal-access endoscopic cranial base surgery. Neurosurgery 2008;62(5 Suppl 2): ONSE342–3 [discussion: ONSE343].

45. Tabaee A, Placantonakis DG, Schwartz TH, et al. Intrathecal fluorescein in endo-scopic skull base surgery. Otolaryngol Head Neck Surg 2007;137(2):316–20.

46. Janecka IP, Sen C, Sekhar L, et al. Treatment of paranasal sinus cancer with cra-nial base surgery: results. Laryngoscope 1994;104(5 Pt 1):553–5.

47. Origitano TC, al-Mefty O, Leonetti JP, et al. En bloc resection of an ethmoid car-cinoma involving the orbit and medial wall of the cavernous sinus. Neurosurgery 1992;31(6):1126–30 [discussion: 1130–1].

48. Gormley WB, Sekhar LN, Wright DC, et al. Management and long-term outcome of adenoid cystic carcinoma with intracranial extension: a neurosurgical perspec-tive. Neurosurgery 1996;38(6):1105–12 [discussion: 1112–3].

49. Bumpous JM, Maves MD, Gomez SM, et al. Cavernous sinus involvement in head and neck cancer. Head Neck 1993;15(1):62–6.

50. Brennan JA, Jafek BW. Elective carotid artery resection for advanced squamous cell carcinoma of the neck. Laryngoscope 1994;104(3 Pt 1):259–63.

51. Meleca RJ, Marks SC. Carotid artery resection for cancer of the head and neck. Arch Otolaryngol Head Neck Surg 1994;120(9):974–8.

52. Okamoto Y, Inugami A, Matsuzaki Z, et al. Carotid artery resection for head and neck cancer. Surgery 1996;120(1):54–9.

53. Origitano TC, al-Mefty O, Leonetti JP, et al. Vascular considerations and compli-cations in cranial base surgery. Neurosurgery 1994;35(3):351–62 [discussion: 362–3].

54. Snyderman CH, D'Amico F. Outcome of carotid artery resection for neoplastic disease: a meta-analysis. Am J Otolaryngol 1992;13(6):373–80.

55. Wright JG, Nicholson R, Schuller DE, et al. Resection of the internal carotid artery and replacement with greater saphenous vein: a safe procedure for en bloc can-cer resections with carotid involvement. J Vasc Surg 1996;23(5):775–80 [discus-sion: 781–2].

56. Lawton MT, Spetzler RF. Internal carotid artery sacrifice for radical resection of skull base tumors. Skull Base Surg 1996;6(2):119–23.

57. Liu JK, Couldwell WT. Interpositional carotid artery bypass strategies in the sur-gical management of aneurysms and tumors of the skull base. Neurosurg Focus 2003;14(3):e2.

58. Yang T, Tariq F, Chabot J, et al. Cerebral revascularization for difficult skull base tumors: a contemporary series of 18 patients. World Neurosurg 2014;82(5): 660–71.

59. Pieper DR, LaRouere M, Jackson IT. Operative management of skull base malig-nancies: choosing the appropriate approach. Neurosurg Focus 2002;12(5):e6.

60. Couldwell WT, Taussky P, Sivakumar W. Submandibular high-flow bypass in the treatment of skull base lesions: an analysis of long-term outcome. Neurosurgery 2012;71(3):645–50 [discussion: 650–1].

61. Couldwell WT, Liu JK, Amini A, et al. Submandibular-infratemporal interpositional carotid artery bypass for cranial base tumors and giant aneurysms. Neurosurgery 2006;59(4 Suppl 2):ONS353–9 [discussion: ONS359–60].

The Role of Robotic Surgery in Sinonasal and Ventral Skull Base Malignancy

Ralph Abi Hachem, MD[a], Sanjeet Rangarajan, MD[a],
Andre Beer-Furlan, MD[b], Daniel Prevedello, MD[a,b],
Enver Ozer, MD[a], Ricardo L. Carrau, MD[a,b],*

KEYWORDS

• Robotic surgery • Sinonasal • Skull base • Malignancies • Ventral skull base

KEY POINTS

- Multiple extended approaches have been described to optimize access and surgery through the confines of the sinonasal cavities and skull base.
- Robotic surgery offers several advantages over conventional, endoscopic, or endoscopic-assisted surgery including 3-dimensional visualization, tremor-free surgery, fine precise dissection, and bimanual surgery.
- Robotic surgery also presents disadvantages, such as the lack of haptic feedback, absence of drills, bone cutting or any other power instrumentation, and relatively large size of the instruments.
- Despite very active research in this regard, the current indication for robotic sinonasal and ventral skull base surgery is the resection of recurrent nasopharyngeal carcinoma or the primary resection of malignancies of salivary origin.
- Transoral robotic surgery (TORS) can be combined with an expanded endonasal approach to resect large malignant lesions extending inferiorly below the level of the hard palate. These 2 techniques are complementary in their anatomic reach and available instrumentation.

 Video content accompanies this article at http://www.oto.theclinics.com.

INTRODUCTION

Over the past decade, robotic surgery has gained wide popularity, making a significant impact on multiple surgical specialties, such as gynecology, urology, abdominal

---

Disclosure: None.
[a] Department of Otolaryngology - Head and Neck Surgery, The Ohio State University Wexner Medical Center, Starling Loving Hall – Room B221, 320 West 10th Avenue, Columbus, OH 43210, USA; [b] Department of Neurological Surgery, The Ohio State University Wexner Medical Center, Doan Hall 410 West 10th Avenue, Room N1011-A, Columbus, OH 43210, USA
* Corresponding author. Department of Otolaryngology - Head and Neck Surgery, The Ohio State University Wexner Medical Center, Starling Loving Hall – Room B221, 320 West 10th Avenue, Columbus, OH 43210.
E-mail address: Ricardo.Carrau@osumc.edu

Otolaryngol Clin N Am 50 (2017) 385–395
http://dx.doi.org/10.1016/j.otc.2016.12.012
0030-6665/17/© 2016 Elsevier Inc. All rights reserved.

surgery, and cardiac surgery. In the head and neck arena, transoral robotic surgery (TORS) has proven to be safe and associated with acceptable oncological and superior functional outcomes for surgery of the oropharynx, hypopharynx, supraglottis, and glottis; thus, changing the paradigm for the management of tumors in these anatomic locations. Robotic surgery of the ventral skull base is still at an early stage of development; however, some case series have been published over the past few years. In this article, we review the literature discussing the role of robotic surgery in managing sinonasal and ventral skull base malignant lesions.

AVAILABLE ROBOTS AND INSTRUMENTATION

Currently, there are only 2 surgical robotic systems approved by the Food and Drug Administration that have been used to perform endoscopic ventral skull base surgical procedures: the da Vinci Surgical System (Intuitive Surgical, Inc, Sunnyvale, CA) and the Medrobotics Flex Robotic System (Medrobotics Corp, Raynham, MA). We will describe each in the following section.

The da Vinci Surgical System is the most widely used robotic surgical system in the United States and its applications have been well documented in the otolaryngology literature. It consists of a console that serves as the surgeon control center, a patient-side surgical robot with a 3-dimensional (3D) rigid endoscope, and a video display cart. The endoscopes for use in the newest version of the system is 8.5 mm in diameter and has 0° and 30° viewing angles available. The entire endoscope arm can pivot, rotate, and translate to change the operator's view; however, it is rigid and cannot change its trajectory within the surgical field. The endoscope, which is fit with a dual-lens, 3-charge-coupled device camera, gives the operating surgeon a high-definition, stereoscopic view of the surgical field. Various instrument attachments, as small as 5 mm in diameter, are designed to operate with 7° of freedom, based on the "wristed" movements of the operating surgeon.

The da Vinci system has been used in head and neck surgery since 2005[1] and has gone through several product cycles since its initial launch. This affords a level of relative maturity for the da Vinci product line when compared with the only other surgical robot system cleared for use in the United States. The newest version of the da Vinci Surgical System is the da Vinci Xi, which offers several improvements over its predecessors.[2] One of these is the automatic configuration of its boom arms based on endoscopic and laser guidance, a feature that reduces the set-up time, which has been a common source of criticism.[3] Nonetheless, even this current iteration does not provide the surgeon with haptic feedback or stereotactic navigation features.

The Medrobotics Flex Robotic System was approved for use in the United States in July 2015 and was specifically designed for use in the oropharynx, hypopharynx, and larynx. The primary advantage of the Flex system lies in the maneuverability of its endoscope and accompanying instrumentation, offering a flexible system capable of steering around obstructing anatomy (**Fig. 1**). In spite of its flexible, steerable configuration, the large diameter of the endoscope and instrumentation preclude a purely endonasal approach to the ventral skull base. Schuler and colleagues[4] demonstrated a successful endoscopic visualization of the anterior ventral skull base using the Flex system; however, a midfacial degloving was required to accommodate the robotic arms. In their study, the Flex endoscope was used for visualization, whereas the actual surgical maneuvers were performed using standard, conventional instrumentation. The robotic arms were able to reach pertinent anatomic features; however, they did not perform any actual procedural tasks.

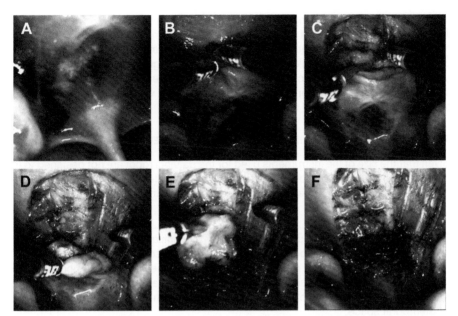

Fig. 1. This figure shows the different steps to performing a nasopharyngectomy by using the Medrobotics Flex on a cadaver. (*A*) Endonasal view of the nasopharynx. (*B, C*) Subperiosteal dissection (*D*) and resection (*E, F*) of the median nasopharynx.

Like the da Vinci system, the Flex does not provide haptic feedback or stereotactic navigation features.

Neither robotic system is able to access the sinonasal cavity or ventral skull base using a purely endonasal approach, instead requiring additional morbidity through traditional open approaches. A common limiting factor of both systems is the size of their endoscopes and instrumentation. A typical endonasal endoscope is only 4 mm in diameter, and the size of endonasal instruments is only on the order of millimeters. Further limitations of both systems are the lack of a high-speed drill, which is required to remove the hard bone of the sinonasal cavity and ventral skull base and the lack of adequate suctions to handle the typical bleeding arising from the sinonasal corridor and surgical field. In addition, the lack of tactile feedback is a significant barrier to the practical use of either robotic system in sinonasal and ventral skull base surgery. Alternatives to overcome these hurdles are being actively investigated by teams across the world. Haptics is of utmost importance in dissection within anatomically critical areas, such as the ventral skull base, and its study is a subject of high interest within robotics. A feasibility study to investigate haptic feedback in TORS was recently performed by the University of Pennsylvania, and this concept may transfer to endonasal surgery in the near future.[5]

To create steerable robotic instrumentation capable of navigating the sinonasal cavity, a team at Vanderbilt has developed a prototype system using concentric tube robotic arms, allowing tentaclelike motion and manipulation.[6] These advances, when combined, will help to expand the indications and relevance of robotic-assisted ventral skull base surgery.

In addition to the systems discussed, there are several automated endoscope holders and positioning systems that allow for hands-free visualization, but do not have instrumented arms to enable a truly robotic-assisted solution.[7] The neurosurgical literature describes the use of several other robotic systems, including the stereotactic navigation-enabled NeuroMate (NeuroMate PLC, Gloucestershire, UK), which can be used for functional neurosurgical procedures[8] and the BrightMatter Drive by Synaptive Medical Inc (Synaptive Medical, Toronto, Canada). These robots, however, have designs that are physically incompatible with an endonasal ventral skull base approach and are outside the scope of this article.

SURGICAL ROUTES TO THE SINONASAL CAVITIES AND VENTRAL SKULL BASE

Given that the size of the instruments used for the da Vinci robot are not designed to fit the sinonasal cavities, additional augmented surgical routes have been developed on cadaveric models to optimize access and reach the ventral skull base.

Purely Transoral Approach

Transoral robotic skull base surgery was among the initial approaches to the ventral skull base and was developed by the University of Pennsylvania group in 2007.[9] This approach was aimed at dissecting the parapharyngeal and infratemporal space and was initially tested on cadaveric specimens and on a live mongrel dog model. It was then applied on a patient with a benign cystic lesion of the parapharyngeal and infratemporal space.

Technique: The da Vinci robot is docked at the head of the bed. A Crowe-Davis mouth gag retractor (Storz, Heidelberg, Germany) is used to open the oral cavity and expose the oropharynx. The camera and both robotic arms are introduced transorally. The procedure starts with incisions lateral to the anterior tonsillar pillar, followed by dissection of the branches of the external carotid; the jugular vein; internal carotid; and cranial nerves IX, X, XI, and XII. The styloid and pterygoid musculatures are released to gain lateral access within the infratemporal fossa.

Although this proved the feasibility of robotic surgery of the parapharyngeal space and infratemporal fossa, there were major limitations noted and reproduced throughout other experimental studies, including the lack of drills and rongeurs to remove the ventral skull base bone and the inability to complete a wide resection, thus precluding its use for malignant lesions. The transoral approach was also described to access the craniocervical junction; however, drilling of the odontoid and arch of C1 was done by an assistant using a conventional technique.[10]

Combined Transnasal and Transantral Approach

In 2007, Hanna and colleagues,[11] using a cadaveric model, described a surgical approach to the cranial fossa using the da Vinci robot via combined transnasal-transantral approach.

Technique: Access to the sinonasal cavities is gained through bilateral, superior, vestibular/sublabial incisions followed by wide anterior and middle maxillary antrostomies (Caldwell-Luc–like). A posterior septectomy is done joining both sinonasal cavities into one surgical field. Then the da Vinci robot is docked at the head of the bed, the camera arm port is introduced through the nostril and the right and left robotic arm ports through the respective anterior and middle antrostomies into the nasal cavity. Then a total ethmoidectomy, wide common sphenoidotomy, resection of the middle and superior turbinates are performed, providing access to the anterior and middle cranial fossa. The cribriform plate is resected and the dural incision is then repaired, suturing a graft in a watertight fashion. This approach provides excellent access to the anterior and central skull base. The investigators emphasized the ability to perform

2-handed tremor-free suturing of dural defects.[11,12] Cho and colleagues[13] described a similar combined endonasal-transantral approach for robotic nasopharyngectomy.

Combined Transcervical and Transoral Approach

O'Malley and Weinstein[14] described the cervical-TORS (C-TORS) approach of the skull base on a cadaveric model.

Technique: The approach entails placement of a 30-degree angled lens endoscope transorally and the effector robotic arms transcervically. The da Vinci robotic arms are introduced via bilateral incisions along the posterior margin of the submandibular glands, followed by the blind blunt placement of trocars that are directed supero-medially into the oral cavity; thus, accessing the ventral skull base and nasopharynx through the oropharynx. This technique enables surgical dissection in the sphenoid sinus, clivus, sella, and suprasellar fossa with improved instrument angulation and access.

Combined Transoral and Midline Suprahyoid Approach

McCool and colleagues[15] described a cadaveric dissection using a midline supra-hyoid approach to the infratemporal fossa with the da Vinci robot.

Technique: The approach entails a midline 15-mm incision at the level of the hyoid bone with blunt dissection to gain access into the vallecula. The midline port is placed through the suprahyoid incision, a 30-degree camera is placed transorally in the midline, and the second robotic arm is placed transorally contralateral to the site of dissection. An incision is made in the posterior tonsillar pillar and carried superiorly along the salpingopharyngeal fold. The superior pharyngeal constrictor and the medial pterygoid muscle are divided, identifying the lingual and inferior alveolar nerve. The internal and external carotid arteries are identified posterior and medial to cranial nerve V3 and the middle meningeal artery is dissected up to the foramen spinosum. The dissection is extended posteriorly to the jugular foramen, identifying the internal jugular vein and cranial nerves IX to XII. The da Vinci robot was used to place surgical clips using an 8-mm clip applier. The combined transoral-suprahyoid approach provides a central port with low risk of damaging neurovascular structures; thus, allowing dissection of the central and lateral skull base.

Combined Transnasal and Transoral Approach

Combined transnasal and transoral approaches were described by Dallan and colleagues[16] in 2012 and Ozer and colleagues[17] in 2013. Ozer and colleagues[17] gained further anterior access using a mucoperiosteal flap to allow an approach through the hard palate.

Technique: The setting includes docking the da Vinci robot cranially at the head of the cadaver with a transnasal 30° lens endoscope facing upward. For dissection, a Maryland dissector (Intuitive Surgical, Inc) and a cauterization device with a spatula tip are placed transorally. The dissection starts with a midline incision in the posterior nasopharyngeal wall followed by bilateral medial to lateral hemi-nasopharyngectomy, including resection of the Eustachian tube. This technique provides an optimal approach to the nasopharynx and posterior skull base, especially in patients who are edentulous, given the transoral access without the need to split the palate. Furthermore, the dissection work is done under typical endonasal endoscopic vision, thus providing the surgeon a more familiar anatomy compared with the purely transoral technique, in which dissection occurs in inferior to superior fashion. As described by Ozer and colleagues,[17] this approach can be augmented by removing the bony hard palate (transpalatal approach) after elevation of a posteriorly based U-shaped palatal flap (**Fig. 2**).

Combined Transnasal and Transcervical Approach

The combined transnasal and transcervical approach was developed by Dallan and colleagues[18] to avoid damage to the teeth in dentate patients when using a transoral port.

Technique: Similar to the C-TORS, it involves the placement of transcervical paramandibular trocars by performing a small cervical incision at the angle of the mandible, then reaching the oral cavity through blunt subperiosteal dissection. The trocars are directed through the oropharynx superiorly into the nasopharynx (**Fig. 3**). Then a posterior septectomy is performed to improve visualization of the operative field, reduce conflict between the instruments, and increase maneuverability. The skull base is removed using conventional endonasal technique with drills and rongeurs, then the da Vinci robot is used to dissect the posterior cranial fossa and pituitary region. This approach provides a superior access to the sella, suprasellar region, clivus, optic chiasm, and pons with the ability to perform a robotic pituitary transposition.

Combined Expanded Endonasal Approach and Transoral Approach

The combined expanded endonasal approach and transoral approach (EEA-TORS) was described by Carrau and colleagues[19] in 2013, initially developed in a cadaveric model and subsequently applied on 2 patients.

Technique: The first step of the dissection is to provide a sinonasal corridor using an endoscopic endonasal technique. This includes the ipsilateral resection of the infero-posterior half of the middle turbinate, maxillary antrostomy, total ethmoidectomy, and a wide sphenoidotomy. The next step is an ipsilateral Denker approach

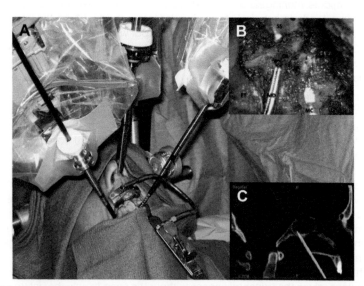

Fig. 2. (*A*) Combined transnasal-transoral technique in a cadaveric model. The camera is introduced via the left nostril and the instrument ports are placed transorally. (*B*) Camera image of the surgical field. CR, clival recess; ET, Eustachian tube; MC, monopolar cautery; MD, Maryland dissector; SS, sphenoid sinus. (*C*) Sagittal navigation image of the working corridor to the upper clivus, which constitutes the ventral limit of the exposure.

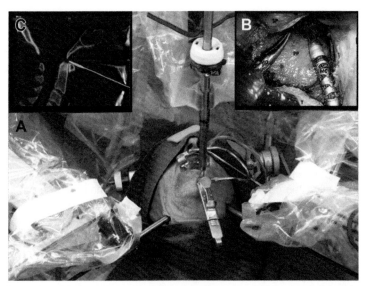

Fig. 3. (*A*) Combined transoral-transcervical technique on a cadaveric model with a camera placed transorally and instrument ports introduced transcervically. (*B*) Camera image of the surgical field. MC, monopolar cautery; MD, Maryland dissector; PP, posterior pharyngeal wall; SP, soft palate; T, tongue. (*C*) Sagittal computed tomography scan navigation image showing the working corridor to the anterior arch of C1.

(ie, Sturman-Canfield approach), which entails removal of the pyriform aperture and anterior maxillary wall; thus, providing full access to the ipsilateral posterior and lateral maxillary wall. A posterior septectomy is done to optimize binostril access. The sphenoid floor is drilled to be flush with the clivus. The vidian nerve and maxillary nerve (V2) are followed proximally to identify the junction of the paraclival and petrous carotid artery. The pterygoid process is drilled exposing the Eustachian tube, mandibular nerve (V3), and middle cranial fossa. The pterygoid and tensor veli palatine muscles are resected or mobilized exposing the parapharyngeal internal carotid artery (ICA), which constitutes the "danger zone" and lateral limit of dissection in endoscopic nasopharyngectomy. Once the inferior-most limit using EEA is reached at the level of the Eustachian tube, the da Vinci robot is brought into position. A Crowe-Davis mouth gag is inserted. The soft palate is retracted using a red rubber catheter inserted into the nose and pulled through the mouth. A Maryland dissector, a spatula-tip monopolar cautery, and a 0-degree endoscopic camera are inserted into the mouth. The superior aspect of the palatoglossal arch is incised and the infero-medial border of the medial pterygoid muscle is dissected, identifying the parapharyngeal fat and ICA. The styloid process and musculature are identified. Further dissection lateral to the parapharyngeal ICA exposes cranial nerves IX to XII and the internal jugular vein. The pterygoid muscles are transected at their mandibular insertion. Then, the dissection is extended medially, connecting it with the inferior border of the EEA dissection and completing the nasopharyngectomy with resection of the Eustachian tube.

The EEA-TORS approach provides excellent exposure to the posterior ventral skull base, nasopharynx, and infratemporal fossa. The main benefits of combining TORS to EEA to manage skull base tumors is the ability to reach the posterior ventral skull base below the level of the Eustachian tube, which is the inferior limit of EEA, and subsequently achieve a complete resection of the tumor's inferior margin with potential en bloc resection.

APPLICATION OF ROBOTIC SURGERY IN SINONASAL AND VENTRAL SKULL BASE MALIGNANCIES

Nasopharynx

Robotic surgery of the nasopharynx was initially described in a cadaveric model in 2008,[20] followed by subsequent case reports of robotic or robotic-assisted nasopharyngectomy. Tsang and colleagues[21] published a case series of 12 patients who underwent TORS/TORS-assisted nasopharyngectomy. The current indication for robotic nasopharyngectomy is small recurrent nasopharyngeal carcinoma involving the roof or posterior wall of the nasopharynx or the fossa of Rosenmuller, without intranasal or pterygopalatine fossa extension and more than 1 cm away from the ICA. The course of the ICA should not be medial to the medial pterygoid plate.

In this approach, tumors abutting or invading the floor of the sphenoid sinus require an additional endoscopic endonasal approach to achieve gross total resection with negative margins. Contraindications to robotic nasopharyngectomy include tumors extending into the pterygopalatine and infratemporal fossa, or less than 1 cm from the ICA, or with retropharyngeal lymph node metastasis or maxillary sinus invasion.

Technique: The patient is orally intubated using a nonkinking endotracheal tube placed over the central lower lip and placed in Trendelenburg position with the head slightly extended. A Dingman mouth gag retractor is used to expose the palate and oropharynx. The soft palate is divided under direct visualization and retracted laterally. The da Vinci robot is docked at the head of the bed and a 0-degree or 30-degree 8-mm dual channel camera is introduced transorally. Then, using the 5-mm Maryland grasping forceps mounted to the left robotic arm and a monopolar diathermy mounted to the right robotic arm, the nasopharyngeal soft tissue is dissected laterally between the carotid arteries, in an inferior to superior direction. The medial crus of the torus tubarius can be included in the specimen if needed. The dissection is carried through the soft tissue down to clival bone. Peripheral margins are checked intraoperatively with frozen section. The defect can be covered using a free mucosal graft or a nasoseptal flap if the carotid is exposed.[21,22]

The major advantages of TORS compared with endoscopic endonasal techniques are as follows:

- The 3D magnified endoscopic view provides excellent visualization of the surgical field.
- The Endowrist of the robot allows complex fine maneuvers in a narrow space.
- It can be performed by 1 main surgeon with an experienced first assistant sitting at the head of the bed to suction and report tactile feedback if needed.
- No need to resect the pterygoid plates.

A major disadvantage is the lack of tactile feedback. Another potential disadvantage is brought by the need for a lateral palatal incision to optimize exposure (select cases), which carries the risk of oronasal fistula. In the series by Tsang and colleagues,[21] the 2-year local control rate was 86% with acceptable functional outcomes.

Parapharyngeal Space

Recently, several case series have been published regarding the use of the da Vinci robot to resect transorally parapharyngeal space masses.[23,24] Parapharyngeal space tumors can be approached through a transcervical or transparotid approach;

however, these are not the most direct approach. The transoral approach provides a straight access to the parapharyngeal space but is limited mostly by the lack of visualization with decreased maneuverability leading to a higher risk of tumor spillage. It is relatively contraindicated to treat malignant lesions given the difficulty of obtaining a cuff of normal tissue and achieving negative margins within the parapharyngeal space. TORS provides improved illumination and 3D visualization with increased maneuverability using tremor-free wristed instruments. TORS to the parapharyngeal space can be augmented by using a transcervical approach to complete the resection and for carotid artery control.

Most of the case series include patients with benign tumors, the most common being pleomorphic adenoma. Boyce and colleagues[25] reported 1 case of low-grade mucoepidermoid carcinoma of the parapharyngeal space resected using TORS with no recurrence at 50 months of follow-up.

Expanded Endonasal Approach and Transoral Approach

Carrau and colleagues[19] reported their combined EEA-TORS technique and used it to resect an adenoid cystic carcinoma of the nasopharynx with extension laterally into the infratemporal fossa and inferiorly below the level of the hard palate, and a clival chordoma with extension into the craniocervical junction down to C2. Both patients had gross total resection with no complications and minimal postoperative morbidity (Video 1).

SUMMARY

Currently, robotic skull base surgery for sinonasal and ventral skull base malignancies is still at an early stage. Robotic surgery has many advantages, including 3D visualization, tremor-free surgery with ability to translate large macro-movement into fine precise dissection, and bimanual surgery, all of which are advantageous to resect malignant tumors in a confined space such as the sinonasal cavities and ventral skull base. However, the lack of haptic feedback, the absence of drills and bone-cutting instruments, the bulkiness of the instruments, the advanced technical skills required, and the cost are still major drawbacks to popularizing robotic sinonasal and ventral skull base surgery. The only accepted current indication is select nasopharyngeal malignancies. However, robotic surgery can be combined with EEA to resect large lesions extending inferiorly and laterally into the ventral skull base. The role of robotic skull base surgery in treating malignancies is evolving, and the refinement in surgical instrumentation will offer a great potential in the near future.

SUPPLEMENTARY DATA

Supplementary data related to this article can be found at http://dx.doi.org/10.1016/j.otc.2016.12.012.

REFERENCE

1. McLeod IK, Melder PC. Da Vinci robot-assisted excision of a vallecular cyst: a case report. Ear Nose Throat J 2005;84(3):170–2.
2. Available at: http://www.intuitivesurgical.com/products/da-vinci-xi/.
3. Gettman M. Innovations in robotic surgery. Curr Opin Urol 2016;26(3):271–6.
4. Schuler PJ, Scheithauer M, Rotter N, et al. A single-port operator-controlled flexible endoscope system for endoscopic skull base surgery. HNO 2015;63(3): 189–94.

5. Bur AM, Gomez ED, Newman JG, et al. Haptic feedback in transoral robotic surgery: a feasibility study. Annual Meeting of the Triologic Society at the Combined Otolaryngology Spring Meetings. Boston, April 24-25, 2015

6. Swaney PJ, Gilbert HB, Webster RJ 3rd, et al. Endonasal skull base tumor removal using concentric tube continuum robots: a phantom study. J Neurol Surg B Skull Base 2015;76(2):145–9.

7. Kristin J. Assessment of the endoscopic range of motion for head and neck surgery using the SOLOASSIST endoscope holder. Int J Med Robot 2015;11(4): 418–23.

8. Xia T, Baird C, Jallo G, et al. An integrated system for planning, navigation and robotic assistance for skull base surgery. Int J Med Robot 2008;4(4):321–30.

9. O'Malley BW Jr, Weinstein GS. Robotic skull base surgery: preclinical investigations to human clinical application. Arch Otolaryngol Head Neck Surg 2007; 133(12):1215–9.

10. Lee JY, O'Malley BW, Newman JG, et al. Transoral robotic surgery of craniocervical junction and atlantoaxial spine: a cadaveric study. J Neurosurg Spine 2010;12:13–8.

11. Hanna EY, Holsinger C, DeMonte F, et al. Robotic endoscopic surgery of the skull base. A novel surgical approach. Arch Otolaryngol Head Neck Surg 2007;133: 1209–14.

12. Kupferman ME, Demonte F, Levine N, et al. Feasibility of a robotic surgical approach to reconstruct the skull base. Skull Base 2011;21(2):79–82.

13. Cho HJ, Kang JW, Min HJ, et al. Robotic nasopharyngectomy via combined endonasal and transantral port: a preliminary cadaveric study. Laryngoscope 2015; 125(8):1839–43.

14. O'Malley BW Jr, Weinstein GS. Robotic anterior and midline skull base surgery: preclinical investigations. Int J Radiat Oncol Biol Phys 2007;69(2 Suppl):S125–8.

15. McCool RR, Warren FM, Wiggins RH, et al. Robotic surgery of the infratemporal fossa utilizing novel suprahyoid port. Laryngoscope 2010;120:1738–43.

16. Dallan I, Castelnuovo P, Montevecchi F, et al. Combined transoral transnasal robotic-assisted nasopharyngectomy: a cadaveric feasibility study. Eur Arch Otorhinolaryngol 2012;269(1):235–9.

17. Ozer E, Durmus K, Carrau RL, et al. Applications of transoral, transcervical, transnasal, and transpalatal corridors for robotic surgery of the skull base. Laryngoscope 2013;123(9):2176–9.

18. Dallan I, Castelnuovo P, Seccia V, et al. Combined transnasal transcervical robotic dissection of posterior skull base: feasibility in a cadaveric model. Rhinology 2012;50(2):165–70.

19. Carrau RL, Prevedello DM, de Lara D, et al. Combined transoral robotic surgery and endoscopic endonasal approach for the resection of extensive malignancies of the skull base. Head Neck 2013;35(11):E351–8.

20. Ozer E, Waltonen J. Transoral robotic nasopharyngectomy: a novel approach for nasopharyngeal lesions. Laryngoscope 2008;118:1613–6.

21. Tsang RK, To VS, Ho AC, et al. Early results of robotic assisted nasopharyngectomy for recurrent nasopharyngeal carcinoma. Head Neck 2015;37(6):788–93.

22. Wei WI, Ho WK. Transoral robotic resection of recurrent nasopharyngeal carcinoma. Laryngoscope 2010;120(10):2011–4.

23. O'Malley BW Jr, Quon H, Leonhardt FD, et al. Transoral robotic surgery for parapharyngeal space tumors. ORL J Otorhinolaryngol Relat Spec 2010;72:332–6.

24. Chan JY, Tsang RK, Eisele DW, et al. Transoral robotic surgery of the paraphar-yngeal space: a case series and systematic review. Head Neck 2015;37(2): 293–8.
25. Boyce BJ, Curry JM, Luginbuhl A, et al. Transoral robotic approach to paraphar-yngeal space tumors: case series and technical limitations. Laryngoscope 2016; 126(8):1776–82.

Management of Skull Base Defects After Surgical Resection of Sinonasal and Ventral Skull Base Malignancies

 CrossMark

Jean Anderson Eloy, MD[a,b,c,d,*], Emily Marchiano, MD[e],
Alejandro Vázquez, MD[a], Michael J. Pfisterer, MD[a],
Leila J. Mady, MD, PhD, MPH[f], Soly Baredes, MD[a,b], James K. Liu, MD[a,b,c]

KEYWORDS

- Skull base defects • Cerebrospinal fluid rhinorrhea • Endoscopic skull base surgery
- Dural defect • Nasoseptal flap • Expanded skull base approaches
- Endoscopic repair techniques • Skull base repair

KEY POINTS

- Recently, the vascularized pedicled nasoseptal flap has emerged as the workhorse for reconstruction of ventral skull base defects after endoscopic skull base surgery. However, for repair of skull base defects after resection of sinonasal and ventral skull base malignancies, extreme care should be taken to assure the flap is not involved with cancer cells.

Continued

Financial Disclosures and Conflicts of Interest: None.
Presented in part at the 2015 American Rhinologic Society Annual Meeting, Dallas, TX on September 26, 2015.
[a] Department of Otolaryngology – Head and Neck Surgery, Rutgers New Jersey Medical School, Newark, New Jersey, USA; [b] Center for Skull Base and Pituitary Surgery, Neurological Institute of New Jersey, Rutgers New Jersey Medical School, Newark, New Jersey, USA; [c] Department of Neurological Surgery, Rutgers New Jersey Medical School, Newark, New Jersey, USA; [d] Department of Ophthalmology and Visual Science, Rutgers New Jersey Medical School, 90 Bergen Street, Suite 8100, Newark, NJ 07103, USA; [e] Department of Otolaryngology – Head and Neck Surgery, University of Michigan Health System, Ann Arbor, Michigan, USA; [f] Department of Otolaryngology – Head and Neck Surgery, University of Pittsburgh Medical Center, 203 Lothrop Street, Suite 500, Pittsburgh, PA 15213, USA
* Corresponding author. Endoscopic Skull Base Surgery Program, Department of Otolaryngology – Head and Neck Surgery, Rhinology and Sinus Surgery, Otolaryngology Research, Neurological Institute of New Jersey, Rutgers New Jersey Medical School, 90 Bergen Street, Suite 8100, Newark, NJ 07103.
E-mail address: jean.anderson.eloy@gmail.com

Otolaryngol Clin N Am 50 (2017) 397–417
http://dx.doi.org/10.1016/j.otc.2016.12.013

Continued

- Although free grafts and single-layer repair techniques have been used to repair large skull base defects, multilayer closure with the inclusion of vascularized tissue may provide a stronger repair option.
- If postoperative radiotherapy is expected after resection of a ventral skull base malignancy, the use of vascularized tissue may help decrease the likelihood of dehiscence of the repair during radiotherapy.
- In cases where a combined endoscopic and open approach is performed for resection of a malignant ventral skull base lesion, a double-flap technique consisting of a vascularized pericranial flap and a vascularized pedicled nasoseptal flap can be used simultaneously to decrease the chance of failure.

Abbreviations

CSF	Cerebrospinal fluid
PCF	Pericranial flap
PNSF	Pedicled nasoseptal flap

 Video content accompanies this article at http://www.oto.theclinics.com.

INTRODUCTION

Over the past 2 decades, the management of patients with sinonasal and ventral skull base malignancies has changed with more aggressive surgical resection being performed. One of the main factors facilitating aggressive surgical resection has been the improvement in ventral skull base repair techniques (open transcranial, combined open transcranial and endoscopic endonasal, or purely endoscopic endonasal) with decreasing rates of postoperative cerebrospinal fluid (CSF) rhinorrhea and associated intracranial complications. The decrease in postoperative CSF leak paralleled the emergence of the vascularized pedicled nasoseptal flap (PNSF) as the workhorse for reconstruction of ventral skull base defects after combined and endoscopic endonasal ventral skull base surgery.[1-15] Some of these ventral skull base defects extend from the cribriform plate to the craniocervical junction in the sagittal plane and orbit to orbit and as far lateral as the infratemporal fossae and middle cranial fossae in the coronal plane,[6,16,17] presenting a significant challenge for repair.[16,18,19] A tight seal along the entire margin of a ventral skull base defect is necessary for successful repair. Inadequate repair can result in postoperative sequelae, such as CSF leak, meningitis, or intracranial abscess.[6,10,20,21] Hence, it is of utmost importance to use the available repair methods as effectively as possible, with a significant emphasis placed on maximizing the surface area of the grafts used. This review discusses some of the more common techniques currently used for repair of these ventral skull base defects with an emphasis on the senior authors' (J.A.E. and J.K.L.) preferred closure techniques. As one of the most commonly used options for ventral skull base defect repairs, nuances and pearls on the vascularized PNSF are emphasized in this article.

REPAIR AFTER OPEN TRANSCRANIAL SURGERY

In patients undergoing bifrontal transbasal approaches and craniofacial resection, the vascularized pedicled pericranial flap (PCF) has been the gold standard for repair

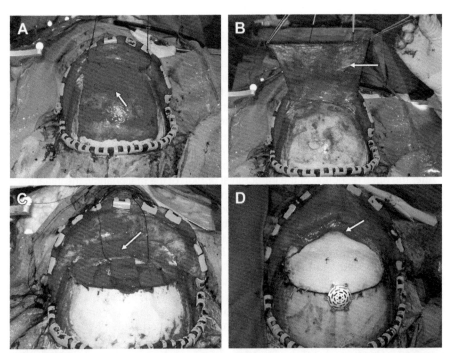

Fig. 1. Intraoperative photograph of a patient who underwent bifrontal transbasal approach and craniofacial resection of a sinonasal malignant lesion. The ventral skull base defect was repaired with the vascularized pedicled PCF (*arrow*). (*A, B*) PCF after elevation. (*C*) The PCF is layered along the floor of the ventral skull base and tucked underneath the dura. Several sutures are used to anchor the pericranium to the dura in this location. (*D*) Replacement of the bony flap after ventral skull base repair.

(**Fig. 1**).[22,23] A bicoronal scalp incision is performed from ear to ear and the scalp flap is elevated in a 2-layer fashion. The galeal flap is elevated with the skin as one layer while leaving the pericranium on the skull. Undermining the galea posterior to the skin incision is performed in order to obtain a larger surface area of pericranium. The PCF is subsequently elevated as a second layer and rotated anteriorly where it is pedicled. The transbasal cranial approach is then performed for resection of the sinonasal/ventral skull base malignancy.[24–26] The frontal sinus mucosa is exenterated and the sinus cranialized. After this approach and resection of the sinonasal and ventral skull base malignancy and the cribriform plate, the dura is typically repaired by suturing a dural patch graft (usually from a dural substitute) to close the intracranial dural defect in a watertight fashion. The PCF is subsequently layered along the floor of the ventral skull base and tucked underneath the dura overlying the planum sphenoidale. Several sutures may be used to anchor the pericranium to the dura in this location. The distal end of the PCF is then folded on itself to provide coverage along the frontobasal dural closure. The closure of the transbasal approach is performed in the standard fashion.

REPAIR AFTER COMBINED OPEN TRANSCRANIAL AND ENDOSCOPIC ENDONASAL SURGERY

The vascularized PCF is the gold standard for repair after bifrontal transbasal approaches and craniofacial resection.[22,23] Likewise, the vascularized PNSF has emerged as the workhorse for reconstruction of ventral skull base defects after endoscopic endonasal approaches.[6,27] In the authors' practice, they sometimes use a combined bifrontal transbasal approach and endoscopic endonasal approach to resect large anterior ventral skull base malignancies with significant sinonasal and intracranial extension or in some cases with significant neurovascular involvement. For these lesions, postoperative radiation therapy is anticipated, which can predispose patients to delayed flap necrosis and secondary CSF leakage. In these instances, the authors reconstruct the ventral skull base defect using a double-flap repair, which is composed of 2 vascularized pedicled tissue flaps: the PCF harvested from the transbasal approach from above augmented by a PNSF harvested from an endoscopic endonasal approach from below (**Figs. 2–4**).[28–30]

After the open resection of the intracranial portion of the malignancy, the initial dural and ventral skull base defect is repaired using a dural patch and a vascularized PCF as previously described. An endoscopic endonasal approach is then performed from below to remove tumor in the nasal cavity and paranasal sinuses. After complete resection of the intranasal portion of the lesion and achievement of intraoperative negative margins, a vascularized PNSF is harvested from the nasal septum as described by Hadad and colleagues[1] and Kassam and colleagues.[27] As part of the preparation for flap placement, an extended sphenoid sinusotomy (opening and combining the 2 sphenoid sinuses into a single cavity) is typically performed and the sinus mucosa completely removed to prevent the development of intracranial mucocele formation[31,32] and to allow for proper adherence of the PNSF to the ventral

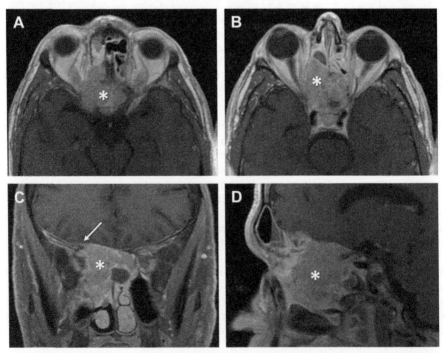

Fig. 2. Preoperative axial (*A*, *B*), coronal (*C*), and sagittal (*D*) T1-weighted gadolinium-enhanced MRI of a patient with a large sinonasal and ventral skull base moderately differentiated invasive squamous cell carcinoma with right optic canal and orbital apex involvement (*arrow*) treated with combined bifrontal transbasal and endoscopic endonasal approach. The asterisk depicts lesion.

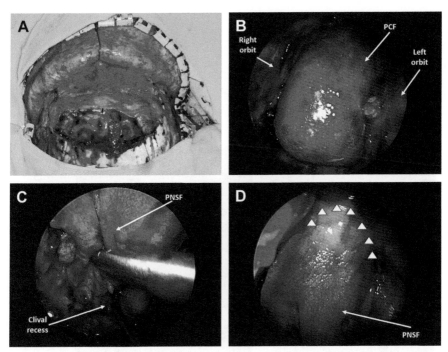

Fig. 3. Intraoperative photograph of the patient in **Fig. 2** who underwent combined bifrontal transbasal and endoscopic endonasal approach for resection of sinonasal and ventral skull base moderately differentiated squamous cell carcinoma. The ventral skull base defect was repaired with a double-flap technique using the vascularized pedicled PCF from above (*A, B*) and augmented with a vascularized PNSF from below (*C, D*). Arrowheads depict anterior limit of the PNSF reach.

skull base. It is much preferred to use the contralateral PNSF for repair of ventral skull base defects after resection of a sinonasal and ventral skull base malignancy in order to prevent placing a flap involved with cancer in the repair. Frozen section of the PNSF edges should be taken to rule out cancer involvement. In the authors' institution, they use the ipsilateral PNSF only if no other repair option is available, and when the likelihood of the ipsilateral flap involvement with cancer cell is unlikely. When this has to be performed, they usually harvest the flap as far away from the tumor as feasible and typically involve the mucosa of the hard palate in the flap. The PNSF is rotated to cover the ventral skull base defect endonasally. This endonasal repair is then bolstered with gentamicin-soaked absorbable gelatin sponge pledgets followed by an expandable Merocel (Medtronic Xomed, Jacksonville, Florida, USA) nasal packing. Postoperatively, patients are kept on antibiotics for approximately 10 days until endoscopic removal of the nasal tampon in the outpatient setting.

The combination of the vascularized PCF and PNSF offers several advantages. Each flap complements the other at its weakest point. In a PCF repair alone, the weakest point and likely failure site is the region of the planum sphenoidale at the posterior suture line. The PNSF provides robust coverage of that area to strengthen the PCF's point of weakness. Conversely, the PNSF's weakest point is anteriorly near the region of the frontal sinus because of its maximal reach. This fact is particularly true if portions of the PNSF are involved by tumor and need to be excised, which compromises the surface area and reach of the flap. In such a situation, the PNSF's point of weakness can be bolstered by the PCF because coverage of the cranialized frontal sinuses is quite robust.[28]

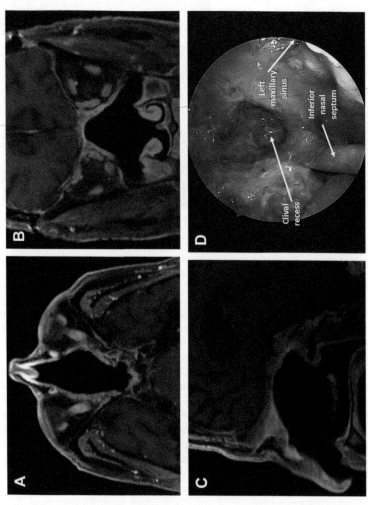

Fig. 4. Postoperative axial (A), coronal (B), and sagittal (C) T1-weighted gadolinium enhanced MRI of the patient in **Figs. 2** and **3** approximately 18 months after combined bifrontal transbasal and endoscopic endonasal approach for resection of the sinonasal and ventral skull base moderately differentiated squamous cell carcinoma and repair of the ventral skull base defects with the double-flap technique. (D) In-office endoscopic view of the ventral skull base in approximately the same time period after postoperative chemoradiotherapy.

REPAIR AFTER PURELY ENDOSCOPIC ENDONASAL SURGERY

In patients undergoing purely endoscopic endonasal resection of sinonasal/ventral skull base malignancies, repair of the ventral skull base defect can be performed using a variety of donor graft materials (middle turbinate, temporalis fascia, fascia lata, palatal mucosal, septal mucosa), flaps (PNSF, inferior turbinate flap, middle turbinate flap, and so forth), synthetic materials (acellular dermal allograft), and surgical techniques (Video 1). Some techniques involve a single-layer closure, whereas others involve the use of a multilayer closure. Some investigators advocate for rigid reconstructive techniques, whereas others think such an option to be unwise. Although still controversial, what has emerged as the most commonly used technique in major endoscopic skull base centers (including the senior authors' clinical practice) is the use of a multilayer closure with vascularized tissue when available without rigid reconstruction. However, other commonly used techniques are important to discuss.

Single-Layer Acellular Dermal Allograft Reconstruction

Casiano and colleagues have described the endoscopic repair of large ventral skull base defects using a single layer of thick acellular dermal allograft[33] or 2- to 3-ply lyophilized dura. For large defects extending the full length of the anterior ventral skull base (approximately 2 × 3 cm), the lyophilized dura or acellular dermal allograft is tucked at least 1 cm circumferentially between the remaining dura and the orbital roof (**Fig. 5**). Further discussion of this repair technique is provided in Ghassan Alokby and Roy R. Casiano's article, "Endoscopic Resection of Sinonasal and Ventral Skull Base Malignancies," in this issue.

Vascularized Pedicled Nasoseptal Flap Reconstruction

Vascularized pedicled nasoseptal flap reconstruction based on ventral skull base regions

The vascularized PNSF has become an essential component for repair of large ventral skull base defects after endoscopic endonasal skull base surgery.[1,2,6,28,34,35] The PNSF has become a mainstay technique because of its high success rate based on

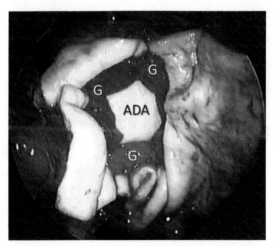

Fig. 5. Intraoperative photograph of a large ventral skull base defect repaired using a single layer of thick acellular dermal allograft. ADA, acellular dermal allograft; G, absorbable gelatin sponge.

its ability to be specifically tailored on a case-by-case basis. The dimensions of the PNSF are largely determined by the ventral skull base defect site/size. The ventral skull base can be divided into 5 broad regions: (1) the cribriform region; (2) the planum sphenoidale/tuberculum sellae region; (3) the sella; (4) the clival/odontoid region; and (5) the lateral corridors. Each region requires unique PNSF dimensions to achieve a successful repair. Endoscopic ventral skull base surgery can involve one or more of these regions, creating a large spectrum of potential defects.[3,4,14,16,18,19,36,37] Fortunately, the versatility of the PNSF allows this repair option to be an almost universal repair material for large and complex ventral skull base defects.[1,3,13,28,35] Below are specific PNSF designs that are individually fashioned for ideal coverage of each of the 5 distinct regions of the ventral skull base.[38] These designs can be customized/combined based on the regions involved.

Cribriform region Defects in the cribriform area (**Fig. 6**A) necessitate a maximization of the PNSF length. To this end, the anterior limit of the PNSF needs to be extended to the limen nasi (**Fig. 6**B). The inferior longitudinal incision is created just deep to the nasal vestibule at the limen nasi. PNSFs with these boundaries may provide sufficient coverage of a standard surgical defect of the cribriform region. When the defect is

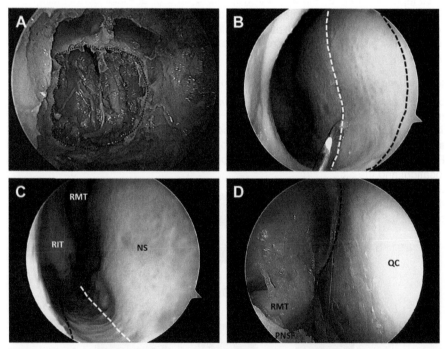

Fig. 6. (A) Endoscopic cadaveric dissection depicting a large cribriform region defect extending to the posterior table of the frontal sinus. (B) Depiction of the typical location for the anterior incision for an average length PNSF design (*white dotted line*) and a longer PNSF design (*black dotted line*). Note that the longer PNSF require an incision placed near or at the level of the columella. (C) Depiction of the typical location for the inferolateral incision for an average PNSF (*white dotted line*) and a wider PNSF (*black dotted line*). (D) In order to increase the width of the PNSF, the superior incision is placed near or up to the level of the nasoseptal angle (*black dotted line*). NS, nasal septum; QC, quadrangular cartilage; RIT, right inferior turbinate; RMT, right middle turbinate.

widened from medial orbital wall to medial orbital wall, full coverage requires a much broader flap; this is accomplished by placing the inferior longitudinal incision underneath the inferior turbinate (**Fig. 6**C) and the superior incision near or up to the level of the nasoseptal angle (**Fig. 6**D).

Planum sphenoidale/tuberculum sellae region After creation of a planum sphenoidale/tuberculum sellae defect, a long PNSF is required, given that the flap has to lie on the inferior and posterior walls of the sphenoid sinus (clival recess) before arching back onto the planum sphenoidale/tuberculum sellae region (**Fig. 7**).

Sella region Coverage of a standard sellar defect requires a relatively shorter flap than the previous two regions. Positioning the anterior vertical incision at approximately the junction of the anterior and middle one-third of the nasal septum provides sufficient flap length to reach the limit of the sellar defect (**Fig. 8**). Flap width is not an issue, and placing the inferior longitudinal incision at the junction of the nasal floor and nasal septum provides a sufficiently broad flap. There is also no need to place the superior incision as high as the nasoseptal angle.

Clival/odontoid region Considering sphenoid rostrum resection and subsequent shortening of the PNSF rotational arc, the clival/odontoid region typically necessitates relatively shorter flaps for adequate repair (**Fig. 9**).

Lateral corridor regions A relatively short PNSF is able to reach the limit of the defect if it did not extend far laterally (ie, past the midpoint of the posterior wall of the maxillary sinus) (**Fig. 10**). However, in cases where the defect is more laterally placed and a large middle cranial fossa defect is created, a much longer and larger PNSF is necessary for adequate coverage. This process entails placing the anterior incision at the level of the columella, the lateral incision under the inferior turbinate, and the superior incision at the level of the nasoseptal angle in a similar fashion to a large cribriform region defect.

The authors divide the ventral skull base into 5 general regions and determine the minimum PNSF requirements in an effort to avoid a situation of flap insufficiency. Longer flaps are required in the repair of cribriform region defects (given the anterior location) and the planum/tuberculum sellae area (given the need to lay this flap along the inferior and posterior sphenoid sinus in the clival recess). Small to average length flaps are sufficient for repair of sellar defects, given the anatomic proximity of the sella to the PNSF vascular pedicle and the ability to reach it without excessive rotation.

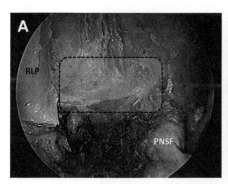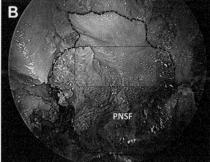

Fig. 7. (*A*) Endoscopic cadaveric dissection showing the location of the planum sphenoidale/tuberculum sellae region defect (*blue rectangle with dotted border*). (*B*) Endoscopic view of the corrected defect (*blue rectangle with dotted border*) with a left vascularized PNSF (*black dotted line*). RLP, right lamina papyracea.

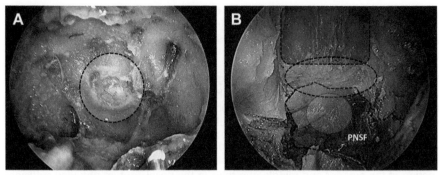

Fig. 8. (*A*) Endoscopic cadaveric dissection depicting the location of the sella region defect (*yellow circle with dotted border*). (*B*) Endoscopic view of the corrected defect (*yellow circle with dotted border*) with a left vascularized PNSF. Note the location of the cribriform (*red rectangle with dotted border*) and planum sphenoidale/tuberculum sellae region defect (*blue oval with dotted border*).

Short flaps are adequate reconstructive options for clival/odontoid and lateral corridor defects. In the case of the latter, however, a broad flap may be required for the repair of a large infratemporal fossa corridor defect. If the defect is quite expansive and extends far laterally and superiorly with a large middle cranial fossa defect, a long and wide PNSF (similar to what would be needed for a large cribriform defect) may be necessary for adequate coverage.

Pearls for maximizing the reach of the vascularized pedicled nasoseptal flap

Because it is of utmost importance to use the available repair methods as effectively as possible, significant emphasis needs to be placed on maximizing the surface area of the PNSF during ventral skull base defect repairs. Some technical pearls to maximize the reach of the PNSF are describe later.[39] The authors detail 6 separate maneuvers that can be used to maximize the surface coverage of a PNSF for ventral skull base repair after endoscopic endonasal ventral skull base approaches. Each maneuver can significantly extend the reach of the PNSF and when used in combination can provide maximum tensionless flap coverage. The individual maneuvers can be customized

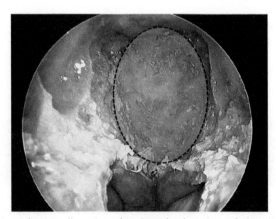

Fig. 9. Endoscopic cadaveric dissection showing the location of the clival region defect (*green oval with dotted border*).

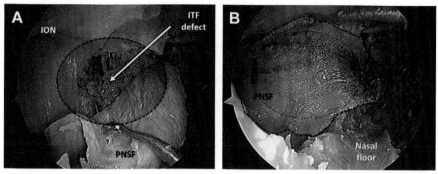

Fig. 10. (*A*) Endoscopic cadaveric dissection depicting the location of the infratemporal fossa defect (*purple oval with dotted border*). (*B*) Endoscopic view of the repaired defect (*purple oval with dotted border*) with a right vascularized PNSF (*black dotted line*). ION, infraorbital nerve; ITF, infratemporal fossa.

on a case-by-case basis depending on the complexity and size of the ventral skull base defect. These maneuvers include (1) maximally placed anterior incision near or at the columella; (2) laterally placed incision under the inferior turbinate to include the hard palate mucoperiosteum or over the inferior turbinate to include the inferior turbinate mucoperiosteum; (3) choanal releasing incision for flap rotation; (4) relaxing transverse incision at the level of the pedicle for anterior elongation; (5) resection of the sphenoid rostrum and sinus septi; and (6) initial lateral placement of the flap pedicle in select defects. All of the following maneuvers are designed to be simple yet effective.

Maneuver 1: maximally placed anterior incision at or near the columella The initial anterior incision can be placed at or near the columella to maximize the sagittal length of the PNSF (**Fig. 11**A). The anterior limit of the incision is directly responsible for the length of the PNSF. In cases where a very long PNSF is necessary, such as an anterior cribriform defect that extends to the posterior table of the frontal sinus (**Fig. 11**B), it is recommended to make the incision as anteriorly as feasible.

Maneuver 2: laterally placed incision under the inferior turbinate to include the hard palate mucoperiosteum or over the inferior turbinate to include the inferior turbinate mucoperiosteum The inferior incision can be placed laterally away from the junction of the nasal septum and nasal floor. This incision can be extended laterally either under (**Fig. 12**A) or over (**Fig. 12**B) the inferior turbinate to include the respective mucoperiosteum. The mucoperiosteum is included for the purpose of maximizing the coronal width of the flap. Similarly, the superior incision can be placed very high on the nasal septum to maximize the width of the PNSF. This placement is important in cases with very wide cribriform defects (ie, from one lamina papyracea to the next) or large defects of the infratemporal/middle cranial fossa region (**Fig. 12**C, D). The inclusion of the septal mucoperichondrial/mucoperiosteal, the hard and soft palate mucoperiosteal, and the inferior turbinate mucoperiosteal coverage in continuity results in a very large flap with the width to cover most ventral skull base defects (**Fig. 13**).

Maneuver 3: choanal releasing incision for flap rotation After the superior and inferior incisions are extended posteriorly to the levels of the anterior face of the sphenoid sinus and choana, respectively, creating the sagittal length of the PNSF from the

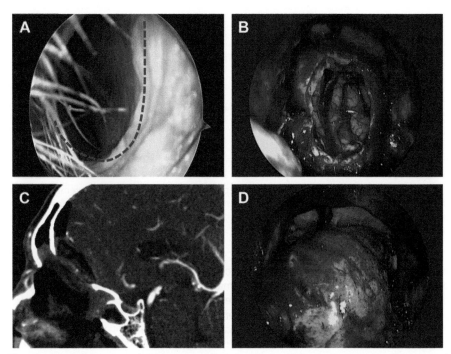

Fig. 11. (*A*) Endoscopic cadaveric image depicting the initial anterior incision (*red dotted line*) placed at the columella for maximum vascularized PNSF length. (*B*) Intraoperative 30° endoscopic view of a patient after tumor resection showing a large ventral skull base defect extending to the posterior table of the frontal sinus. (*C*) Sagittal CT scan demonstrating the anterior extent of the defect. (*D*) Intraoperative 30° endoscopic view after PNSF placement. The flap adequately reaches the posterior table of the frontal sinus with sufficient coverage.

columella to the choana, a releasing incision along the choanal arch is then performed (**Fig. 14**A). This incision is made beginning from the inferior choanal arch and progressing superiorly and laterally (**Fig. 14**B). It is important to preserve the integrity of the posterior septal branch of the sphenopalatine artery in order to maintain vascularization of the PNSF. The farther lateral this incision is carried out, the more release and rotation are achieved.

Maneuver 4: relaxing transverse incision at the level of the pedicle for anterior elongation A relaxing slit incision is made across the sphenoidal segment of the PNSF, which is the segment of flap that bridges the sphenoid sinus once the flap is rotated into position (**Fig. 15**A–C; Video 1). This maneuver is important in providing additional sagittal reach to the PNSF. In the case of a large defect that reaches the posterior table of the frontal sinus and where the PNSF is just short of the defect's edge, this releasing maneuver can increase the anterior reach of the flap to cover the posterior table of the frontal sinus. The remaining sphenoidal flap (mud flap) can be positioned superiorly and posteriorly to cover the defect if it extends to the planum sphenoidale. An illustrative case is depicted in **Fig. 15**D–E.

Maneuver 5: resection of the sphenoid rostrum and sinus septations For defects in the sella, clivus, superior cervical spine, and tuberculum sellae/planum sphenoidale region,

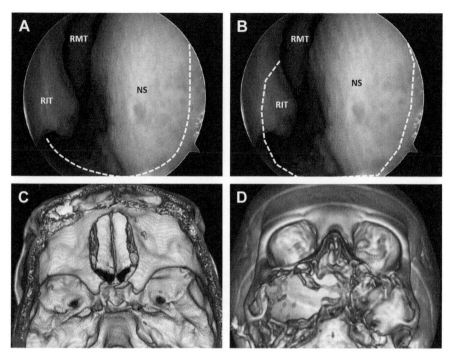

Fig. 12. Endoscopic cadaveric image depicting the inferior incision position (*dotted line*) placed laterally away from the junction of the nasal septum and nasal floor. The incision can be extended laterally under (*A*) or over (*B*) the inferior turbinate to include the respective mucoperiosteum. (*C*) A 3-dimensional (3D) CT scan depicting a large anterior skull base defect that can benefit from extending the vascularized PNSF as described in (*A*). A 3D CT scan showing a large right infratemporal/middle cranial fossa defect that may benefit from the PNSF extension described in (*D*). NS, nasal septum; RIT, right inferior turbinate; RMT, right middle turbinate.

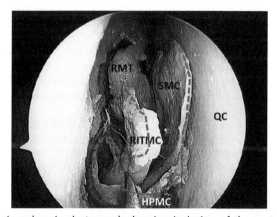

Fig. 13. Endoscopic cadaveric photograph showing inclusion of the septal mucoperichon-drial/mucoperiosteal, the hard and soft palate mucoperiosteal, and the inferior turbinate mucoperiosteal coverage in continuity for elevation of a very large flap (*dotted line*). The resulting flap has the width to cover most ventral skull base defects. HPMC, hard palate mucosal coverage; QC, quadrangular cartilage; RITMC, right inferior turbinate mucosal coverage; RMT, right middle turbinate; SMC, septal mucosal coverage.

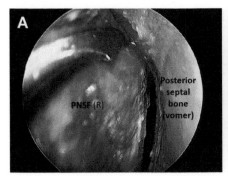
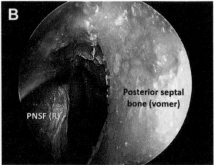

Fig. 14. Endoscopic cadaveric photograph depicting the site of the releasing incision (*dotted line*) along the choanal arch (*A*). This incision is made beginning from the inferior choanal arch and progressing superiorly and laterally (*B*). R, right.

the sphenoid sinus rostrum and sphenoid sinus septations (partitions) can serve as ledges of bone that can prevent adequate placement of the PNSF. The sphenoid rostrum may require additional flap coverage that may prevent the flap from reaching the defect site. This area may also cause significant tension in a PNSF, specifically in the case of a small flap. The sphenoid septations may prevent the placement of the PNSF on a flat surface and subsequently can lead to inadequate skull base repair. By resecting the sphenoid sinus rostrum (**Fig. 16**A) and septations (**Fig. 16**B), the path to the defect is significantly shortened and a more ergonomic rotation and flap positioning can be achieved. Consequently, some defects in these areas may be repaired with smaller flaps if adequate sphenoid rostral resection is performed. Caution should be taken in cases of tuberculum sellae/planum sphenoidale defects because this region is significantly less forgiving and may still necessitate a larger PNSF for adequate repair.

Maneuver 6: initial lateral placement of the flap pedicle in select defects One way to maximize the reach of the PNSF involves the proper positioning of the PNSF in order to decrease unnecessary placement of a portion of the flap in an unimportant location (**Fig. 17**). In cases of anterior cribriform defects, instead of placing the flap in the sphenoid sinus and cover the clival recess, sella, and planum sphenoidale/tuberculum sellae before reaching the cribriform defects, the PNSF can be positioned laterally over the area of the orbital apex/medial orbital wall and then positioned over the cribriform defects. This positioning bypasses the clival recess, sella, and part of the planum sphenoidale/tuberculum sellae and may render a potentially shorter PNSF adequate for these repairs.

These 6 maneuvers can be divided into 3 categories of modifiable variables: (1) length determinant, (2) width determinant, and (3) tension reduction with proper placement. Maneuver 1 largely determines the sagittal length of the PNSF, whereas maneuver 2 creates the coronal/transverse width of the PNSF. The goal of maneuvers 3 through 6 is to augment the length and width created by the first 2 maneuvers to maximize flap coverage. These last 4 maneuvers focus on reducing flap tension and providing the most efficient placement of the flap. Maneuver 3 completes the sagittal length of the PNSF, releases the flap, and most importantly maximizes the release and subsequent rotation of the flap. By advancing the choanal releasing incision in a superolateral direction (**Fig. 14**), tension is reduced so that the flap can be freely released and rotated into the plane of the defect. Therefore, maneuver 3 allows the flap to lie flat in the transverse/coronal plane and make even contact with the entire

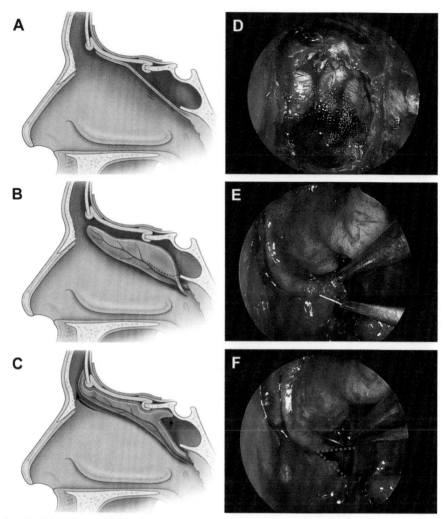

Fig. 15. (*A*) A short PNSF under tension and not reaching the anterior edge of a cribriform defect. (*B*) Site of relaxing slit incision for additional length. (*C*) Placement of the vascularized PNSF after the relaxing incision with adequate coverage of the anterior edge of the defect. (*D*) Intraoperative endoscopic view of a patient with a large anterior ventral skull base/cribriform defect. (*E*) Relaxing incision (*dotted line*) with microscissors. (*F*) Flap placement with the gap/rotation created (*dotted line*) from the releasing incision. (*Courtesy of* Chris Gralapp, MA, CMI, Fairfax, CA.)

border of the defect. A proper releasing incision and flap rotation are both essential to achieving an adequate ventral skull base repair. Similarly, maneuver 4 is also used to reduce tension in the flap but specifically to allow for a far anterior reach while maintaining the ability to lie flat over the defect. Ventral skull base defects that involve the cribriform plate can be difficult to repair because of the challenge of achieving sufficient anterior reach of the PNSF. When attempting to cover a far anterior ventral skull base defect, tension often builds in the sphenoidal portion of the PNSF, which can restrict the simultaneous full anterior reach and flat coverage (**Fig. 15**) necessary for

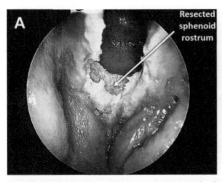
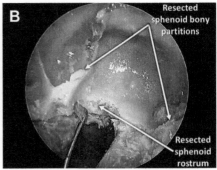

Fig. 16. Endoscopic cadaveric photograph showing the resected sphenoid rostrum (*A*) and septations (*B*).

a proper repair. Hence, maneuver 4 is specifically used to augment maneuver 1 in order to achieve the maximum sagittal length possible.

Maneuver 5 is unique in that it does not involve modifying the PNSF itself but instead focuses on altering the surrounding bony anatomy to reduce the distance the PNSF must traverse and the surface area the PNSF must cover (**Fig. 16**). The sphenoid sinus rostrum and sphenoid sinus septations (partitions) can represent increased surface area for flap coverage, which can create a significant amount of restrictive tension. Resection of the sphenoid sinus rostrum allows for a more direct path for the PNSF, which further reduces tension and maintains maximum reach. The sphenoid septations may present an uneven surface for the PNSF to lie on, which makes forming a circumferential tight seal difficult. Resection of the sphenoid septations allows for a smoother surface for the PNSF to be positioned over, making an adequate repair more achievable. Maneuver 5 can potentially obviate large PNSFs and allow for the harvest/use of smaller flaps. However, caution should be taken in cases of tuberculum sellae/planum sphenoidale defects because this region is significantly less forgiving and may still necessitate a larger PNSF for adequate repair. Lastly, maneuver 6 aims to achieve ideal positioning of the PNSF to avoid placement of the flap in an insignificant location.

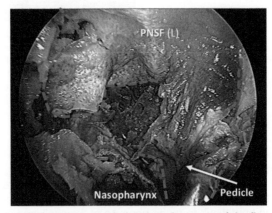

Fig. 17. Endoscopic cadaveric photograph showing placement of the flap pedicle positioned laterally over the area of the left orbital apex/medial orbital wall area and then positioned over a cribriform defects. This positioning bypasses the clival recess, sella, and part of the planum sphenoidale/tuberculum sellae. (*blue dotted line* depicts flap edge). L, left.

Depending on the site of the defect, the PNSF can be positioned in specific ways that can extend its reach. For example, in the repair of certain cribriform defects, the PNSF does not have to be placed in the sphenoid sinus, unnecessarily covering the clival recess, sella, and planum sphenoidale/tuberculum sellae before reaching the cribriform defect. Instead the PNSF can be more directly positioned laterally over the area of the orbital apex/medial orbital wall and then positioned over the cribriform defects.

SPECIAL CONSIDERATIONS AFTER VENTRAL SKULL BASE DEFECT RECONSTRUCTION
Rigid Reconstruction Techniques

With the improved access for tumor resection seen in the last 2 decades, larger cranial base defects are being created and repaired with the potential for higher postoperative CSF leaks and ventral skull base sagging.[10,40] In order to decrease postoperative CSF leakage and encephalocele formation after repair of these large skull base defects, the vascularized PNSF was introduced, and some authors have advocated the use of rigid reconstructive options. Some centers have reported the use of cartilage, vomeric bone, or synthetic material, such as a titanium plate to reinforce these repairs.[14,41,42] The autologous grafts are often reabsorbed from the chronic pulsation of the brain, and the synthetic materials carry the risk of extrusion and constitute a significant challenge in case of an infection. In a recent study, the authors examined the degree of frontal lobe descent after reconstruction of large ventral skull base defects without rigid structural grafting techniques.[43] Although all the patients studied had a ventral skull base and dural defect size of 5.0 cm^2 or greater with a mean defect size of 9.1 cm^2, no significant frontal lobe sagging was found. Therefore, the authors concluded that rigid structural reconstruction of the ventral skull base may not be necessary when performing multilayer reconstruction.[43] Other studies have noted no frontal lobe sagging using a single layer of thick acellular dermal allograft.[33,44–46]

Use of Dural Sealants

Dural sealants are commonly used in repair of ventral skull base defects. The authors used these materials in the past. However, in a recent study, they found no significant difference when a dural sealant was added to the PNSF for repair of ventral skull base defects in their skull base center.[2] Based on these findings, the authors think that the addition of a dural sealant to the PNSF repair is not warranted and have discontinued the use of dural sealant in ventral skull base defect reconstruction. Given the current climate with medical costs continuously increasing, the need for cost-effective medical techniques and practices is important. There are significant costs associated with the use of dural sealants.[47] The authors, however, think that endoscopic skull base surgeons who find these materials useful should not change their practice based solely on the authors' experience.

Use of Cerebrospinal Fluid Diversion

Until recently, the use of CSF diversion (typically a lumbar drain) was routinely used after repair of ventral skull base defects. However, with the use of the vascularized PNSF, multilayer closures, and improved repair techniques, many studies have shown that CSF diversion is not necessary in most CSF leaks encountered during ventral skull base surgery.[6,48] Casiano and Jassir[49] retrospectively reviewed the effectiveness of endoscopic repair of CSF leaks of iatrogenic or spontaneous origin without the use of lumbar drains and noted a 97% success rate in 33 patients. Burns and colleagues[50] and Hughes and colleagues[51] found CSF leak rates of 16.7% and 5.9%, respectively. The authors previously published their early institution's experience in 59 patients who underwent ventral skull base defect repair using a PNSF without diversion and experienced no postoperative CSF leaks.[13] Studies in which postoperative lumbar drainage was used by Anand and colleagues[52] and Lanza and colleagues[53] described a leak rate of 8.3% and 5.5%, respectively. Hence, no definitive data demonstrate whether postoperative lumbar drainage or other methods of CSF diversion minimize the rate of postoperative CSF leakage. In a recent evidence-based report on the use of CSF diversion after endoscopic ventral skull base reconstruction, Tien and colleagues[48] noted that the use of lumbar drains was not necessary in the management of most CSF leaks. These investigators concluded that the use of a lumbar drain should be reserved for high-risk patients with high-flow CSF leaks and significant risk factors for failure.[48] Currently, in the authors' clinical practice, postoperative lumbar drainage is not routinely used in order to avoid complications related to intracranial hypotension and to facilitate earlier mobilization of the patients. The authors reserve the use of CSF diversion for patients with defects in the planum sphenoidale/tuberculum sellae region because of the known higher risk of postoperative CSF leak in this area.[5]

Microvascular Free Flap Reconstruction

Historically, free microvascular tissue transfer was a cornerstone of reconstruction after ventral skull base surgery. However, with the increased use of local and regional pedicled vascularized flaps, such as the PCF and the PNSF, as well as more efficient synthetic materials, the need for free microvascular tissue transfer for repair of ventral skull base defects has markedly diminished. Nonetheless, free microvascular tissue transfer remains a viable option in previously irradiated patients or when radiotherapy is expected and local or regional vascularized flaps are not available.[54,55]

SUMMARY

There has been a significant increase in the resection of larger and more complex ventral skull base malignancies. The resection of these lesions has led to the creation of more complex ventral skull base defects with associated increased difficulty in repair. Many available options for ventral skull base reconstruction exist; the ideal method for repair of these defects depends on the extent of resection, surgical approach (open vs endoscopic), histology, and surgical preference. Despite the many reconstructive options, the key objective is to eliminate any communication between the intracranial space and the sinonasal cavity.

SUPPLEMENTARY DATA

Supplementary video related to this article can be found at http://dx.doi.org/10.1016/j.otc.2016.12.013.

REFERENCES

1. Hadad G, Bassagasteguy L, Carrau RL, et al. A novel reconstructive technique after endoscopic expanded endonasal approaches: vascular pedicle nasoseptal flap. Laryngoscope 2006;116:1882–6.
2. Eloy JA, Choudhry OJ, Friedel ME, et al. Endoscopic nasoseptal flap repair of skull base defects: is addition of a dural sealant necessary? Otolaryngol Head Neck Surg 2012;147:161–6.
3. Eloy JA, Choudhry OJ, Shukla PA, et al. Nasoseptal flap repair after endoscopic transsellar versus expanded endonasal approaches: is there an increased risk of postoperative cerebrospinal fluid leak? Laryngoscope 2012;122:1219–25.

4. Eloy JA, Patel SK, Shukla PA, et al. Triple-layer reconstruction technique for large cribriform defects after endoscopic endonasal resection of anterior skull base tumors. Int Forum Allergy Rhinol 2013;3:204–11.
5. Eloy JA, Shukla PA, Choudhry OJ, et al. Challenges and surgical nuances in reconstruction of large planum sphenoidale tuberculum sellae defects after endoscopic endonasal resection of parasellar skull base tumors. Laryngoscope 2013;123:1353–60.
6. Liu JK, Schmidt RF, Choudhry OJ, et al. Surgical nuances for nasoseptal flap reconstruction of cranial base defects with high-flow cerebrospinal fluid leaks after endoscopic skull base surgery. Neurosurg Focus 2012;32:E7.
7. Mammis A, Agarwal N, Eloy JA, et al. Intraventricular tension pneumocephalus after endoscopic skull base surgery. J Neurol Surg A Cent Eur Neurosurg 2013;74(Suppl 1):e96–9.
8. Eloy JA, Vivero RJ, Hoang K, et al. Comparison of transnasal endoscopic and open craniofacial resection for malignant tumors of the anterior skull base. Laryngoscope 2009;119:834–40.
9. Husain Q, Patel SK, Soni RS, et al. Celebrating the golden anniversary of anterior skull base surgery: reflections on the past 50 years and its historical evolution. Laryngoscope 2013;123:64–72.
10. Kassam AB, Prevedello DM, Carrau RL, et al. Endoscopic endonasal skull base surgery: analysis of complications in the authors' initial 800 patients. J Neurosurg 2011;114:1544–68.
11. Couldwell WT, Weiss MH, Rabb C, et al. Variations on the standard transsphenoidal approach to the sellar region, with emphasis on the extended approaches and parasellar approaches: surgical experience in 105 cases. Neurosurgery 2004;55:539–47 [discussion: 547–50].
12. Eloy JA, Kalyoussef E, Choudhry OJ, et al. Salvage endoscopic nasoseptal flap repair of persistent cerebrospinal fluid leak after open skull base surgery. Am J Otol 2012;33:735–40.
13. Eloy JA, Kuperan AB, Choudhry OJ, et al. Efficacy of the pedicled nasoseptal flap without cerebrospinal fluid (CSF) diversion for repair of skull base defects: incidence of postoperative CSF leaks. Int Forum Allergy Rhinol 2012;2:397–401.
14. Greenfield JP, Anand VK, Kacker A, et al. Endoscopic endonasal transethmoidal transcribriform transfovea ethmoidalis approach to the anterior cranial fossa and skull base. Neurosurgery 2010;66:883–92 [discussion: 892].
15. Wood JW, Eloy JA, Vivero RJ, et al. Efficacy of transnasal endoscopic resection for malignant anterior skull-base tumors. Int Forum Allergy Rhinol 2012;2:487–95.
16. Liu JK, Eloy JA. Expanded endoscopic endonasal transcribriform approach for resection of anterior skull base olfactory schwannoma. J Neurosurg 2012; 32(Suppl):E3.
17. Liu JK, Eloy JA. Expanded endoscopic endonasal transcribriform approach for resection of anterior skull base olfactory schwannoma. Neurosurg Focus 2012; 32(Suppl 1):E3.
18. Liu JK, Christiano LD, Patel SK, et al. Surgical nuances for removal of olfactory groove meningiomas using the endoscopic endonasal transcribriform approach. Neurosurg focus 2011;30:E3.
19. Verillaud B, Bresson D, Sauvaget E, et al. Transcribriform and transplanum endoscopic approach for skull-base tumors. Eur Ann Otorhinolaryngol Head Neck Dis 2013;130:233–6.
20. Kovalerchik O, Mady LJ, Svider PF, et al. Physician accountability in iatrogenic cerebrospinal fluid leak litigation. Int Forum Allergy Rhinol 2013;3:722–5.

21. Nadimi S, Caballero N, Carpenter P, et al. Immediate postoperative imaging after uncomplicated endoscopic approach to the anterior skull base: is it necessary? Int Forum Allergy Rhinol 2014;4:1024–9.

22. Price JC, Loury M, Carson B, et al. The pericranial flap for reconstruction of anterior skull base defects. Laryngoscope 1988;98:1159–64.

23. Johns ME, Winn HR, McLean WC, et al. Pericranial flap for the closure of defects of craniofacial resection. Laryngoscope 1981;91:952–9.

24. Liu JK, Decker D, Schaefer SD, et al. Zones of approach for craniofacial resection: minimizing facial incisions for resection of anterior cranial base and paranasal sinus tumors. Neurosurgery 2003;53:1126–35 [discussion: 1127–35].

25. Liu JK, O'Neill B, Orlandi RR, et al. Endoscopic-assisted craniofacial resection of esthesioneuroblastoma: minimizing facial incisions–technical note and report of 3 cases. Minim Invasive Neurosurg 2003;46:310–5.

26. Liu JK, Eloy JA. Modified one-piece extended transbasal approach for resection of giant anterior skull base sinonasal teratocarcinosarcoma. J Neurosurg 2012; 32(Suppl):E4.

27. Kassam AB, Thomas A, Carrau RL, et al. Endoscopic reconstruction of the cranial base using a pedicled nasoseptal flap. Neurosurgery 2008;63:ONS44–52 [discussion: ONS52–3].

28. Eloy JA, Choudhry OJ, Christiano LD, et al. Double flap technique for reconstruction of anterior skull base defects after craniofacial tumor resection: technical note. Int Forum Allergy Rhinol 2013;3:425–30.

29. Chaaban MR, Chaudhry A, Riley KO, et al. Simultaneous pericranial and nasoseptal flap reconstruction of anterior skull base defects following endoscopic-assisted craniofacial resection. Laryngoscope 2013;123:2383–6.

30. Eloy JA, Liu JK. In reference to simultaneous pericranial and nasoseptal flap reconstruction of anterior skull base defects following endoscopic-assisted craniofacial resection. Laryngoscope 2014;124:E149.

31. Eloy JA, Fatterpekar GM, Bederson JB, et al. Intracranial mucocele: an unusual complication of cerebrospinal fluid leakage repair with middle turbinate mucosal graft. Otolaryngol Head Neck Surg 2007;137:350–2.

32. Husain Q, Sanghvi S, Kovalerchik O, et al. Assessment of mucocele formation after endoscopic nasoseptal flap reconstruction of skull base defects. Allergy Rhinol (Providence) 2013;4:e27–31.

33. Germani RM, Vivero R, Herzallah IR, et al. Endoscopic reconstruction of large anterior skull base defects using acellular dermal allograft. Am J Rhinol 2007; 21:615–8.

34. Peris-Celda M, Pinheiro-Neto CD, Funaki T, et al. The extended nasoseptal flap for skull base reconstruction of the clival region: an anatomical and radiological study. J Neurol Surg B Skull Base 2013;74:369–85.

35. Eloy JA, Patel AA, Shukla PA, et al. Early harvesting of the vascularized pedicled nasoseptal flap during endoscopic skull base surgery. Am J Otol 2013;34: 188–94.

36. Kassam A, Snyderman CH, Mintz A, et al. Expanded endonasal approach: the rostrocaudal axis. Part I. Crista galli to the sella turcica. Neurosurg Focus 2005; 19:E3.

37. Snyderman CH, Pant H, Carrau RL, et al. What are the limits of endoscopic sinus surgery?: the expanded endonasal approach to the skull base. Keio J Med 2009; 58:152–60.

38. Eloy JA, Vazquez A, Marchiano E, et al. Zones of endoscopic pedicled nasoseptal flap reconstruction: a paradigm for site-directed flap design American Rhinologic Society Annual Fall Meeting. Dallas, Texas, September 25-26, 2015.

39. Eloy JA, Mendelson ZS, Marchiano E, et al. Maximizing the reach of the vascularized pedicled nasoseptal flap: a cadaveric study with clinical correlates American Rhinologic Society Annual Fall Meeting. Dallas, Texas, September 25-26, 2015.

40. Zanation AM, Carrau RL, Snyderman CH, et al. Nasoseptal flap reconstruction of high flow intraoperative cerebral spinal fluid leaks during endoscopic skull base surgery. Am J Rhinol Allergy 2009;23:518–21.

41. Leng LZ, Brown S, Anand VK, et al. "Gasket-seal" watertight closure in minimal-access endoscopic cranial base surgery. Neurosurgery 2008;62:ONSE342-3 [discussion: ONSE343].

42. Garcia-Navarro V, Anand VK, Schwartz TH. Gasket seal closure for extended endonasal endoscopic skull base surgery: efficacy in a large case series. World Neurosurg 2011;80(5):563–8.

43. Eloy JA, Shukla PA, Choudhry OJ, et al. Assessment of frontal lobe sagging after endoscopic endonasal transcribriform resection of anterior skull base tumors: is rigid structural reconstruction of the cranial base defect necessary? Laryngoscope 2012;122:2652–7.

44. Casiano RR, Numa WA, Falquez AM. Endoscopic resection of esthesioneuroblastoma. Am J Rhinol 2001;15:271–9.

45. Har-El G, Casiano RR. Endoscopic management of anterior skull base tumors. Otolaryngol Clin North Am 2005;38:133–44, ix.

46. Dave SP, Bared A, Casiano RR. Surgical outcomes and safety of transnasal endoscopic resection for anterior skull tumors. Otolaryngol Head Neck Surg 2007;136: 920–7.

47. Kus LH, Rotenberg BW, Duggal N. Use of tissue glues in endoscopic pituitary surgery: a cost comparison. Can J Neurol Sci 2010;37:650–5.

48. Tien DA, Stokken JK, Recinos PF, et al. Cerebrospinal fluid diversion in endoscopic skull base reconstruction: an evidence-based approach to the use of lumbar drains. Otolaryngol Clin North Am 2016;49:119–29.

49. Casiano RR, Jassir D. Endoscopic cerebrospinal fluid rhinorrhea repair: is a lumbar drain necessary? Otolaryngol Head Neck Surg 1999;121:745–50.

50. Burns JA, Dodson EE, Gross CW. Transnasal endoscopic repair of cranionasal fistulae: a refined technique with long-term follow-up. Laryngoscope 1996;106: 1080–3.

51. Hughes RG, Jones NS, Robertson IJ. The endoscopic treatment of cerebrospinal fluid rhinorrhoea: the Nottingham experience. J Laryngol Otol 1997;111:125–8.

52. Anand VK, Murali RK, Glasgold MJ. Surgical decisions in the management of cerebrospinal fluid rhinorrhoea. Rhinology 1995;33:212–8.

53. Lanza DC, O'Brien DA, Kennedy DW. Endoscopic repair of cerebrospinal fluid fistulae and encephaloceles. Laryngoscope 1996;106:1119–25.

54. Hachem RA, Elkhatib A, Beer-Furlan A, et al. Reconstructive techniques in skull base surgery after resection of malignant lesions: a wide array of choices. Curr Opin Otolaryngol Head Neck Surg 2016;24:91–7.

55. Reyes C, Mason E, Solares CA. Panorama of reconstruction of skull base defects: from traditional open to endonasal endoscopic approaches, from free grafts to microvascular flaps. Int Arch Otorhinolaryngol 2014;18:S179–86.

The Role of Radiation Therapy in the Management of Sinonasal and Ventral Skull Base Malignancies

Kyle Wang, MD[a], Adam M. Zanation, MD[b],
Bhishamjit S. Chera, MD[a],*

KEYWORDS

- Nasal cavity • Sinonasal • Paranasal • Sinus • Skull base • Radiation

KEY POINTS

- Sinonasal and ventral skull base cancers encompass a variety of rare "orphan" tumors. Existing evidence is predominantly from retrospective single-institution series.
- Multimodality treatment with surgery and postoperative radiation therapy is the standard paradigm.
- Advances including intensity-modulated radiation therapy and charged particle therapy have allowed for improved oncologic outcomes and reduced toxicity.
- Radiation oncologists must balance target coverage and critical structure dose to maximize tumor control while minimizing severe toxicity.
- Specific radiotherapy considerations vary by histology and location and are important for optimal management.

INTRODUCTION

Sinonasal and ventral skull base malignancies are rare tumors; therefore, evidence for optimal management is limited primarily to single-institution retrospective series and population-based registry studies. Initial management is usually maximal surgical resection. Although no randomized trials exist, high rates of local failure have led to the wide adoption of postoperative radiation therapy for all except early-stage tumors without adverse pathologic risk factors. Numerous institutions published their

Disclosure Statement: The authors have nothing to disclose.
[a] Department of Radiation Oncology, University of North Carolina Hospitals, 101 Manning Drive, CB #7512, Chapel Hill, NC 27599-7512, USA; [b] Division of Head and Neck Surgery, Department of Otolaryngology, University of North Carolina Hospitals, 170 Manning Drive, CB #7070, Chapel Hill, NC 27599-7070, USA
* Corresponding author.
E-mail address: bchera@med.unc.edu

Table 1
Select large institutional series using RT for sinonasal cancer

Series	Years Treated	n	% Surgery	Results	Conclusions/Toxicity
Blanco et al,[1] 2004 (WashU)	1960–1998	106	65	5-y OS 27%, DFS 33%, LC 58%	Better outcomes in those who had surgery
Hoppe et al,[2] 2007 (MSKCC)	1987–2005	85	100	5-y OS 67%, DFS 55%, LC 62%	Only 1 G3+ ocular toxicity using mostly modern techniques (3DCRT, IMRT)
Dulguerov et al,[3] 2001 (UCLA, Switzerland)	1975–1994	220	71	5-y OS 40%, LC 57%	Better outcomes in those who had surgery
Chen et al,[4] 2007 (UCSF)	1960–2005	127	84	5-y OS 52%, DFS 62%, LC 54%	Decreased toxicity across decade treated due to advances in RT technique
Dirix et al,[5] 2007 (Belgium)	1976–2003	127	88	5-y OS 54%, DFS 37%, LC 53%	15 patients with RT retinopathy, 2 patients with severe optic neuropathy
Bristol et al,[6] 2007 (MDACC)	1969–2002	146	100	5-y OS 55%, DFS 53%, LC 74%	34% G3+ toxicity if treated before 1991 vs 8% if treated after 1991
Mendenhall et al,[7] 2009 (UF)	1964–2005	109	49	(Excluded maxillary tumors) 5-y OS 55%, LC 63%	20% severe complications, including 19 patients with at least ipsilateral blindness
Duprez et al,[8] 2012 (Belgium)	1998–2009	130	78	5-y OS 52%, DFS 39%, LC 59%	G3+ ocular toxicity in 11 patients, but no blindness in patients who had IMRT
Al-Mamgani et al,[9] 2012 (Netherlands)	1999–2010	82	78	5-y OS 54%, DFS 56%, LC 74%	Decreased late toxicity and increased vision preservation with IMRT vs 3DCRT

Abbreviations: DFS, disease-free survival; IMRT, intensity-modulated radiation therapy; LC, local control; MDACC, MD Anderson Cancer Center; MSKCC, Memorial Sloan Kettering Cancer Center; RT, radiation therapy; UCLA, University of California, Los Angeles; UCSF, University of California, San Francisco; UF, University of Florida; WashU, Washington University in St. Louis.

experiences with this approach (**Table 1**), with most reports spanning at least several decades and encompassing a mix of tumor stages and histologies. These series report 5-year overall survival (OS) rates of roughly 50% and local control (LC) of 50% to 70%.[1–9] When patients present with unresectable disease or comorbidities precluding surgery, definitive radiotherapy or chemoradiation are used. In these cases, outcomes are suboptimal and toxicities significant as higher doses are needed to control gross disease.[10–12] In select patients, a reassessment of resectability may occur after completion of definitive radiotherapy.

The combination of aggressive surgical resection and radiation therapy comes at the price of significant toxicity, particular to ocular structures and brain (eg, blindness, brain necrosis, cerebrospinal fluid leak, infection). Clinicians often face the decision of whether to sacrifice vision for cancer control, whether through orbital exenteration or radiation coverage. Conversely, surgeons may leave behind gross residual disease or positive margins adjacent to the orbit and base of skull, and radiation oncologists frequently reduce treatment volumes around these organs to prioritize sparing of vision.

RADIATION THERAPY: INDICATIONS AND TECHNIQUES

Postoperative radiation therapy is indicated when adverse features are found at the time of surgery. These include advanced T stage, high tumor grade or high-risk histology, perineural invasion, lymphovascular space invasion, positive lymph nodes, positive margins, and surgeon concern about the adequacy of resection or tumor spillage. One could consider radiation therapy for most patients, as margin status may always be considered close because of the "close quarters" and anatomic constraints in which these operations are performed and surgical techniques used, that is, piecemeal resection in a difficult anatomic area. Postoperative doses typically range from 50 to 66 Gy, but doses of 70 to 74.4 Gy or higher may be necessary to control gross residual or unresectable disease. Fraction size is usually 1.8 Gy or 2 Gy using once-daily fractionation or 1.2 Gy twice daily.

The necessity for high-dose for disease control and the sensitivity of adjacent structures presents challenges to the treating radiation oncologist. Advances in radiotherapy technique have altered the therapeutic ratio and allowed better coverage of tumors and increased sparing of these normal structures. Historically, sinonasal radiation was delivered using 2-dimensional portals using a 3-field technique drawn based on skull radiograph anatomy. Three-dimensional conformal radiotherapy (3DCRT) allowed planning based on computed tomography anatomy and led to improvements in target coverage and normal tissue sparing. In most modern centers, however, these techniques are no longer used for sinonasal and ventral skull base cancer.

Intensity-Modulated Radiation Therapy

Intensity-modulated radiation therapy (IMRT) was one of the most important advances in modern radiotherapy planning and is the most common technique used for the treatment of sinonasal and ventral skull base malignancies in the United States. IMRT uses computational mathematics and inverse radiation planning combined with multiple beams of varying shapes and intensities to create an optimal radiation plan that conforms around irregular targets and avoids critical structures. Dosimetric studies have found that IMRT allows for better sparing of optic and brain structures and improved coverage of tumor.[13] **Fig. 1** shows an example of an IMRT plan.

Multiple studies report reduced toxicities with the use of IMRT compared with older techniques.[4,6,8,9,14] Perhaps most striking are the studies that show reductions in toxicity across decades of treatment alongside advances in radiotherapy technique. Chen and colleagues[4] reported the University of California, San Francisco experience over 5 decades and found a linear decrease in grade 3/4 late toxicities from 53% in the

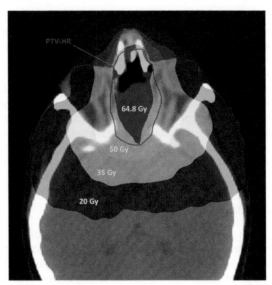

Fig. 1. An example of an IMRT plan in a patient with resected pT4 sinonasal adenocarcinoma. The high-risk planning target volume (PTV-HR) is shown as a nonshaded contour, and the doses delivered are shown shaded. Underdosing of the PTV is allowed to spare the bilateral optic nerves to less than 60 Gy and maximize vision preservation.

1960s to 16% in the 2000s, with most of the latter patients treated with IMRT. Similarly, Dirix and colleagues[14] compared patients treated with postoperative 3DCRT before 2003 versus postoperative IMRT after 2003 and found better disease-free survival and reduced cutaneous, salivary, and ocular toxicity in the patients treated with IMRT.

Charged Particles

Charged particle therapy using protons or carbon ions have garnered particular interest in the treatment of sinonasal and ventral skull base cancer. Charged particles are characterized by maximal dose deposition at an energy-specific depth (the "Bragg

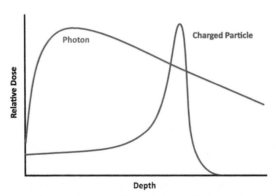

Fig. 2. Photon beams (*red*) typically reach their maximum dose at a lower depth followed by a slow fall-off region. Charged particles (*blue*) may improve normal tissue sparing because most of the dose is deposited at a characteristic depth, the "Bragg peak."

peak") with minimal dose within the build-up and fall-off regions characteristic of photon beams (**Fig. 2**). Therefore, charged particles have the potential to maintain target coverage and further lower dose to surrounding normal organs. Protons may be delivered via 2 techniques: passive scanning 3-dimensional conformal proton therapy and pencil beam scanning intensity-modulated proton therapy.

Dosimetric studies have found better normal tissue sparing with protons versus photon techniques.[15–17] An example of proton versus IMRT dosimetry is shown in **Fig. 3**. Mock and colleagues[15] compared protons with conventional, 3-dimensional, and IMRT photon plans in 5 patients with paranasal sinus carcinoma. Protons reduced the mean dose to all normal structures compared with photon techniques, but the maximum dose to ipsilateral critical structures (adjacent to the postoperative bed) was not significantly different. Similarly, Lomax and colleagues[16] and Chera and colleagues[17] compared IMRT and photon plans in patients with paranasal sinus cancer. Protons and IMRT delivered similar maximum doses to adjacent critical structures, but protons were superior in lowering mean dose to more distant normal tissues. These findings suggest that charged particles may provide significant advantages over IMRT in reducing regions of low dose (eg, 20–50 Gy) but may not have the same perceived advantage for sparing brain and visual pathway structures adjacent to target. Thus, the long-term toxicities of vision loss and other central nervous system (CNS) toxicities may not be significantly reduced with protons compared with IMRT. In addition, sinonasal anatomy constitutes a mixture of air, fluid, and bone that may confound the robustness of proton radiotherapy plans, which are inherently more sensitive to daily changes in tissue heterogeneity. For example, a proton beam planned through a fluid-filled obstructed sinus may unintentionally overdose organs downstream of the target if that obstruction were relieved and that sinus filled with air.[18]

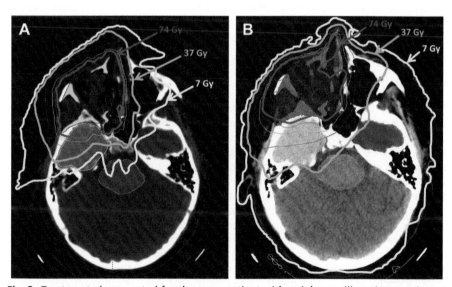

Fig. 3. Treatment plans created for the same patient with a right maxillary sinus carcinoma using 3-dimensional conformal proton therapy (A) versus intensity-modulated photon radiotherapy (B). The high-risk target is shown in shaded blue, with the brainstem and temporal lobes also shown shaded. Dose coverage is shown as labeled contours. Protons reduced average dose to contralateral organs at risk but not maximum dose to ipsilateral structures adjacent to target.

Nonetheless, several centers report promising clinical results using charged particle therapy for sinonasal cancers.[12,19] In addition, charged particle therapy has an established role in skull base chondrosarcoma and chordoma, which are discussed in further detail below. Of note, a large systematic review of single-institutional retrospective studies suggested that charged particle therapy improved survival and cancer control compared with photon therapy in patients with sinonasal tumors, although this analysis is limited by the heterogeneity of patients and inclusion of studies with older (2-dimensional, 3DCRT) radiation techniques in the photon group.[20] Although data for charged particles are encouraging, the lack of widespread access and high cost associated with these facilities limits their routine use.

Stereotactic Body Radiation Therapy

Conceptually, stereotactic body radiation therapy (SBRT) and stereotactic radiosurgery are similar to IMRT but with sharper dose gradients and higher dose per fraction delivered in only 1 to 5 treatments. These highly conformal treatments historically were limited to specialized platforms such as Gamma Knife (Elekta, Stockholm, Sweden) and Cyberknife (Accuray, Sunnyvale, CA, USA), but modern linear accelerators are now capable of similar precision. The use of SBRT is not indicated in the primary treatment of most sinonasal and ventral skull base cancers because of the need to cover large elective regions and concern for excess late toxicity with higher dose per fraction, that is, hypofractionation. However, SBRT may have a role in the setting of reirradiation[21,22] and for small ventral skull base tumors.[23,24]

Reirradiation

Reirradiation for recurrent sinonasal tumors is not usually performed because of the potential for excessive ocular and neurologic toxicities along with poor prognosis; the chance for severe toxicity is often equivalent or even greater than the chance for cure.[25] Nonetheless, there are reports on reirradiation with acceptable toxicity using modern techniques capable of maximal normal tissue sparing such as IMRT,[26] SBRT,[21,22] and charged particles.[27]

RADIATION TOXICITY

Radiotherapy toxicities are divided into acute and late effects. Patients commonly experience acute toxicities that improve after treatment completion such as fatigue, radiation dermatitis, dysgeusia, and mucositis. Late ocular and neurologic toxicity are of particular concern in sinonasal cancer management. **Table 2** shows select studies with detailed late toxicity reporting for relevant normal tissues.[28–34] Critical structures including the retina, optic nerves, chiasm, brain, brainstem, and spinal cord are standardly avoided during radiation therapy planning. Based on dose and volume parameters generated from studies such as those in **Table 2**, radiation therapy plans are optimized to achieve both acceptable normal tissue dose and adequate target coverage. In addition to ocular and neurologic toxicity, long-term survivors may also experience dry mouth, hearing loss, and hypopituitarism. Modern radiotherapy techniques also allow the delineation and sparing of major salivary glands, vestibulocochlear structures, and the hypothalamic-pituitary axis in an effort to reduce these sequelae. Simple measures such as the use of a "bite block" in the mouth during treatment may further reduce toxicity (oral cavity mucositis and xerostomia) by increasing the distance between sinonasal targets and the inferior oral cavity.

Hyperfractionated radiotherapy has been observed to decrease late toxicity. Hyperfractionation typically replaces the once-daily fraction of 1.8 to 2.0 Gy with 2 smaller

Table 2
Select series with detailed reporting of relevant normal tissue dose and toxicity

Series	n	Disease Site	RT Technique	Toxicity
Mayo et al,[28] 2010	Review	Multiple	All	Optic nerve: Significant increase in optic nerve and chiasm toxicity at optic nerve doses >60 Gy (1.8 Gy/fx) and >12 Gy (one fx)
Parsons et al,[29] 1994	131	Head and neck	Non-IMRT	Optic nerve: No toxicity if <59 Gy. In patients receiving ≥60 Gy to nerve, 11% rate of optic neuropathy if <1.9 Gy/fx vs 47% if ≥1.9 Gy/fx
Monroe et al,[30] 2005	186	Sinonasal, nasopharynx	Non-IMRT	Retina: 83% of retinopathy cases occurred with retina doses >60 Gy. Lower rate of retinopathy with hyperfractionation (1.1–1.2 Gy/fx)
Parsons et al,[31] 1994	64	Head and neck	Non-IMRT	Retina: Progressive increase in retinopathy after retina dose 45–55 Gy. More retinopathy if ≥1.9 Gy/fx
McDonald et al,[32] 2015	66	Skull base	Protons	CNS: Temporal lobe V60 Gy >5.5 mL or V70 Gy >1.7 mL predicted 15% 3-y rate of temporal lobe necrosis (any grade)
Shaw et al,[33] 2002	203	Low-grade glioma	Non-IMRT	CNS: Grade 3–5 radiation necrosis occurred in 5% of patients randomized to 64.8 Gy vs 2.5% of patients randomized to 50.4 Gy at 2 y
Hitchcock et al,[34] 2009	66	Head and neck	3DCRT, IMRT	Cochlea: Sensorineural hearing loss increases with cochlea dose >40 Gy

Abbreviations: fx, fraction; V(x)Gy, volume receiving at least (x) Gy.

twice-daily fractions of 1.1 to 1.2 Gy. The rationale behind its use lies in the radiobiologic principle that slow-dividing cells (ie, neurons) are more sensitive to large fraction size, whereas tumor cells respond equally as long as total dose is maintained. In a study of 186 patients with retinal exposure to radiotherapy, those with retina dose greater than 50 Gy receiving hyperfractionation had a 13% rate of radiation retinopathy versus 37% with conventional fractionation. Fractionation schedule and retinal dose were the 2 most significant factors on multivariate analysis.[30] Similarly, Parsons and colleagues[29,31] reported increased optic nerve and retinal toxicity with dose per fraction greater than 1.9 Gy.

RADIOTHERAPY PLANNING

Radiation targets for head and neck cancer typically consist of (1) a high-risk clinical target volume receiving 60 to 74.4 Gy that encompasses gross tumor, postoperative bed, regions of positive margin, and regions with nodal extracapsular extension and (2) an elective standard-risk target volume receiving 45 to 54 Gy that encompasses regions at risk for microscopic disease spread. To account for setup error and motion, each clinical target volume is expanded around 3 to 5 mm to create the final planning target volume (PTV).

Target Delineation

For sinonasal and ventral skull base cancer specifically, the authors recommend creating 2 target volumes and 2 separate IMRT plans. The high-risk volume includes gross tumor or postoperative bed with an additional margin, and should be treated to 60 to 74.4 Gy using 1.2 Gy fractions twice daily: 60 to 64.6 Gy for margin-negative resections, 64.6 to 69.6 Gy for close or positive margins, and 74.4 Gy for gross disease. The standard-risk volume includes adjacent sinuses (eg, maxillary, ethmoid, frontal, sphenoid) with associated sinonasal passages and base of skull (eg, clivus and cribriform plate) and is prescribed 45.6 Gy using 1.2 Gy fractions twice daily. In cases of substantial perineural invasion, the cavernous sinus and Meckel's cave may be included, with the elective volume sometimes extending to the brainstem. **Fig. 4** shows an example of clinical target volume delineation for IMRT planning. Given the priority placed on sparing critical structures discussed above, patients are at risk for marginal failures adjacent to or outside of carefully designed radiotherapy target volumes. In a patterns of failure analysis of patients at our institution who had local failure after treatment for sinonasal cancer, more than half failed marginally or out of field, with all such failures overlapping less than 39% with the prescribed dose volume. Most of these failures were above the original tumor location at or superior to eye level, suggesting that they were related to efforts to preserve vision during surgery or radiation therapy.[35] Given that doses of 45 to 54 Gy (less than optic pathway and brainstem tolerance) are used for standard-risk volumes, it may be reasonable to extend these volumes into the superior sinuses and ventral skull base to prevent such recurrences.

Elective Nodal Irradiation

The benefit of elective nodal irradiation (ENI) is unclear, as most disease progresses or recurs locally.[35] Although some studies suggest minimal benefit for elective neck treatment,[5] others report regional failure rates between 10% and 20% if ENI is omitted in the N0 neck, with the ipsilateral level 1 to 2 neck the most common sites of

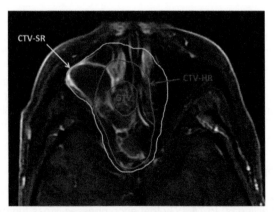

Fig. 4. Clinical target volume delineation using MRI in a patient with T4 ethmoid squamous cell carcinoma treated with definitive IMRT using twice-daily hyperfractionation. The gross target volume (GTV) is delineated in the center. The high-risk clinical target volume (CTV-HR) prescribed 74.4 Gy is delineated in pink and includes GTV and adjacent regions. The elective standard risk clinical target volume (CTV-SR) prescribed 45.6 Gy is delineated in green and includes an additional margin and extension to cover unilateral sinuses.

failure.[36,37] Many of the series reporting high rates of neck failures included patients with mostly maxillary sinus squamous cell carcinoma.[36–38] One large series of 704 patients reported an 8% nodal positivity at presentation and 13% 5-year nodal failure rate for maxillary tumors versus only 2% and 4%, respectively, for ethmoid tumors.[39] There are also reports of frequent neck failures in patients with other histologies, such as esthesioneuroblastoma.[40,41] Elective nodal irradiation is, therefore, indicated for all maxillary sinus squamous cell carcinomas and may be considered for other tumor histologies and locations. In these cases, we usually treat the retropharyngeal nodes and level 1 to 3 neck, covering bilateral nodes if the primary tumor approaches or crosses midline. As elective neck radiation appears to be efficacious, neck dissection may not be needed for the radiographically node-negative neck.

Balancing Target Coverage Versus Normal Tissue Sparing

Radiotherapy treatment planning for sinonasal and ventral skull base malignancies is challenging. The dilemma is whether to sacrifice important organs for maximization of tumor control probability or vice versa. The high-risk PTV for sinonasal tumors frequently abuts or overlaps critical organs including optic nerve, chiasm, and brainstem. The degree of compromise on target coverage depends on the magnitude of deficit expected if severe toxicity occurs; the risk of some unilateral vision loss may be tolerated, but spinal cord/brainstem paralysis and bilateral blindness are always unacceptable. The authors, therefore, compromise on target volume coverage by underdosing or adjusting the PTVs to not overlap with the brainstem, spinal cord, and optic chiasm. The maximum dose is limited to 60 Gy (to 0.1 mL) for brainstem and optic chiasm and 50 Gy for spinal cord. In cases in which the PTV abuts these critical structures, it is not uncommon for only 80% to 90% of the PTV to receive the full prescription dose. For the temporal lobes, we minimize dose heterogeneity, limiting the maximum temporal lobe dose to the prescription dose. Generally, doses greater than the tolerance limits to ipsilateral optic nerve and retina are allowed, with the trade-off being improvement in target coverage but acceptance of increased risk of unilateral vision loss. The authors council patients that this risk is a real possibility and that the compromise is necessary to improve tumor control. As discussed above, the authors recommend hyperfractionation using twice-daily fractions of 1.2 Gy for most cases to minimize the chance of vision loss.[29–31]

SPECIFIC CONSIDERATIONS
Nasal Cavity Tumors

Nasal cavity tumors are subject to the same concerns as other paranasal sinus cancers. Although surgery with postoperative radiotherapy is the standard, radiotherapy alone may be used successfully in stage I to II (T1–T2, N0) tumors and may be considered when there are concerns about cosmesis or operability. Allen and colleagues[42] reported their experience with 32 patients treated with definitive radiation therapy alone to a median dose of 65 Gy. With median follow-up of 11 years, 5-year locoregional control was 81% and OS was 94%, with few serious adverse events.

Adenoid Cystic Carcinoma

Adenoid cystic carcinomas are a subset of minor salivary gland carcinomas and are characterized by their propensity to spread along nerves and recur both locally and distally. In a report on 208 patients with paranasal sinus cancer, the rate of perineural invasion was 55% for adenoid cystic carcinomas and 60% for sinonasal undifferentiated carcinomas but less than 25% for all other histologies.[43] Because adenoid cystic carcinoma may have a prolonged natural history, prevention of potentially symptomatic local recurrence is paramount.[19,44] The authors recommend postoperative radiotherapy for all resected adenoid cystic carcinomas regardless of stage, with coverage of involved or nearby cranial nerves to at least the ventral skull base foramina, often tracking back to the cavernous sinus and surface of the brainstem. The authors do not electively treat neck nodes in patients with sinonasal adenoid cystic carcinoma.

Esthesioneuroblastoma

Esthesioneuroblastomas are tumors that arise from olfactory epithelium and are treated with a combination of surgery and radiation therapy. A systematic review of 26 studies and 390 patients reported superior survival in patients who received both surgery and radiation therapy versus either modality alone.[45] A recent population-based analysis also showed an overall survival benefit of radiation therapy for high-grade tumors, although no such benefit was seen for low-grade tumors.[46] Radiation doses greater than 54 Gy may be associated with improved outcomes.[47] Several studies also suggest that regional failures are common, supporting consideration of elective nodal irradiation for esthesioneuroblastoma. MD Anderson reported an 18% rate of nodal failure in 49 patients who did not receive ENI, versus no nodal relapses in 22 patients who received ENI.[40] Similarly, the University of Michigan reported a 27% rate of regional nodal failure without elective neck treatment.[41] In these series, salvage was successfully performed in only 60% of those who presented with isolated relapses.

Sinonasal Undifferentiated Carcinoma

Sinonasal undifferentiated carcinoma has been recognized as a distinct neuroendocrine tumor subtype characterized by aggressive behavior and poor outcomes. These tumors often present with extensive intracranial extension and are often unresectable at presentation. In a meta-analysis of 167 cases treated between 1986 and 2009, only around 26% of patients remained disease free at a median follow-up of 15 months.[48] Prognosis is especially poor if patients are unable to receive a gross total resection. The authors recently reported promising results with a strategy incorporating preoperative chemoradiation, with 3 of 7 patients having a complete pathologic response at the time of surgery.[49] Given the importance of multidisciplinary management, it may be reasonable to consider neoadjuvant treatment to maximize resectability.

Chondrosarcoma and Chordoma

Chondrosarcomas and chordomas are locally aggressive tumors that present similarly in the ventral skull base. Because of their unfavorable location, gross total resection is often difficult and most patients have residual macroscopic disease after surgery.[50–52] Chordomas have a significantly worse prognosis than chondrosarcomas and are therefore usually managed with postoperative radiation therapy. Adjuvant radiotherapy for chondrosarcomas is also effective, but its use is more controversial because of the generally favorable prognosis and success of surgical salvage. For both, the radiotherapy target includes the tumor bed and areas of gross disease plus a margin to account for local microscopic spread.

Most studies supporting the use of radiotherapy for chondrosarcoma and chondroma used protons or carbon ions. Several large European series report long-term control of more than 90% for chondrosarcomas and 60% for chordomas, and a randomized trial is ongoing comparing protons and carbon ions.[50–52] The lack of comparable data for photons may be attributable to the inability to safely use adequate doses in the ventral skull base region with older radiation techniques. One such study used photons delivering 50 Gy in the treatment of chordoma and reported only 27% local control.[53]

However, modern series using IMRT and SBRT to deliver higher doses report rates of control approaching those achieved with charged particle therapy.[23,24,54]

Inverted Papilloma

The role of radiation therapy for inverted papillomas is limited to patients with carcinoma in situ or invasive features found after resection. Although little data exist to support the practice, radiotherapy is recommended in these cases to prevent progression to frank invasive sinonasal cancer. The importance of prevention is supported by a recent Chinese study that reviewed 213 patients with inverted papilloma diagnosed over several decades. Eighty-seven (40%) of these patients eventually had malignant transformation, which was associated with a 5-year OS of only 40%.[55]

Nasal Natural Killer T-Cell Lymphoma

Nasal-type natural killer T-cell lymphoma is an Epstein-Barr virus–associated non-Hodgkin lymphoma and is treated nonsurgically. Radiotherapy is a critical component of curative treatment in patients who present with localized disease, with studies reporting long-term survival of roughly 70%.[56] A recent study that included 1273 early-stage patients reported that definitive radiation therapy with or without chemotherapy was more effective than strategies that used induction or primary chemotherapy.[57] Consistent with the involved field technique used for most lymphomas, the radiotherapy target volume should include the entire nasal cavity and adjacent structures including adjacent sinuses and occasionally the nasopharynx. The cervical nodes are included when patients present with positive lymph nodes. In contrast to the lower radiation doses needed for most other lymphomas, doses for definitive treatment of nasal-type natural killer T-cell lymphoma should be on the order of 50 Gy or higher.[56]

SUMMARY

Sinonasal and ventral skull base cancers present significant challenges because of their proximity to critical structures, and multimodality treatments incorporating both surgery and radiation are indicated. Good communication between surgeons and radiation oncologists is necessary for optimal patient care. Modern radiotherapy techniques such as IMRT and charged particle therapy have improved outcomes, but efforts to balance local control with acceptable morbidity may result in marginal and out-of-field failures. Detailed knowledge of anatomy, routes of perineural and sinonasal spread, normal tissue tolerance, and considerations unique to different histologies is critical for safe and effective radiotherapy planning.

REFERENCES

1. Blanco AI, Chao KS, Ozyigit G, et al. Carcinoma of paranasal sinuses: long-term outcomes with radiotherapy. Int J Radiat Oncol Biol Phys 2004;59:51–8.
2. Hoppe BS, Stegman LD, Zelefsky MJ, et al. Treatment of nasal cavity and paranasal sinus cancer with modern radiotherapy techniques in the postoperative setting–the MSKCC experience. Int J Radiat Oncol Biol Phys 2007;67:691–702.
3. Dulguerov P, Jacobsen MS, Allal AS, et al. Nasal and paranasal sinus carcinoma: are we making progress? A series of 220 patients and a systematic review. Cancer 2001;92:3012–29.
4. Chen AM, Daly ME, Bucci MK, et al. Carcinomas of the paranasal sinuses and nasal cavity treated with radiotherapy at a single institution over five decades: are we making improvement? Int J Radiat Oncol Biol Phys 2007;69:141–7.

5. Dirix P, Nuyts S, Geussens Y, et al. Malignancies of the nasal cavity and paranasal sinuses: long-term outcome with conventional or three-dimensional conformal radiotherapy. Int J Radiat Oncol Biol Phys 2007;69:1042–50.

6. Bristol IJ, Ahamad A, Garden AS, et al. Postoperative radiotherapy for maxillary sinus cancer: long-term outcomes and toxicities of treatment. Int J Radiat Oncol Biol Phys 2007;68:719–30.

7. Mendenhall WM, Amdur RJ, Morris CG, et al. Carcinoma of the nasal cavity and paranasal sinuses. Laryngoscope 2009;119:899–906.

8. Duprez F, Madani I, Morbée L, et al. IMRT for sinonasal tumors minimizes severe late ocular toxicity and preserves disease control and survival. Int J Radiat Oncol Biol Phys 2012;83:252–9.

9. Al-Mamgani A, Monserez D, Rooij Pv, et al. Highly-conformal intensity-modulated radiotherapy reduced toxicity without jeopardizing outcome in patients with paranasal sinus cancer treated by surgery and radiotherapy or (chemo)radiation. Oral Oncol 2012;48:905–11.

10. Guntinas-Lichius O, Kreppel MP, Stuetzer H, et al. Single modality and multimodality treatment of nasal and paranasal sinuses cancer: a single institution experience of 229 patients. Eur J Surg Oncol 2007;33:222–8.

11. Hoppe BS, Nelson CJ, Gomez DR, et al. Unresectable carcinoma of the paranasal sinuses: outcomes and toxicities. Int J Radiat Oncol Biol Phys 2008;72:763–9.

12. Zenda S, Kohno R, Kawashima M, et al. Proton beam therapy for unresectable malignancies of the nasal cavity and paranasal sinuses. Int J Radiat Oncol Biol Phys 2011;81:1473–8.

13. Huang D, Xia P, Akazawa P, et al. Comparison of treatment plans using intensity-modulated radiotherapy and three-dimensional conformal radiotherapy for paranasal sinus carcinoma. Int J Radiat Oncol Biol Phys 2003;56:158–68.

14. Dirix P, Vanstraelen B, Jorissen M, et al. Intensity-modulated radiotherapy for sinonasal cancer: improved outcome compared to conventional radiotherapy. Int J Radiat Oncol Biol Phys 2010;78:998–1004.

15. Mock U, Georg D, Bogner J, et al. Treatment planning comparison of conventional, 3D conformal, and intensity-modulated photon (IMRT) and proton therapy for paranasal sinus carcinoma. Int J Radiat Oncol Biol Phys 2004;58:147–54.

16. Lomax AJ, Goitein M, Adams J. Intensity modulation in radiotherapy: photons versus protons in the paranasal sinus. Radiother Oncol 2003;66:11–8.

17. Chera BS, Malyapa R, Louis D, et al. Proton therapy for maxillary sinus carcinoma. Am J Clin Oncol 2009;32:296–303.

18. Park PC, Zhu XR, Lee AK, et al. A beam-specific planning target volume (PTV) design for proton therapy to account for setup and range uncertainties. Int J Radiat Oncol Biol Phys 2012;82:e329–36.

19. Jensen AD, Poulakis M, Nikoghosyan AV, et al. High-LET radiotherapy for adenoid cystic carcinoma of the head and neck: 15 years' experience with raster-scanned carbon ion therapy. Radiother Oncol 2016;118:272–80.

20. Patel SH, Wang Z, Wong WW, et al. Charged particle therapy versus photon therapy for paranasal sinus and nasal cavity malignant diseases: a systematic review and meta-analysis. Lancet Oncol 2014;15:1027–38.

21. Unger KR, Lominska CE, Deeken JF, et al. Fractionated stereotactic radiosurgery for reirradiation of head-and-neck cancer. Int J Radiat Oncol Biol Phys 2010;77:1411–9.

22. Xu KM, Quan K, Clump DA, et al. Stereotactic ablative radiosurgery for locally advanced or recurrent skull base malignancies with prior external beam radiation therapy. Front Oncol 2015;5:65.
23. Kano H, Iqbal FO, Sheehan J, et al. Stereotactic radiosurgery for chordoma: a report from the North American Gamma Knife Consortium. Neurosurgery 2011; 68:379–89.
24. Kano H, Sheehan J, Sneed PK, et al. Skull base chondrosarcoma radiosurgery: report of the North American Gamma Knife Consortium. J Neurosurg 2015;123: 1268–75.
25. De Crevoisier R, Bourhis J, Domenge C, et al. Full-dose reirradiation for unresectable head and neck carcinoma: experience at the Gustave-Roussy Institute in a series of 169 patients. J Clin Oncol 1998;16:3556–62.
26. Duprez F, Madani I, Bonte K, et al. Intensity-modulated radiotherapy for recurrent and second primary head and neck cancer in previously irradiated territory. Radiother Oncol 2009;93:563–9.
27. McDonald MW, Linton OR, Shah MV. Proton therapy for reirradiation of progressive or recurrent chordoma. Int J Radiat Oncol Biol Phys 2013;87:1107–14.
28. Mayo C, Martel MK, Marks LB, et al. Radiation dose-volume effects of optic nerves and chiasm. Int J Radiat Oncol Biol Phys 2010;76:S28–35.
29. Parsons JT, Bova FJ, Fitzgerald CR, et al. Radiation optic neuropathy after megavoltage external-beam irradiation: analysis of time-dose factors. Int J Radiat Oncol Biol Phys 1994;30:755–63.
30. Monroe AT, Bhandare N, Morris CG, et al. Preventing radiation retinopathy with hyperfractionation. Int J Radiat Oncol Biol Phys 2005;61:856–64.
31. Parsons JT, Bova FJ, Fitzgerald CR, et al. Radiation retinopathy after external-beam irradiation: analysis of time-dose factors. Int J Radiat Oncol Biol Phys 1994;30:765–73.
32. McDonald MW, Linton OR, Calley CS. Dose-volume relationships associated with temporal lobe radiation necrosis after skull base proton beam therapy. Int J Radiat Oncol Biol Phys 2015;91:261–7.
33. Shaw E, Arusell R, Scheithauer B. Prospective randomized trial of low- versus high-dose radiation therapy in adults with supratentorial low-grade glioma: initial report of a North Central Cancer Treatment Group/Radiation Therapy Oncology Group/Eastern Cooperative Oncology Group study. J Clin Oncol 2002;20: 2267–76.
34. Hitchcock YJ, Tward JD, Szabo A, et al. Relative contributions of radiation and cisplatin-based chemotherapy to sensorineural hearing loss in head-and-neck cancer patients. Int J Radiat Oncol Biol Phys 2009;73:779–88.
35. Fried DV, Zanation AM, Huang B, et al. Patterns of local failure for sinonasal malignancies. Pract Radiat Oncol 2013;3:e113–20.
36. Le QT, Fu KK, Kaplan MJ, et al. Lymph node metastasis in maxillary sinus carcinoma. Int J Radiat Oncol Biol Phys 2000;46:541–9.
37. Guan X, Wang X, Liu Y, et al. Lymph node metastasis in sinonasal squamous cell carcinoma treated with IMRT/3D-CRT. Oral Oncol 2013;49:60–5.
38. Abu-Ghanem S, Horowitz G, Abergel A, et al. Elective neck irradiation versus observation in squamous cell carcinoma of the maxillary sinus with N0 neck: A meta-analysis and review of the literature. Head Neck 2015;37:1823–8.
39. Cantù G, Bimbi G, Miceli R, et al. Lymph node metastases in malignant tumors of the paranasal sinuses: prognostic value and treatment. Arch Otolaryngol Head Neck Surg 2008;134:170–7.

40. Jiang W, Mohamed AS, Fuller CD, et al. The role of elective nodal irradiation for esthesioneuroblastoma patients with clinically negative neck. Pract Radiat Oncol 2016;6(4):241–7.
41. Demiroz C, Gutfeld O, Aboziada M, et al. Esthesioneuroblastoma: is there a need for elective neck treatment? Int J Radiat Oncol Biol Phys 2011;81:e255–61.
42. Allen MW, Schwartz DL, Rana V, et al. Long-term radiotherapy outcomes for nasal cavity and septal cancers. Int J Radiat Oncol Biol Phys 2008;71:401–6.
43. Gil Z, Carlson DL, Gupta A, et al. Patterns and incidence of neural invasion in patients with cancers of the paranasal sinuses. Arch Otolaryngol Head Neck Surg 2009;135:173–9.
44. Ramakrishna R, Raza SM, Kupferman M, et al. Adenoid cystic carcinoma of the skull base: results with an aggressive multidisciplinary approach. J Neurosurg 2016;124:115–21.
45. Dulguerov P, Allal AS, Calcaterra TC. Esthesioneuroblastoma: a meta-analysis and review. Lancet Oncol 2001;2:683–90.
46. Tajudeen BA, Arshi A, Suh JD, et al. Importance of tumor grade in esthesioneuroblastoma survival: a population-based analysis. JAMA Otolaryngol Head Neck Surg 2014;140:1124–9.
47. Ozsahin M, Gruber G, Olszyk O, et al. Outcome and prognostic factors in olfactory neuroblastoma: a rare cancer network study. Int J Radiat Oncol Biol Phys 2010;78:992–7.
48. Reiersen DA, Pahilan ME, Devaiah AK. Meta-analysis of treatment outcomes for sinonasal undifferentiated carcinoma. Otolaryngol Head Neck Surg 2012; 147:7–14.
49. Fried D, Zanation AM, Huang B, et al. Management of nonesthesioneuroblastoma sinonasal malignancies with neuroendocrine differentiation. Laryngoscope 2012; 122:2210–5.
50. Feuvret L, Bracci S, Calugaru V, et al. Efficacy and Safety of Adjuvant Proton Therapy Combined With Surgery for Chondrosarcoma of the Skull Base: A Retrospective, Population-Based Study. Int J Radiat Oncol Biol Phys 2016;95:312–21.
51. Uhl M, Mattke M, Welzel T, et al. Highly effective treatment of skull base chordoma with carbon ion irradiation using a raster scan technique in 155 patients: first long-term results. Cancer 2014;120:3410–7.
52. Uhl M, Mattke M, Welzel T, et al. High control rate in patients with chondrosarcoma of the skull base after carbon ion therapy: first report of long-term results. Cancer 2014;120:1579–85.
53. Catton C, O'Sullivan B, Bell R, et al. Chordoma: long-term follow-up after radical photon irradiation. Radiother Oncol 1996;41:67–72.
54. Sahgal A, Chan MW, Atenafu EG, et al. Image-guided, intensity-modulated radiation therapy (IG-IMRT) for skull base chordoma and chondrosarcoma: preliminary outcomes. Neuro Oncol 2015;17:889–94.
55. Liang QZ, Li DZ, Wang XL, et al. Survival Outcome of Squamous Cell Carcinoma Arising from Sinonasal Inverted Papilloma. Chin Med J (Engl) 2015;128:2457–61.
56. Li YX, Liu QF, Wang WH, et al. Failure patterns and clinical implications in early stage nasal natural killer/T-cell lymphoma treated with primary radiotherapy. Cancer 2011;117:5203–11.
57. Yang Y, Zhu Y, Cao JZ, et al. Risk-adapted therapy for early-stage extranodal nasal-type NK/T-cell lymphoma: analysis from a multicenter study. Blood 2015; 126:1424–32.

The Role of Chemotherapy in the Management of Sinonasal and Ventral Skull Base Malignancies

George A. Scangas, MD[a],*, Jean Anderson Eloy, MD[b],
Derrick T. Lin, MD[c]

KEYWORDS

- Chemotherapy • Sinonasal cancer • Sinonasal tumor • Multimodality therapy
- Systemic treatment • Neoadjuvant chemotherapy

KEY POINTS

- In most cases of advanced sinonasal and ventral skull base cancer, a multimodal treatment approach provides the best chance for improved outcomes.
- Depending on the tumor type and extent of disease, systemic chemotherapy has been shown to play an important role in neoadjuvant, concomitant, and adjuvant settings.
- Prospective, high-quality studies are needed to understand ideal chemotherapeutic regimens and their role and sequential timing in sinonasal and ventral skull base cancer.

INTRODUCTION

Sinonasal cancer (SNC) represents less than 3% of all head and neck cancers with an overall incidence of less than 0.001%.[1] Although more than half of tumors originate in the nasal cavity, tumors may also frequently originate in the maxillary or ethmoid sinuses.[2] Due to the wide array of tumor histology and molecular profiles, as well as close proximity of vital structures, such as the brain and orbit, treatment planning can be complex. A multimodality therapeutic approach with complete surgical resection with postoperative radiotherapy remains standard of care.[3] The advancement of

Disclosures: None.
[a] Department of Otolaryngology, Massachusetts Eye and Ear Infirmary, Harvard Medical School, 243 Charles Street, Boston, MA 02114, USA; [b] Endoscopic Skull Base Surgery Program, Department of Otolaryngology - Head and Neck Surgery, Rhinology and Sinus Surgery, Otolaryngology Research, Neurological Institute of New Jersey, Rutgers New Jersey Medical School, 185 South Orange Avenue, Newark, NJ 07103, USA; [c] Division of Head and Neck Oncology, Massachusetts Eye and Ear Infirmary, Massachusetts General Hospital, Harvard Medical School, 243 Charles Street, Boston, MA 02114, USA
* Corresponding author.
E-mail address: George_Scangas@meei.harvard.edu

endoscopic approaches as well as intensity-modulated radiation and proton therapy has improved survival and outcomes.[4-6]

Despite these advances, the overall prognosis of patients with advanced SNC remains poor, with a reported 5-year survival rate of 30%.[2] Following the treatment paradigm of other head and neck cancers, physicians have investigated the hypothesis that the inclusion of chemotherapy in the treatment of SNC may improve locoregional control rates and reduce the frequency of metastasis, ultimately resulting in improved survival. Classically, the role of chemotherapy in SNC has been limited to palliative treatment of locally advanced or metastatic SNC.[3] This role has expanded, however, to neoadjuvant, concurrent, or adjuvant settings in appropriate patient cohorts. This article explores the role of systemic therapy in the management of SNC.

NEOADJUVANT CHEMOTHERAPY

Due primarily to the rare nature of SNC, no prospective, randomized trials have been performed examining the efficacy of neoadjuvant chemotherapy. Single-center studies have used chemotherapy protocols extrapolated from the head and neck literature, such as the larynx preservation studies. In addition, interpretation of such studies has been complicated by the inclusion of patient cohorts with varying histologic tumor types.[2] As in all cases of neoadjuvant therapy, the potential benefit of optimal drug delivery through an intact tumor blood supply is weighed against the potential of delaying multimodal locoregional treatment due to systemic toxicity.[7] Despite these limitations, single-center studies on neoadjuvant chemotherapy for advanced SNC have shown promising results (**Table 1**).

A 2003 study from Licitra and colleagues[8] investigated neoadjuvant 5-fluorouracil, cisplatin, and leucovorin in 49 patients with resectable paranasal sinus tumors. Although the 3-year overall survival rate was 69% and the achievement of a pathologic complete response predicted a favorable outcome, significant morbidity was reported. Namely, 2 deaths due to thromboembolic events as well as 8 cases of cardiac complications resulting in discontinued therapy were reported. In 2011, Hanna and colleagues[9] published a retrospective series of 46 patients with sinonasal squamous cell carcinoma treated with a combination of neoadjuvant platinum and taxane or taxane and 5-fluorouracil followed by either chemoradiation or surgery and radiotherapy; 80% of patients had stage IV disease. Despite this advanced disease stage at presentation, response to neoadjuvant chemotherapy was reported in 67% of patients and predicted treatment outcome and prognosis. This effect was independent of subsequent choice of locoregional therapy.

Although these studies analyzed SNCs with differing histologies, the results highlight the potential benefit of neoadjuvant chemotherapy in the multimodal treatment of advanced SNC. In the future, efforts should focus on elucidating the effect of induction chemotherapy on varying tumor types to allow for development of disease-specific protocols.

CONCURRENT CHEMOTHERAPY

Advanced head and neck cancer has been successfully treated with concurrent chemoradiotherapy,[10] but data regarding its use in SNC remain less robust. Recent evidence suggests that concomitant chemotherapy and radiotherapy can achieve promising survival and locoregional control rates in certain cases of SNC.[11] Protocols typically describe weekly carboplatin regimens.[12-14] Individualized concurrent chemotherapy with cetuximab has been described in patients whose tumors overexpress epidermal growth factor receptor.[15]

Table 1
Trials of systemic therapy by histologic subtype

Tumor Type	Study	Stage of Tumors	Chemotherapy Regimen	N	Outcomes
PSSCC	Rosen et al,[13] 1993	Stage IV	NA 5-fluorouracil and cisplatin	9	2-y DFS 92%
	Björk-Eriksson et al,[22] 1992	Stages III and IV	NA 5-fluorouracil and cisplatin	8	4-y DFS 83%
Adenocarcinoma	Licitra et al,[28] 2004	AJCC I–IVb	NA cisplatin, 5-fluorouracil, and leucovorin	30	55-mo DFS in pCR 100%
SNUC	Musy et al,[32] 2002	Kadish B and C	Variable NA regimens	10	2-y OS 64%
	Rischin et al,[33] 2004	Stage 4	NA platinum and 5-Fluorouracil	7	2-y OS 64%
SNEC	Rosenthal et al,[35] 2004	Stages II–IV	NA	8	5-y OS 64% DMR 14%
ONB	Loy et al,[39] 2006	Kadish C	NA vincristine and cyclophosphamide	50	5-y DFS 87% 15-y DFS 83%
SNPMM	Lian et al,[49] 2013	Stage II–III	Adjuvant temozolomide and cisplatin	63	Significant improvement in DFS over surgery alone
Sarcoma	Callender et al,[53] 1995	Various stages	Various regimens	24	5-y OS 60%

Abbreviations: AJCC, American Joint Committee on Cancer; DFS, disease-free survival; DMR, distant metastasis rate; NA, neoadjuvant; OS, overall survival rate; pCR, pathologic complete responders.

Comparative studies demonstrating a statistically significant survival benefit for concurrent chemoradiotherapy compared with neoadjuvant chemotherapy, however, have not yet been performed. A 2008 retrospective study by Hoppe and colleagues[12] analyzed survival in 39 patients with unresectable stage IVB SNC, 35 of whom received concurrent chemoradiotherapy (82% with cisplatin). With a median follow-up of 90 months, overall survival rate was only 15%. Furthermore, the importance of surgical resection was highlighted in a 2012 retrospective review of resectable maxillary sinus tumors treated with either surgery with adjuvant chemoradiation or concurrent primary chemoradiotherapy alone. Patients in the surgical arm had statistically significant better progression-free survival as well as overall survival. Ultimately, prospective, comparative studies are needed to further inform physicians on the role of concurrent chemoradiotherapy in advanced cases of SNC.

INTRA-ARTERIAL CHEMOTHERAPY

The intra-arterial approach to directly delivering chemotherapy to advanced SNC remains largely an experimental option. In 2004, Samant and colleagues[16] examined the long-term efficacy of intra-arterial cisplatin and concomitant radiotherapy followed by organ-preserving surgery in 19 patients. Of those patients, there were 14 with squamous cell carcinoma, 2 with adenocarcinoma, 2 with adenoid cystic carcinoma, and 1 with undifferentiated carcinoma. They reported that overall survival rates at 2 and 5 years were 68% and 53%, respectively, and concluded that despite the advanced level of the SNC, intra-arterial chemotherapy holds promise as a treatment option. Despite exciting organ-preservation rates, intra-arterial chemotherapy carries substantial risk of toxicity,[11,17] including brain necrosis, osteonecrosis, and ocular complications, including loss of vision, which have limited its application in the treatment of advanced SNC.

THE ROLE OF CHEMOTHERAPY IN SPECIFIC TUMOR TYPES

Depending on the tumor type and extent of disease, systemic chemotherapy has been shown to play an important role in various phases of care including neoadjuvant, concomitant, and adjuvant settings (see **Table 1**).

Squamous Cell Carcinoma

Although paranasal sinus squamous cell carcinoma (PSSCC) accounts for 3% of all head and neck malignancies, no randomized trials have been conducted to guide management decisions.[18] Reported prognostic factors for PSSCC include disease stage, site of origin, histopathology, and patient characteristics.[19] The combination of radiation therapy and surgery has demonstrated superiority compared with radiotherapy alone, which was the original treatment of choice.[20,21] For PSSCC involving the orbit, dura, or brain, induction chemotherapy followed by concurrent chemoradiation or surgery followed by radiation therapy remain the considered options.[20,22] Degree of response to chemotherapy can also be used to direct chemotherapy/radiation therapy before surgery.[23] The decision to undergo adjuvant therapy is based on extent of tumor, stage, subsite, and various prognostic indicators, including orbital involvement, perineural invasion, and dural involvement.[24] If nonsurgical treatment is chosen, post-treatment biopsy and PET scanning can be used to assess persistent disease, recurrent disease, and distant metastasis.[20,25] Despite these guidelines, disease-free survival for advanced (stage III or IV) PSSCC is reported as low as 25% to 30%,[14] underscoring the importance of early detection and aggressive treatment.

Adenocarcinoma

Adenocarcinoma is reported as 1 of the 3 most common tumor types within the sino-nasal passages.[20] Normally classified as a primary SNC of minor salivary origin, this tumor is classically treated with surgery followed by radiation therapy in the setting of high-grade disease or positive margins[24,26] Chemotherapy has not been shown to provide a survival advantage for sinonasal adenocarcinoma.[26] Studies out of Italy have shown, however, that the use of cisplatin, 5-fluorouracil, and leucovorin induction chemotherapy can be justified in a specific subset of patients with advanced sinonasal intestinal-type adenocarcinoma with functional p53 status.[27,28]

Sinonasal Undifferentiated Carcinoma

Sinonasal undifferentiated carcinomas (SNUCs) are characterized by very aggressive local destruction, high rates of regional and distant metastasis, and poor overall sur-vival.[29] Although optimum treatment varies from patient to patient, multimodality ther-apy has been reported as the preferred approach.[29,30] Several studies have focused on establishing the chemosensitivity of SNUC. A 2012 meta-analysis of data from 167 SNUC patients reported improved patient survival with the addition of systemic ther-apy to surgery.[31]

Induction and concomitant chemoradiotherapy for SNUCs have yielded reasonable locoregional control rates. In 2002, Musy and colleagues[32] demonstrated a 2-year overall survival rate of 64% with the addition of induction chemotherapy and radiation therapy prior to anterior craniofacial resection. A 2004 study by Rischin and col-leagues[33] reported a 2-year overall survival rate of 64% in 10 patients treated with in-duction chemotherapy followed by chemoradiotherapy. Although these and other single-institution reviews need confirmation by prospective studies, they suggest that SNUC may be a chemosensitive disease with potential to improve local control and decrease the rate of distant metastasis through the addition of systemic therapy.[2,20]

SINONASAL NEUROENDOCRINE CARCINOMA

Although considered a separate entity from SNUC, sinonasal neuroendocrine carci-nomas (SNECs) are similarly considered susceptible to systemic therapy as part of multimodal treatment.[34] Specific reported protocols include cisplatin plus etoposide or 5-fluorouracil and carboplatin plus etoposide or docetaxel.[2] In a 2004 study by Rosenthal and colleagues,[35] 18 patients with SNEC were treated with multimodality therapy, including induction chemotherapy, in 8 of 18 patients, with encouraging out-comes of 64% 5-year overall survival rate and 14% distant metastasis rate. A pro-spective study by Fitzek and colleagues[36] of 18 patients with a mixture of SNEC and olfactory neuroblastoma (ONB) concluded that neoadjuvant chemotherapy plus high-dose proton therapy remains a successful treatment approach. Until larger studies are conducted, multimodality therapy should be favored in the treatment of advanced SNEC.

Olfactory Neuroblastoma/Esthesioneuroblastoma

ONB is a rare tumor arising from the olfactory neuroepithelium that is typically locally aggressive with an overall better prognosis than other SNCs.[2,37] Surgery followed by radiation therapy and upfront chemoradiotherapy with planned or surgical salvage remain the 2 most common treatment options. Eich and colleagues[38] reported superior 5-year event-free survival rates for patients with advanced ONB treated with multimo-dality therapy (74% vs 41%, respectively), albeit with no difference in overall survival.

Upfront surgical excision with adjuvant radiation therapy has traditionally been the treatment of choice. Rosenthal and colleagues[35] reported a series of 31 patients with ONB treated with upfront surgery from 1982 to 2002 with a 5-year survival rate of 93%, a 5-year local control rate of 96%, and a regional failure rate of only 9%. In comparison, 50 patients with ONB out of the University of Virginia treated with neoadjuvant vincristine and cyclophosphamide achieved 5-year and 15-year disease-free survival rates of 87% and 83%, respectively.[39]

Although cervical lymphatic metastasis is reported as less common in ONB compared with other SNCs, it likely portends an extremely unfavorable prognosis.[40,41] Long-term follow-up remains crucial for these patients; 1 study reported that although less than 10% of patients presented with nodal disease, 25% developed nodal disease at a mean time interval of 6 years post-treatment.[42]

Sinonasal Primary Mucosal Melanoma

Sinonasal primary mucosal melanomas (SNPMMs), which arise from melanocytes located in the nasal cavity, often present with advanced stage and consequently portend a worse prognosis than cutaneous melanomas.[20] Despite aggressive multimodal therapy, local recurrence and distant metastasis rates remain high.[43]

The decision of upfront surgery versus neoadjuvant chemoradiation is usually dictated by the extent of disease at presentation.[44] The current role of chemotherapy in the treatment of SNPMM includes palliative treatment and for patients with metastatic disease.[45] Recent work suggests, however, that multimodal first-line treatment, including chemotherapy, may have a role for locally aggressive forms of SNPMM.[46,47] Specifically, a good response to the use of an upfront chemotherapeutic agent in combination with a biologic agent in patients with metastatic disease, unresectable tumors, or extracapsular spread has been shown to be a favorable prognostic factor for long-term survival.[48]

The role of adjuvant chemotherapy in SNPMM was studied in a phase II randomized trial that reported median relapse-free survival was significantly prolonged with chemotherapy compared with interferon and observation.[49] Finally, targeted therapies, such as imatinib for tumors with KIT mutations, the use of the monoclonal antibody ipilimumab, and anti–PD-1 receptor therapy, may offer viable treatment options in the near future.[50–52]

SARCOMA

The role of chemotherapy in sarcomas depends on the histologic subtype. A retrospective study on rhabdomyosarcomas of the nose and paranasal sinuses reported that a combination of chemotherapy and radiotherapy provided the best locoregional control, with a 5-year overall survival rate of 60%.[53] In comparison, chemotherapy remains experimental in adult soft tissue sarcomas, because studies have shown inconclusive or poor results for both neoadjuvant and adjuvant therapy.[54,55] The role of chemotherapy is inconclusive in sinonasal chondrosarcoma,[56] whereas surgery and adjuvant chemotherapy remain the most common multimodal treatments of sinonasal osteosarcoma.[57]

SUMMARY

In most cases of advanced SNC, a multimodal treatment approach provides the best chance for improved outcomes. Depending on the tumor type and extent of disease, systemic chemotherapy has been shown to play an important role in various phases of care, including neoadjuvant, concomitant, and adjuvant settings. The lack of randomized trials continues to limit its indications. Further high-quality studies are needed to understand ideal chemotherapeutic regimens and their role and sequential timing in SNC.

REFERENCES

1. Turner JH, Reh DD. Incidence and survival in patients with sinonasal cancer: a historical analysis of population-based data. Head Neck 2012;34:877–85.
2. Bossi P, Saba NF, Vermorken JB, et al. The role of systemic therapy in the management of sinonasal cancer: a critical review. Cancer Treat Rev 2015;41:836–43.
3. Llorente JL, López F, Suárez C, et al. Sinonasal carcinoma: clinical, pathological, genetic and therapeutic advances. Nat Rev Clin Oncol 2014;11:460–72.
4. Su SY, Kupferman ME, DeMonte F, et al. Endoscopic resection of sinonasal cancers. Curr Oncol Rep 2014;16:369.
5. Duprez F, Madani I, Morbée L, et al. IMRT for sinonasal tumors minimizes severe late ocular toxicity and preserves disease control and survival. Int J Radiat Oncol Biol Phys 2012;83:252–9.
6. Alonso-Basanta M, Lustig RA, Kennedy DW. Proton beam therapy in skull base pathology. Otolaryngol Clin North Am 2011;44:1173–83.
7. Hoffmann TK. Systemic therapy strategies for head-neck carcinomas: current status. Laryngorhinootologie 2012;91(Suppl 1):S123–43 [in German].
8. Licitra L, Locati LD, Cavina R, et al. Primary chemotherapy followed by anterior craniofacial resection and radiotherapy for paranasal cancer. Ann Oncol 2003; 14:367–72.
9. Hanna EY, Cardenas AD, DeMonte F, et al. Induction chemotherapy for advanced squamous cell carcinoma of the paranasal sinuses. Arch Otolaryngol Head Neck Surg 2011;137:78–81.
10. Forastiere AA, Goepfert H, Maor M, et al. Concurrent chemotherapy and radiotherapy for organ preservation in advanced laryngeal cancer. N Engl J Med 2003;349:2091–8.
11. Homma A, Oridate N, Suzuki F, et al. Superselective high-dose cisplatin infusion with concomitant radiotherapy in patients with advanced cancer of the nasal cavity and paranasal sinuses: a single institution experience. Cancer 2009;115: 4705–14.
12. Hoppe BS, Nelson CJ, Gomez DR, et al. Unresectable carcinoma of the paranasal sinuses: outcomes and toxicities. Int J Radiat Oncol Biol Phys 2008;72: 763–9.
13. Rosen A, Vokes EE, Scher N, et al. Locoregionally advanced paranasal sinus carcinoma. Favorable survival with multimodality therapy. Arch Otolaryngol Head Neck Surg 1993;119:743–6.
14. Lee MM, Vokes EE, Rosen A, et al. Multimodality therapy in advanced paranasal sinus carcinoma: superior long-term results. Cancer J Sci Am 1999;5:219–23.
15. Kies MS, Holsinger FC, Lee JJ, et al. Induction chemotherapy and cetuximab for locally advanced squamous cell carcinoma of the head and neck: results from a phase II prospective trial. J Clin Oncol 2010;28:8–14.
16. Samant S, Robbins KT, Vang M, et al. Intra-arterial cisplatin and concomitant radiation therapy followed by surgery for advanced paranasal sinus cancer. Arch Otolaryngol Head Neck Surg 2004;130:948–55.
17. Papadimitrakopoulou VA, Ginsberg LE, Garden AS, et al. Intraarterial cisplatin with intravenous paclitaxel and ifosfamide as an organ-preservation approach in patients with paranasal sinus carcinoma. Cancer 2003;98:2214–23.

18. Ansa B, Goodman M, Ward K, et al. Paranasal sinus squamous cell carcinoma incidence and survival based on surveillance, epidemiology, and end results data, 1973 to 2009. Cancer 2013;119:2602–10.
19. Waldron J, Witterick I. Paranasal sinus cancer: caveats and controversies. World J Surg 2003;27:849–55.
20. Day TA, Beas RA, Schlosser RJ, et al. Management of paranasal sinus malignancy. Curr Treat Options Oncol 2005;6:3–18.
21. Norlander T, Frödin J-E, Silfverswärd C, et al. Decreasing incidence of malignant tumors of the paranasal sinuses in Sweden. An analysis of 141 consecutive cases at Karolinska Hospital from 1960 to 1980. Ann Otol Rhinol Laryngol 2003;112: 236–41.
22. Björk-Eriksson T, Mercke C, Petruson B, et al. Potential impact on tumor control and organ preservation with cisplatin and 5-fluorouracil for patients with advanced tumors of the paranasal sinuses and nasal fossa. A prospective pilot study. Cancer 1992;70:2615–20.
23. Pfister DG, Ang K, Brockstein B, et al. NCCN Practice Guidelines for Head and Neck Cancers. Oncology (Williston Park) 2000;14:163–94.
24. Suarez C, Llorente JL, Fernandez De Leon R, et al. Prognostic factors in sinonasal tumors involving the anterior skull base. Head Neck 2004;26:136–44.
25. Pfister DG, Spencer S, Brizel DM, et al. Head and neck cancers, Version 2.2014. Clinical practice guidelines in oncology. J Natl Compr Canc Netw 2014;12: 1454–87.
26. Porceddu S, Martin J, Shanker G, et al. Paranasal sinus tumors: Peter MacCallum Cancer Institute experience. Head Neck 2004;26:322–30.
27. Bossi P, Perrone F, Miceli R, et al. Tp53 status as guide for the management of ethmoid sinus intestinal-type adenocarcinoma. Oral Oncol 2013;49:413–9.
28. Licitra L, Suardi S, Bossi P, et al. Prediction of TP53 status for primary cisplatin, fluorouracil, and leucovorin chemotherapy in ethmoid sinus intestinal-type adenocarcinoma. J Clin Oncol 2004;22:4901–6.
29. Kim BS, Vongtama R, Juillard G. Sinonasal undifferentiated carcinoma: case series and literature review. Am J Otolaryngol 2004;25:162–6.
30. Jeng Y-M, Sung MT, Fang CL, et al. Sinonasal undifferentiated carcinoma and nasopharyngeal-type undifferentiated carcinoma: two clinically, biologically, and histopathologically distinct entities. Am J Surg Pathol 2002;26:371–6.
31. Reiersen DA, Pahilan ME, Devaiah AK. Meta-analysis of treatment outcomes for sinonasal undifferentiated carcinoma. Otolaryngol Head Neck Surg 2012;147:7–14.
32. Musy PY, Reibel JF, Levine PA. Sinonasal undifferentiated carcinoma: the search for a better outcome. Laryngoscope 2002;112:1450–5.
33. Rischin D, Porceddu S, Peters L, et al. Promising results with chemoradiation in patients with sinonasal undifferentiated carcinoma. Head Neck 2004;26:435–41.
34. Likhacheva A, Rosenthal DI, Hanna E, et al. Sinonasal neuroendocrine carcinoma: impact of differentiation status on response and outcome. Head Neck Oncol 2011;3:32.
35. Rosenthal DI, Barker JL Jr, El-Naggar AK, et al. Sinonasal malignancies with neuroendocrine differentiation: patterns of failure according to histologic phenotype. Cancer 2004;101:2567–73.
36. Fitzek MM, Thornton AF, Varvares M, et al. Neuroendocrine tumors of the sinonasal tract. Results of a prospective study incorporating chemotherapy, surgery, and combined proton-photon radiotherapy. Cancer 2002;94:2623–34.
37. Dulguerov P, Calcaterra T. Esthesioneuroblastoma: the UCLA experience 1970-1990. Laryngoscope 1992;102:843–9.

38. Eich HT, Hero B, Staar S, et al. Multimodality therapy including radiotherapy and chemotherapy improves event-free survival in stage C esthesioneuroblastoma. Strahlenther Onkol 2003;179:233–40.
39. Loy AH, Reibel JF, Read PW, et al. Esthesioneuroblastoma: continued follow-up of a single institution's experience. Arch Otolaryngol Head Neck Surg 2006;132:134–8.
40. Koka VN, Julieron M, Bourhis J, et al. Aesthesioneuroblastoma. J Laryngol Otol 1998;112:628–33.
41. Ow TJ, Bell D, Kupferman ME, et al. Esthesioneuroblastoma. Neurosurg Clin N Am 2013;24:51–65.
42. Levine PA, Gallagher R, Cantrell RW. Esthesioneuroblastoma: reflections of a 21-year experience. Laryngoscope 1999;109:1539–43.
43. Thompson LDR, Wieneke JA, Miettinen M. Sinonasal tract and nasopharyngeal melanomas: a clinicopathologic study of 115 cases with a proposed staging system. Am J Surg Pathol 2003;27:594–611.
44. Breik O, Sim F, Wong T, et al. Survival Outcomes of Mucosal Melanoma in the Head and Neck: Case Series and Review of Current Treatment Guidelines. J Oral Maxillofac Surg 2016;74(9):1859–71.
45. Roth TN, Gengler C, Huber GF, et al. Outcome of sinonasal melanoma: clinical experience and review of the literature. Head Neck 2010;32:1385–92.
46. Gore MR, Zanation AM. Survival in Sinonasal Melanoma: A Meta-analysis. J Neurol Surg B Skull Base 2012;73:157–62.
47. Bartell HL, Bedikian AY, Papadopoulos NE, et al. Biochemotherapy in patients with advanced head and neck mucosal melanoma. Head Neck 2008;30:1592–8.
48. Bedikian AY, Johnson MM, Warneke CL, et al. Prognostic factors that determine the long-term survival of patients with unresectable metastatic melanoma. Cancer Invest 2008;26:624–33.
49. Lian B, Si L, Cui C, et al. Phase II randomized trial comparing high-dose IFN-α2b with temozolomide plus cisplatin as systemic adjuvant therapy for resected mucosal melanoma. Clin Cancer Res 2013;19:4488–98.
50. Hodi FS, Friedlander P, Corless CL, et al. Major response to imatinib mesylate in KIT-mutated melanoma. J Clin Oncol 2008;26:2046–51.
51. Del Vecchio M, Di Guardo L, Ascierto PA, et al. Efficacy and safety of ipilimumab 3mg/kg in patients with pretreated, metastatic, mucosal melanoma. Eur J Cancer 2014;1990(50):121–7.
52. Min L, Hodi FS. Anti-PD1 following ipilimumab for mucosal melanoma: durable tumor response associated with severe hypothyroidism and rhabdomyolysis. Cancer Immunol Res 2014;2:15–8.
53. Callender TA, Weber RS, Janjan N, et al. Rhabdomyosarcoma of the nose and paranasal sinuses in adults and children. Otolaryngol Head Neck Surg 1995;112:252–7.
54. Edmonson JH. Chemotherapeutic approaches to soft tissue sarcomas. Semin Surg Oncol 1994;10:357–63.
55. Mattavelli D, Miceli R, Radaelli S, et al. Head and neck soft tissue sarcomas: prognostic factors and outcome in a series of patients treated at a single institution. Ann Oncol 2013;24:2181–9.
56. Khan MN, Husain Q, Kanumuri VV, et al. Management of sinonasal chondrosarcoma: a systematic review of 161 patients. Int Forum Allergy Rhinol 2013;3:670–7.
57. van den Berg H, Schreuder WH, de Lange J. Osteosarcoma: a comparison of jaw versus nonjaw localizations and review of the literature. Sarcoma 2013;2013:316123.

The Role of Targeted Therapy in the Management of Sinonasal Malignancies

Lawrence Kashat, MD, MSc, Christopher H. Le, MD,
Alexander G. Chiu, MD*

KEYWORDS

- Targeted therapy • Immunotherapy • Sinonasal malignancy
- Head and neck squamous cell carcinoma • Sinonasal tumors
- Cell-mediated immunity • Head and neck melanoma • Mucosal melanoma

KEY POINTS

- Malignancy arises when cancer cells evade detection and destruction by immune system cells. The cell-mediated immune response, particularly that involving CD8$^+$ cytotoxic T lymphocytes, is a critical component of the antitumor response.
- Activation of the cell-mediated immune response is a complex process involving interactions between tumors and the immune system. This process involves foreign proteins expressed and/or shed by cancer cells (tumor antigens), APCs (including dendritic cells and macrophages), CD4$^+$ helper T lymphocytes, and CD8$^+$ cytotoxic T lymphocytes.
- Cancers evade the immune response by numerous mechanisms, including expression of inhibitory immune checkpoint proteins, release of cytokines, and interactions with inhibitory cells in the tumor microenvironment.
- Cancers may prevent their own destruction through the exploitation of several inhibitory pathways found on T lymphocytes, including the CTLA-4 and PD-1 pathways. These inhibitory cell-surface interactions between cancer cells, APCs, and lymphocytes are an important therapeutic target.
- Several targeted immune therapies that block these inhibitory interactions have resulted in unprecedented clinical efficacy in the treatment of numerous malignancies and may present a novel therapeutic approach to the treatment of sinonasal and ventral skull base malignancies.

Department of Otolaryngology, University of Kansas School of Medicine, 3901 Rainbow Blvd, MS 3010, Kansas City, KS 66160, USA
* Corresponding author.
E-mail address: alexchiumd@gmail.com

Otolaryngol Clin N Am 50 (2017) 443–455
http://dx.doi.org/10.1016/j.otc.2016.12.016
0030-6665/17/© 2016 Elsevier Inc. All rights reserved.

INTRODUCTION

The notion that the immune system is important in defending against malignancy had first been postulated more than 100 years ago by Robert Ehrlich, who suggested that cancer would occur with high frequency if not for host immune defense preventing tumor growth.[1] Cancers arise secondary to genetic and epigenetic changes that provide the cell with a survival advantage that promotes cellular immortality. Cells that undergo these changes often express foreign antigens on their surface that would ordinarily be expected to stimulate a host immune response to destroy them. Malignancy arises when tumors use mechanisms to evade detection and destruction by the immune system.

Following the discovery of T cells in the 1940s came the concept of "immunosurveillance," the process by which the immune system is able to identify and destroy transformed cells to prevent formation of neoplastic disease. For several decades, scientists have worked to find ways to harness the power of the host's own immune system in the fight against cancer.[2] Many malignancies seem to elicit an immune response, yet somehow manage to avoid destruction by the cells of the immune system. For example, several studies have shown that large subsets of head and neck squamous cell carcinomas (HNSCCs) demonstrate the presence of CD8[+] cytotoxic T lymphocytes and that their presence may be associated with improved response to chemotherapy.[3] Because these tumor-infiltrating lymphocytes function in the immune system to destroy abnormal cells, the question arises: how did these cancers avoid destruction by the host immune system? Furthermore, is there a way to exploit this immune response and make it reactive to the malignant cells?

In recent years there have been unprecedented advances in targeted cancer immunotherapy that are dramatically improving outcomes for several different malignancies, including advanced metastatic cancers that previously had minimal hope for long-term survival. This article discusses some of these remarkable clinical findings and explores their potential for use in treatment of various sinonasal and ventral skull base malignancies.

Immunology Basics

To understand the role of the immune system in the development of malignancy and the mechanisms by which tumors evade the immune system, it is important to understand some essential principles of immunology. Broadly, the immune system is divided into innate and adaptive components (**Tables 1** and **2**).

Innate Immunity

Innate immunity refers to an always-present system that can immediately defend against the development of infections and neoplasia. The components of innate immunity include epithelial cells that act as a barrier to infection; complement proteins; and a variety of cell types, such as monocytes, macrophages, dendritic cells, natural killer cells, eosinophils, mast cells, and basophils. Some of these pertinent components are described in more detail in **Table 1**.

Adaptive Immunity

Adaptive immunity specifically refers to lymphocytes and their products, such as antibodies. This powerful component of the immunity system is not immediately available to defend against pathologic states, but requires additional steps to become active. This includes presentation of a foreign antigen to B or T lymphocytes by antigen presenting cells (APCs), such as dendritic cells and macrophages. After antigen

Table 1	
Important components of the innate immune response and their functions	
Components of Innate Immunity	**Function**
Epithelial cells	Act as barrier to infection
Complement proteins	Circulating proteins that can induce a variety of inflammatory response to pathogens
Select Cells of Innate Immunity	**Function**
Monocytes	May differentiated into macrophages or monocytes in response to infection, neoplastic disease, or inflammation
Macrophages	Migrates from blood vessels into tissues, consumption of pathogens and cancerous cells by phagocytosis, may present antigens to activate the adaptive immune response
Dendritic cell	Presents antigens on its surface resulting in activation of the adaptive immune response
Neutrophils	Represent 50%–60% of circulating leukocytes, release products to kill pathogens, stimulate immune response
Natural killer cell	Possess cell-killing ability, can destroy tumor cells and cells infected with viruses

presentation, differentiation and proliferation of lymphocytes results in a specific response to the presented pathology, including infection or the presence of neoplastic cells. Adaptive immunity is separated into two unique types of responses: humoral and cell-mediated (see **Table 2**). Humoral immunity specifically refers to B lymphocytes and the antibodies that they produce. Cell-mediated immunity refers to immunity that is mediated by the many types of T lymphocytes with several different effector functions (see **Table 2**). Cell-mediated immunity is critical to the detection and destruction of malignant cells.

The Immune System and Malignancy

Activation of the adaptive immune response, particularly cell-mediated immunity, is crucial to the body's response to malignancy. Before discussing mechanisms by

Table 2	
Adaptive immunity and functioning of the different types of lymphocytes	
Types of Lymphocytes	**Function**
B lymphocyte	Production of antibodies, neutralization of microbes, facilitates phagocytosis
Helper CD4$^+$ T lymphocyte	Activates a variety of other cell types (B lymphocytes, other T lymphocytes, including cytotoxic T lymphocytes, macrophages) and mediates inflammatory response
Cytotoxic CD8$^+$ T lymphocyte	Kills infected or neoplastic cells
Regulatory T lymphocytes (regulatory T cells)	This is a subset of CD4$^+$ lymphocytes that inhibits the immune response

which cancer cells are able to evade the immune system, we explain how the cell-mediated response becomes activated in the presence of malignancy.

Cancer cells express many different proteins that are recognized as foreign by the immune system. This includes abnormally expressed protein products, oncogenes, mutated tumor-suppressor proteins, and viral antigens that are expressed by virally transformed cancerous cells. Most of these protein products are expressed as part of the class I major histocompatibility complex (MHC) that is found on the cellular surface. When proteins are expressed in association with MHC molecules on the cell surface, they are referred to as antigens. APCs can detect these antigens and present them to T lymphocytes found within lymph nodes to activate the cell-mediated immune response. Following antigen presentation, these antigens are recognized on tumor cells by CD8+ cytotoxic T lymphocytes, which enter the circulation and migrate to the site of the antigen to carry out their effector function and destroy the abnormal cell.

A key method of destroying cancer cells by the immune system relies on the activation of CD8+ cytotoxic T lymphocytes. The process of activating CD8+ cytotoxic T lymphocytes is mediated by APCs and also by CD4+ helper T lymphocytes. A variety of cell types act as APCs, including dendritic cells and macrophages. APCs consume antigens that are produced by the tumor and then present them to T lymphocytes to activate them. The combination of APCs and/or CD4+ helper T-lymphocyte interactions then contributes to the activation of CD8+ cytotoxic T lymphocytes that may migrate to tumor tissues and carry out their effector function: destruction of malignant cells (**Fig. 1**).

Activation of T lymphocytes depends on a two-signal process: interaction between the T-cell receptor and an MHC molecule on an APC; and interaction between

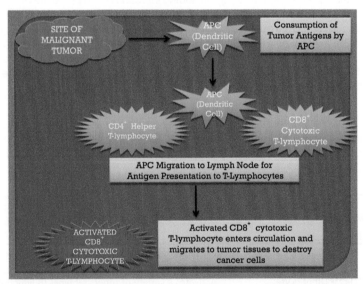

Fig. 1. Summary of the cell-mediated immune response to malignancy. There are several steps involved in the activation of T lymphocytes. Malignant tumors often express and/or release antigens that are consumed by APCs, particularly dendritic cells. These APCs then migrate to lymph nodes and present the antigens to CD8+ cytotoxic T lymphocytes and CD4+ helper T lymphocytes resulting in activation of the cell-mediated immune response. Activated CD8+ cytotoxic T lymphocytes may then migrate to the site of malignant disease and destroy cancer cells. Cancer cells may evade this process using numerous mechanisms.

costimulatory proteins found on APCs, CD4$^+$ T lymphocytes, and/or the cancer cells (**Fig. 2**).[4,5] The first required signal that a T lymphocyte must receive to become active corresponds to the interaction between the T-cell receptor and an MHC molecule that is presenting a peptide antigen on the cell surface of an APC or tumor cell. The second signal corresponds to costimulation, that is, positive signaling by receptors found on the surface of the T lymphocyte and the APC or cancer cell. Many cells of the body express inhibitory proteins, such as B7 and programmed death ligand 1 (PD-L1), which interact with "checkpoint" receptors on the T cell (cytotoxic T-lymphocyte-associated protein [CTLA]-4 and programmed death [PD]-1). These inhibitory interactions compete with the stimulatory "signal 2" required for activation of the T lymphocyte and can inhibit the cell-mediated immune response. Cancer cells may exploit this inhibitory feature of T lymphocytes and often express these inhibitory proteins (PD-L1, B7) as a mechanism by which they are able to evade attack by the immune system. The balance between required stimulatory signals (eg, CD28/B7 interactions) and inhibitory signals (eg, CTLA-4/B7, PD-1/PD-L1, or PD-L2) determines whether a T cell becomes active (**Fig. 3**).

CANCER AND EVASION OF THE IMMUNE SYSTEM

There are several mechanisms used by cancer cells to evade the immune system (**Table 3**).

Some tumor types express checkpoint proteins that bind to receptors on the cell surface of T lymphocytes. The most widely studied of these are the CTLA-4 and PD-1

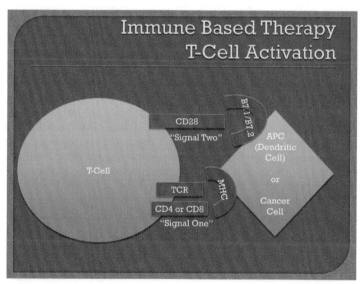

Fig. 2. Two-step model of T-cell activation. In the two-step model of T-cell activation, there are two critical signals required for the activation of T lymphocytes. "Signal One" corresponds to interactions between the T-cell receptor (TCR) and CD4$^+$ or CD8$^+$ coreceptor on the T cell with an MHC molecule found on an APC or cancer cell that is presenting a peptide antigen. The second required signal, "Signal Two," is also referred to as "costimulation." This second signal corresponds to interactions between activating stimulatory molecules on the surface of the T lymphocyte with activating molecules on the APC or cancer cell (eg, CD28/B7 interactions).

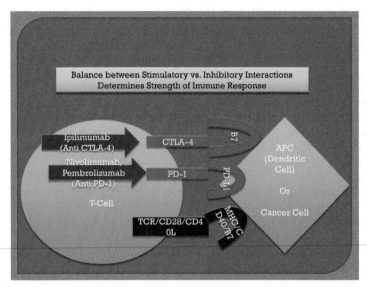

Fig. 3. The balance between costimulatory and coinhibitory interactions determines the strength of the immune response. Numerous coinhibitory signals compete with positive costimulatory signals and may prevent activation of T cells. Among the most widely studied of these inhibitory interactions is that of CTLA-4 or PD-1 (found on the T lymphocyte) with their respective ligands (found on APCs or cancer cells). Several targeted therapies are available that block these inhibitory signals (CTLA-4, PD-1) and enhance the cell-mediated immune response. Many of these agents, including ipilimumab, pembrolizumab, and nivolumab, have shown unprecedented clinical results in the treatment of numerous solid malignancies. TCR, T-cell receptor.

receptors, which act to inhibit the activation of T lymphocytes.[6–10] The CTLA-4 and PD-1 receptors are referred to as immune checkpoint proteins because they provide a mechanism for normal cells in the body to defend against autoimmunity by causing inhibition of the T-cell response. Recall that T-lymphocyte activation and proliferation depends on T-cell receipt of two critical positive signals in its interaction with APCs or with tumor cells (see **Fig. 1**).[4,5] The second of these required signals involves costimulatory interactions between CD28 on the T-cell surface and its ligand on an APC or tumor cell. If the interaction between checkpoint proteins on the surface of a T cell is greater than the costimulatory second signal, then the T cell fails to become activated.

Table 3
Mechanisms by which tumor cells evade immune system detection and prevent lymphocyte activation

Tumor Factors	Tumor Microenvironment Factors
Expression of proteins that inhibit T-lymphocyte response to tumor (eg, PD-L1/PD-1 interaction, B7/CTLA-4 interaction)	Presence of inhibitory immune cells (regulatory T lymphocytes, tumor-promoting [M2] macrophages, myeloid-derived suppressor cells, and Th2 polarized CD4 T cells)
Release of inhibitory cytokines	
Failure to display specific antigens to help initiate an antitumor response	MHC class I downregulation
Growth signals exceed ability of immune response to destroy malignant cells	Physical barriers

Tumors themselves produce numerous cytokines to directly suppress cell-mediated immunity, including transforming growth factor-β and interleukins 6 and 10, and activate signal transducer and activation of transcription-1 suppression.[11]

Some cancer cells stop expressing MHC class I molecules that are required to display antigens to $CD8^+$ cytotoxic T lymphocytes for their cell-killing function. It is known that natural killer cells of innate immunity can recognize when cells do not express MHC class I molecules and thus, possibly may have a role to play in preventing some MHC-negative tumors from developing.

A variety of cells found in the tumor microenvironment and/or in the circulation may inhibit the immune response, including regulatory T lymphocytes. The tumor microenvironment refers to the cellular environment surrounding the tumor cells. It is comprised of a complex mixture of immune cells, fibroblasts, blood vessels, inflammatory cells, signaling molecules, cytokines, and extracellular matrix proteins. Many of the cells within this complex environment act to inhibit the $CD8^+$ cytotoxic T-lymphocyte response to the tumor. Recall that a subset of $CD4^+$ lymphocytes develops into regulatory T cells (Treg) whose function is to inhibit the immune response.[12–14] Expression of checkpoint inhibitors (eg, CTLA-4, PD-1) by Treg cells may directly inhibit the ability of APCs to provide required costimulation for activation of cytotoxic T lymphocytes.[15] Some Treg cells also produce inhibitory cytokines that reduce the activity of cytotoxic T lymphocytes and APCs.[15] In addition to Treg cells, other inhibitors of the antitumor immune response include myeloid-derived suppressor cells, type 2 tumor promoting macrophages (M2), and Treg[12–14] These cells can therefore suppress the antitumor response that would be expected by early infiltration of the malignancy by antitumor macrophages, cytotoxic T lymphocytes, natural killer cells, and dendritic cells.

TARGETED THERAPY FOR THE TREATMENT OF MALIGNANCY: CHECKPOINT INHIBITOR BLOCKADE
Ipilimumab: Anti–Cytotoxic T-Lymphocyte-Associated Protein-4 Antibody

$CD8^+$ cytotoxic T lymphocytes are critical to the antitumor response. These lymphocytes express checkpoint proteins on their cellular surface that may inhibit their antitumor activity. The most widely studied of these checkpoint inhibitors are CTLA-4 and PD-1.

The development of monoclonal antibodies (mABs) that block the interaction between these checkpoint proteins on the cell surface of T lymphocytes and their respective ligands has yielded unprecedented clinical results in clinical trials.[6–10] mABs are antibodies that are highly specific to one antigen alone and can be used to bind to the target with high affinity and specificity. They are generated from immune cells that are all identical clones of a unique parent cell.

CTLA-4 is a checkpoint receptor found on T lymphocytes and it suppresses the early stages of T-cell activation. The first drug to be approved by the Food and Drug Administration within this class is ipilimumab, an mAB that targets CTLA-4. The drug was approved for metastatic or unresectable melanoma after phase III clinical trials showed it to be the first drug to increase overall survival in this disease.[16,17] A pooled meta-analysis of long-term survival data in patients who had received ipilimumab for unresectable or metastatic melanoma found an important plateau in the survival curve at Year 3 with 21% of patients continuing to survive thereafter.[18] Despite these encouraging findings, response to ipilimumab was only seen in a small fraction of the overall patients.

Autoimmune side effects are an important limitation of ipilimumab therapy and have been observed in up to 35% of patients receiving the drug. This is expected because checkpoint inhibitors, such as CTLA-4, act to prevent autoimmunity by attenuating the early T-lymphocyte immune response.

Pembrolizumab and Nivolumab: Anti-Programmed-Death-1 Antibody

Another highly studied checkpoint inhibitor is the PD-1 receptor expressed on T lymphocytes and its ligands, PD-L1/PD-L2. This checkpoint inhibitor is expressed on activated T cells and may be considered an inhibitor of the late/effector activity of the T lymphocyte. As with CTLA-4 interactions with its ligand, the interaction between PD-1 and PD-L1/PD-L2 results in inhibition of cell-mediated immunity.

Pembrolizumab and nivolumab are anti-PD1 mAbs that were approved in 2014 for use in metastatic or unresectable melanoma after clinical trials established improved overall survival in these patients.[19,20] Remarkably, the side effect profile of these drugs was much more favorable in contrast to ipilimumab, with supportive care of immunosuppressive therapy managing most of these patients.[2,21] This more favorable side-effect profile may be related to the role of PD-1 in inhibition of the late T cell response and blockade of this pathway may be causing less nonspecific activation of T lymphocytes.

Since these original clinical trials, the indications for use of pembrolizumab and nivolumab have increased and now include non–small cell lung carcinoma, renal cell carcinoma, bladder carcinoma, recurrent or metastatic HNSCC, and several other solid malignancies.[12]

A head to head randomized phase III clinical trial for patients with advanced melanoma receiving pembrolizumab every 2 weeks, every 3 weeks, or ipilimumab every 3 weeks has been published.[22] Pembrolizumab was found to have a 12-month survival of 74.1% (every 2 weeks) and 68.4% (every 3 weeks) in contrast to 58.2% for ipilimumab. Long-term therapeutic responses have also been reported with recently reported data showing that 34% of patients treated with nivolumab monotherapy for advanced metastatic melanoma are alive 5-years into a phase I study of the drug.[23,24]

COMBINATION IMMUNOTHERAPY: THE WAY OF THE FUTURE

Checkpoint inhibitors represent only one of many possible approaches to targeted immunotherapy, but the clinical data supporting this approach are strong. Other promising approaches are briefly described in **Table 4**.

Combination therapy is broken down into combining different checkpoint inhibitors together or checkpoint inhibitors with other forms of targeted immunotherapies. Recent clinical trials have found combining checkpoint inhibitors to be more effective

Table 4
Summary of different forms of immunotherapy and their mechanisms of action

Type of Immune Therapy	Mechanism of Action
Checkpoint inhibitory blockade	Blockade of inhibitory signals between T lymphocytes and cancer or APCs (eg, anti-CTLA4 or anti-PD1 mAB)
Adoptive cell transfer	Extraction of cancer patient's lymphocytes Ex vivo activation of T lymphocytes followed by transfer back to patient
Tumor microenvironment targeting	Targeting of inhibitory immune cells (Treg, myeloid-derived suppressor cells, M2) Targeting of immune inhibitory or protumor cytokines
Cancer vaccination	Development of vaccines targeting specific tumor antigens to enhance the killing of resistant tumor cells

than monotherapy alone, such as those of patients who received a combination of nivolumab plus ipilimumab.[25,26]

TARGETED THERAPY FOR SINONASAL MALIGNANCY

Cancers of the sinonasal cavity are rare, with an estimated incidence of 0.556 in 100,000 individuals.[27] More than 80% of these malignancies are epithelial in origin, namely, sinonasal squamous cell carcinoma (SNSCC) and adenocarcinoma.[27,28] Less commonly encountered malignancies include adenoid cystic carcinoma; lymphoma; mucosal melanoma; sarcoma; and sinonasal neuroendocrine tumors, such as esthesioneuroblastoma, sinonasal undifferentiated carcinoma, and small cell carcinoma. The rare nature of these malignancies and the significant heterogeneity and genetic variation each of these are associated with contributes to the challenges in devising effective therapies to treat them. Targeted and immune-based therapies offer a new opportunity to potentially revolutionize the treatment of these malignancies.

SQUAMOUS CELL CARCINOMA OF THE SINONASAL CAVITY

Although SCC are genetically heterogeneous,[27–30] there is evidence with respect to the role of the immune system and complex tumor microenvironment in the development and progression of these malignancies.[11,13,31–33] The expression of PD-L1 has been reported in many head and neck tumors, including HNSCC.[34–36] In addition, Udager and colleagues[37] have reported in a study of inverted sinonasal papillomas and SNSCC that activating epidermal growth factor receptor (EGFR) mutations are present in 77% of tumors associated with SNSCC, including identical mutations in matched pairs of inverted sinonasal papilloma associated with SNSCC.

There are several clinical trials currently underway to investigate the potential role of targeted inhibitors, including pembrolizumab, for use in HNSCC. Indeed, cetuximab, an mAb that acts as an antagonist to the EGFR, has already been shown to be effective as an adjunct to standard therapy in several clinical trials for patients with metastatic or recurrent HNSCC.[38] There is evidence that the efficacy of this type of therapy may not only be caused by the direct inhibition of EGFR-induced growth signaling on tumor cells, but also enhanced antibody-dependent cell cytotoxicity because the Fc region of cetuximab has been shown to bind to numerous immune cells, including natural killer cells, thereby promoting direct killing of malignant tissues[39–41]

Efforts to augment this therapeutic strategy have also shown some success. Recently, a phase II study that examined the addition of bevacizumab, an mAb that targets the vascular endothelial growth factor, to a treatment regimen consisting of cetuximab, cisplatin, and concurrent radiation therapy for patients with stage III to IVB HNSCC found the treatment was well tolerated, with 2-year progression-free survival of 88.5% during the median follow-up time of 33.8 months.[42] In addition to targeting of vascular endothelial growth factor, an alternative approach may be to enhance cell-mediated immunity by activation of CD137, a known immune costimulatory molecule, as described in a review by Schoppy and Sunwoo.[41] This has been shown in in vitro studies and in vivo studies on mice.[43–45] This is more evidence for the exciting synergistic potential that combination targeted therapy may hold as a way of treating these malignancies.

INTESTINAL-TYPE ADENOCARCINOMA AND ADENOID CYSTIC CARCINOMA

Because of the rare nature of these malignancies, there is a paucity of evidence to support the use of specific targeted therapeutic agents in their treatment. This does not preclude the potential efficacy of targeted therapies in these malignancies and it is possible that drugs approved for use in other cancers may show similar effects in these malignancies.

For intestinal-type adenocarcinoma, with the exception of the papillary variant, large-scale genomic derangement has been widely reported.[46] Moreover, the immunophenotype has been reported to show immunohistochemical staining for a variety of immune mediators including CK20, CDX2, MUC2, villin, and CK7.[47] Variable expression of EGFR has also been reported.[48,49]

For adenoid cystic carcinoma, c-KIT, a cell-signaling protein that is associated with cellular differentiation and growth, has been reported to be overexpressed in previous studies.[50] Furthermore, recurrent fusion of two transcription factor genes encoding MYB and NFIB has been reported in up to 90% of adenoic cystic carcinomas and seems to be critical in the evolution of the disease.[51,52] There have been numerous clinical trials that have targeted either driver mutations or the immunologic components of this disease. An elegantly written review by Chae and colleagues[53] has summarized the results of these 19 studies with a total of 22 objective responses observed out of 397 patients for all drugs administered.

MUCOSAL MELANOMA

There are limited data regarding the efficacy of targeted therapy in mucosal melanoma, but several studies have shown some promise. Unlike cutaneous malignant melanoma, mucosal melanoma is only rarely associated with activating mutations in the BRAF oncogene at the V600 site, and instead have been associated with higher rates of mutation in the KIT oncogene.[54,55] The use of c-KIT inhibitors is effective in patients with mutations in tumors harboring KIT mutations.[56] It is recommended to test patients for these molecular abnormalities to determine their potential eligibility for these targeted therapies.

Given the remarkable success of immunotherapy for the treatment of cutaneous melanoma, there is a great degree of interest in the potential use of targeted agents, such as ipilimumab, pembrolizumab, and nivolumab, in patients with mucosal melanoma. A study by Del Vecchio and colleagues[57] found that patients receiving ipilimumab for stage III/IV mucosal melanoma who failed other therapies had a 12% response rate and 36% disease control rate. It is possible that anti-PD1 therapy or combination therapy may further improve the response rate in these patients.

SUMMARY

There have been numerous advances in targeted and immune-based therapy. These advances have resulted in unprecedented clinical efficacy for the treatment of numerous malignancies. As more knowledge becomes available with regard to drivers of tumor growth and the important interactions among tumor, tumor microenvironment, and the immune system, it is likely that targeted therapy will gain widespread use in sinonasal and ventral skull base malignancies.

REFERENCES

1. Coffin RS. Oncolytic immunotherapy: an emerging new modality for the treatment of cancer. Ann Oncol 2016;27(9):1805–8.
2. Farkona S, Diamandis EP, Blasutig IM. Cancer immunotherapy: the beginning of the end of cancer? BMC Med 2016;14(1):73.

3. Kim JW, Tsukishiro T, Johnson JT, et al. Expression of pro- and antiapoptotic proteins in circulating CD8+ T cells of patients with squamous cell carcinoma of the head and neck. Clin Cancer Res 2004;10(15):5101–10.

4. Bretscher PA. A two-step, two-signal model for the primary activation of precursor helper T cells. Proc Natl Acad Sci U S A 1999;96(1):185–90.

5. Patel VP, Moran M, Low TA, et al. A molecular framework for two-step T cell signaling: Lck Src homology 3 mutations discriminate distinctly regulated lipid raft reorganization events. J Immunol 2001;166(2):754–64.

6. Murillo O, Arina A, Tirapu I, et al. Potentiation of therapeutic immune responses against malignancies with monoclonal antibodies. Clin Cancer Res 2003;9(15): 5454–64.

7. Leach DR, Krummel MF, Allison JP. Enhancement of antitumor immunity by CTLA-4 blockade. Science 1996;271(5256):1734–6.

8. Dong H, Strome SE, Salomao DR, et al. Tumor-associated B7-H1 promotes T-cell apoptosis: a potential mechanism of immune evasion. Nat Med 2002;8(8): 793–800.

9. Iwai Y, Ishida M, Tanaka Y, et al. Involvement of PD-L1 on tumor cells in the escape from host immune system and tumor immunotherapy by PD-L1 blockade. Proc Natl Acad Sci U S A 2002;99(19):12293–7.

10. Latchman Y, Wood CR, Chernova T, et al. PD-L2 is a second ligand for PD-1 and inhibits T cell activation. Nat Immunol 2001;2(3):261–8.

11. Ferris RL. Immunology and immunotherapy of head and neck cancer. J Clin Oncol 2015;33(29):3293–304.

12. Whiteside TL, Demaria S, Rodriguez-Ruiz ME, et al. Emerging opportunities and challenges in cancer immunotherapy. Clin Cancer Res 2016;22(8):1845–55.

13. Allen CT, Clavijo PE, Van Waes C, et al. Anti-tumor immunity in head and neck cancer: understanding the evidence, how tumors escape and Immunotherapeutic Approaches. Cancers (Basel) 2015;7(4):2397–414.

14. Pitt JM, Marabelle A, Eggermont A, et al. Targeting the tumor microenvironment: removing obstruction to anticancer immune responses and immunotherapy. Ann Oncol 2016;27(8):1482–92.

15. Takeuchi Y, Nishikawa H. Roles of regulatory T cells in cancer immunity. Int Immunol 2016;28(8):401–9.

16. Hodi FS, O'Day SJ, McDermott DF, et al. Improved survival with ipilimumab in patients with metastatic melanoma. N Engl J Med 2010;363(8):711–23.

17. Robert C, Thomas L, Bondarenko I, et al. Ipilimumab plus dacarbazine for previously untreated metastatic melanoma. N Engl J Med 2011;364(26):2517–26.

18. Schadendorf D, Hodi FS, Robert C, et al. Pooled analysis of long-term survival data from phase ii and phase iii trials of ipilimumab in unresectable or metastatic melanoma. J Clin Oncol 2015;33(17):1889–94.

19. Robert C, Ribas A, Wolchok JD, et al. Anti-programmed-death-receptor-1 treatment with pembrolizumab in ipilimumab-refractory advanced melanoma: a randomised dose-comparison cohort of a phase 1 trial. Lancet 2014;384(9948): 1109–17.

20. Topalian SL, Sznol M, McDermott DF, et al. Survival, durable tumor remission, and long-term safety in patients with advanced melanoma receiving nivolumab. J Clin Oncol 2014;32(10):1020–30.

21. Orlov S, Salari F, Kashat L, et al. Induction of painless thyroiditis in patients receiving programmed death 1 receptor immunotherapy for metastatic malignancies. J Clin Endocrinol Metab 2015;100(5):1738–41.

22. Robert C, Schachter J, Long GV, et al. Pembrolizumab versus ipilimumab in advanced melanoma. N Engl J Med 2015;372(26):2521–32.

23. Grossmann KF, Margolin K. Long-term survival as a treatment benchmark in melanoma: latest results and clinical implications. Ther Adv Med Oncol 2015;7(3): 181–91.

24. Dramatic survival benefit with nivolumab in melanoma. Cancer Discov 2016;6(6): OF7.

25. Larkin J, Chiarion-Sileni V, Gonzalez R, et al. Combined nivolumab and ipilimumab or monotherapy in untreated melanoma. N Engl J Med 2015;373(1):23–34.

26. Postow MA, Chesney J, Pavlick AC, et al. Nivolumab and ipilimumab versus ipilimumab in untreated melanoma. N Engl J Med 2015;372(21):2006–17.

27. Turner JH, Reh DD. Incidence and survival in patients with sinonasal cancer: a historical analysis of population-based data. Head Neck 2012;34(6):877–85.

28. Ariza M, Llorente JL, Alvarez-Marcas C, et al. Comparative genomic hybridization in primary sinonasal adenocarcinomas. Cancer 2004;100(2):335–41.

29. Lopez F, Llorente JL, Garcia-Inclan C, et al. Genomic profiling of sinonasal squamous cell carcinoma. Head Neck 2011;33(2):145–53.

30. Perez-Escuredo J, Lopez-Hernandez A, Costales M, et al. Recurrent DNA copy number alterations in intestinal-type sinonasal adenocarcinoma. Rhinology 2016;54(3):278–86.

31. Tilson MP, Gallia GL, Bishop JA. Among sinonasal tumors, CDX-2 immunoexpression is not restricted to intestinal-type adenocarcinomas. Head Neck Pathol 2014; 8(1):59–65.

32. Curry JM, Sprandio J, Cognetti D, et al. Tumor microenvironment in head and neck squamous cell carcinoma. Semin Oncol 2014;41(2):217–34.

33. Re M, Santarelli A, Mascitti M, et al. Trail overexpression inversely correlates with histological differentiation in intestinal-type sinonasal adenocarcinoma. Int J Surg Oncol 2013;2013:203873.

34. Chowdhury S, Veyhl J, Jessa F, et al. Programmed death-ligand 1 overexpression is a prognostic marker for aggressive papillary thyroid cancer and its variants. Oncotarget 2016;7(22):32318–28.

35. Chen MF, Chen PT, Chen WC, et al. The role of PD-L1 in the radiation response and prognosis for esophageal squamous cell carcinoma related to IL-6 and T-cell immunosuppression. Oncotarget 2016;7(7):7913–24.

36. Strome SE, Dong H, Tamura H, et al. B7-H1 blockade augments adoptive T-cell immunotherapy for squamous cell carcinoma. Cancer Res 2003;63(19):6501–5.

37. Udager AM, Rolland DC, McHugh JB, et al. High-frequency targetable EGFR mutations in sinonasal squamous cell carcinomas arising from inverted sinonasal papilloma. Cancer Res 2015;75(13):2600–6.

38. Reeves TD, Hill EG, Armeson KE, et al. Cetuximab therapy for head and neck squamous cell carcinoma: a systematic review of the data. Otolaryngol Head Neck Surg 2011;144(5):676–84.

39. Ferris RL, Jaffee EM, Ferrone S. Tumor antigen-targeted, monoclonal antibody-based immunotherapy: clinical response, cellular immunity, and immunoescape. J Clin Oncol 2010;28(28):4390–9.

40. Taylor RJ, Saloura V, Jain A, et al. Ex vivo antibody-dependent cellular cytotoxicity inducibility predicts efficacy of cetuximab. Cancer Immunol Res 2015;3(5): 567–74.

41. Schoppy DW, Sunwoo JB. Immunotherapy for head and neck squamous cell carcinoma. Hematol Oncol Clin North Am 2015;29(6):1033–43.

42. Fury MG, Xiao H, Sherman EJ, et al. Phase II trial of bevacizumab + cetuximab + cisplatin with concurrent intensity-modulated radiation therapy for patients with stage III/IVB head and neck squamous cell carcinoma. Head Neck 2016; 38(Suppl 1):E566–70.

43. Wilcox RA, Tamada K, Strome SE, et al. Signaling through NK cell-associated CD137 promotes both helper function for CD8+ cytolytic T cells and responsiveness to IL-2 but not cytolytic activity. J Immunol 2002;169(8):4230–6.

44. Kohrt HE, Colevas AD, Houot R, et al. Targeting CD137 enhances the efficacy of cetuximab. J Clin Invest 2014;124(6):2668–82.

45. Makkouk A, Chester C, Kohrt HE. Rationale for anti-CD137 cancer immunotherapy. Eur J Cancer 2016;54:112–9.

46. Persson M, Andren Y, Moskaluk CA, et al. Clinically significant copy number alterations and complex rearrangements of MYB and NFIB in head and neck adenoid cystic carcinoma. Genes Chromosomes Cancer 2012;51(8):805–17.

47. Leivo I. Sinonasal adenocarcinoma: update on classification, immunophenotype and molecular features. Head Neck Pathol 2016;10(1):68–74.

48. Vivanco Allende B, Perez-Escuredo J, Fuentes Martinez N, et al. Intestinal-type sinonasal adenocarcinomas. Immunohistochemical profile of 66 cases. Acta Otorrinolaringol Esp 2013;64(2):115–23.

49. Szablewski V, Solassol J, Poizat F, et al. EGFR Expression and KRAS and BRAF mutational status in intestinal-type sinonasal adenocarcinoma. Int J Mol Sci 2013; 14(3):5170–81.

50. Nishida H, Daa T, Kashima K, et al. KIT (CD117) expression in benign and malignant sweat gland tumors. Am J Dermatopathol 2015;37(12):898–905.

51. Persson M, Andren Y, Mark J, et al. Recurrent fusion of MYB and NFIB transcription factor genes in carcinomas of the breast and head and neck. Proc Natl Acad Sci U S A 2009;106(44):18740–4.

52. Subramaniam T, Lennon P, O'Neill JP. Ongoing challenges in the treatment of adenoid cystic carcinoma of the head and neck. Ir J Med Sci 2015;184(3): 583–90.

53. Chae YK, Chung SY, Davis AA, et al. Adenoid cystic carcinoma: current therapy and potential therapeutic advances based on genomic profiling. Oncotarget 2015;6(35):37117–34.

54. Spencer KR, Mehnert JM. Mucosal melanoma: epidemiology, biology and treatment. Cancer Treat Res 2016;167:295–320.

55. Curtin JA, Busam K, Pinkel D, et al. Somatic activation of KIT in distinct subtypes of melanoma. J Clin Oncol 2006;24(26):4340–6.

56. Hodi FS, Corless CL, Giobbie-Hurder A, et al. Imatinib for melanomas harboring mutationally activated or amplified KIT arising on mucosal, acral, and chronically sun-damaged skin. J Clin Oncol 2013;31(26):3182–90.

57. Del Vecchio M, Di Guardo L, Ascierto PA, et al. Efficacy and safety of ipilimumab 3mg/kg in patients with pretreated, metastatic, mucosal melanoma. Eur J Cancer 2014;50(1):121–7.

The Making of a Skull Base Team and the Value of Multidisciplinary Approach in the Management of Sinonasal and Ventral Skull Base Malignancies

CrossMark

Carl H. Snyderman, MD, MBA[a,*], Eric W. Wang, MD[a],
Juan C. Fernandez-Miranda, MD[b], Paul A. Gardner, MD[b]

KEYWORDS

- Endoscopic endonasal surgery • Sinonasal malignancy • Skull base team • Training

KEY POINTS

- Endoscopic endonasal surgery is true team surgery with concurrent participation of different surgical specialties.
- Benefits of a multidisciplinary team include cross-fertilization of ideas, surgical innovation, and comprehensive patient care.
- Proper training is a key component of building a skull base team.

CONCEPT OF SKULL BASE TEAM

From the beginning, skull base surgery was at the juncture of multiple specialties and borrowed from the domains of neurosurgery, otolaryngology, head and neck surgery, plastic and reconstructive surgery, and maxillofacial surgery. The development of skull base surgery can be roughly divided into 2 eras, those of open and endoscopic skull base surgery.

The concept of team surgery has evolved during these 2 eras. Open cranial base surgery was predominantly a collaboration of neurosurgeons, head and neck surgeons, and plastic or reconstructive surgeons. In contrast, endoscopic endonasal surgery (EES) is predominantly a collaboration of neurosurgeons and rhinologic surgeons. Differences in training are associated with distinct knowledge and skill sets, as well as oncological philosophy. This may be in transition because more head and neck

Disclosure: The authors have no conflicts of interest to disclose.
[a] Department of Otolaryngology, University of Pittsburgh School of Medicine, 200 Lothrop Street, EEI Suite 500, Pittsburgh, PA 15213, USA; [b] Department of Neurological Surgery, University of Pittsburgh School of Medicine, 200 Lothrop Street, PUH B-400, Pittsburgh, PA 15213, USA
* Corresponding author.
E-mail address: snydermanch@upmc.edu

Otolaryngol Clin N Am 50 (2017) 457–465
http://dx.doi.org/10.1016/j.otc.2016.12.017
0030-6665/17/© 2016 Elsevier Inc. All rights reserved.

oto.theclinics.com

oncologists are gaining endoscopic experience with transoral endoscopic resection of pharyngeal and laryngeal malignancies.

Whereas open cranial base surgery can be characterized as sequential team surgery, in which each surgical specialty works somewhat independently, EES is true team surgery, in which there is simultaneous collaboration throughout most of the surgery. This requires a different type of collaboration but offers the possibility of achieving more than either specialty can achieve alone (**Table 1**).

ONCOLOGIC TEAM

Oncologic care of sinonasal and ventral skull base malignancy benefits from the inclusion of other specialties with discussion of patients in a tumor board format. This includes other surgical disciplines such as otology, ophthalmology, pediatric neurosurgery and otolaryngology, neuroradiology and pathology, and medical and radiation oncology. Radiologic interpretation requires expertise in neuroradiology and is critical in establishing a differential diagnosis and assessing extent of tumor. Correct pathologic diagnosis is essential; many tumors are misdiagnosed at presentation. Optimal management of some tumors will require a combination of surgical approaches (endonasal, transoral, transfacial, transcervical, transorbital, transcranial, and transtemporal). High-grade malignancies may need adjunctive radiation therapy or chemotherapy following surgery and advanced planning is helpful, especially when referral to a remote radiation therapy center is anticipated. Advanced stage malignancies may receive induction chemotherapy or radiochemotherapy before considering salvage surgery (**Table 2**).

COMPOSITION OF SURGICAL TEAM

The composition of the skull base team varies depending on the institution, patient population, and type of disease. With EES, the role of the reconstructive surgeon has diminished and the surgical team generally consists of an otolaryngologist (rhinologist) and neurosurgeon. A hybrid team of 2 specialties offers distinct advantages: access to different patient populations and referral sources, different domains of knowledge, and complementary skills. With proper training, however, there is no reason why surgery cannot be performed by 2 neurosurgeons or 2 otolaryngologists working in concert. This may become necessary when surgical specialties are in separate hospitals or there are other disincentives for collaboration.

Who should be performing EES? Ideally, skull base surgeons are trained in all aspects of skull base surgery, including endoscopic and open approaches. Treatment

Table 1		
Comparison of open and endoscopic surgery of the cranial base		
	Open Cranial Base Surgery	**EES of Cranial Base**
Team	Sequential	Concurrent
Visualization	3-dimensional, blind spots	2-dimensional, direct visualization
Approach	Convergent, remove or displace structures, brain retraction	Divergent, minimal displacement, no brain retraction
Resection	En bloc, vascular control	Piecemeal, limited vascular control
Reconstruction	Direct dural repair, bone reconstruction, obliteration of sinuses	Inlay or onlay grafts and flaps, no bone reconstruction, drainage of sinuses
Major morbidity	Craniofacial structures	Sinonasal structures

Table 2
Subspecialty and expertise

Subspecialty	Expertise
Adult neurosurgery	Adult skull base tumors
Pediatric neurosurgery	Pediatric skull base tumors
Head & neck surgery	Head & neck oncology
Otology	Temporal bone surgery
Rhinology	EES
Pediatric otolaryngology	Pediatric tumors
Ophthalmology	Transorbital surgery
Plastic or reconstructive	Complex reconstruction
Neuroradiology	Radiologic diagnosis
Interventional radiology	Embolization, vascular injury, collateral blood flow
Head & neck radiology	Radiologic diagnosis, biopsy
Neuropathology	Intracranial tumors
Head & neck pathology	Sinonasal pathology
Radiation oncology	Radiotherapy
Medical oncology	Chemotherapy

options for the patient are limited if the surgeon is not familiar with all surgical approaches. The alternative is to have a multidisciplinary team that cooperates instead of competing for cases. Due to insufficient volume of pediatric skull base cases, these surgeries are best performed by an adult team in conjunction with pediatric surgeons.

BENEFITS OF TEAM SURGERY

In general, the care of patients is becoming a team sport across multiple disciplines in recognition of the complexity of patient care and the benefits of a multidisciplinary approach:

- Cross-fertilization of ideas
- Surgical innovation
- Comprehensive patient care.

With EES, team surgery provides additional benefits:

- Dynamic endoscopy
  - Improved visualization
  - 3-dimensional (3D) visual cues
  - Introduction of instruments
  - Maintain view during a crisis
- Second opinion (copilot)
- Increased efficiency
- Modulation of enthusiasm.

Improved visualization is the result of dynamic endoscopy.[1] The movement of the endoscope and instruments relative to each other and the environment provides important 3D visual cues. Dynamic endoscopy is especially important in the midst of a crisis such as a vascular injury, in which maintenance of visualization and 2-handed dissection is essential. One of the greatest benefits of team surgery is having a copilot for decision making and problem-solving. Each surgeon concentrates on different features of a case and it is easy to *lose the forest for the trees* when operating. Conversations in the operating room may include interpretation of anatomy ("Where is the carotid?"), selection of tools, surgical technique, differentiation of tissues (tumor margin), and the sequence of surgical steps. Team surgery is also more efficient and helps to modulate extremes of enthusiasm that may occur with a single surgeon.

DEVELOPMENT OF A TEAM

There are many obstacles to the development of a skull base team. Foremost is finding individuals who are committed to working together as a team and willing to make compromises. There needs to be sufficient surgical volume to develop and maintain surgical skills.

- Team of surgeons
  - Attitude
  - Availability
  - Consistency
- Surgical expertise
  - Comfort level
  - Volume of cases
- Institutional resources or equipment
- Financial reimbursement
  - Lack of billing codes
  - Cosurgeons (reduced individual fees)
  - Low return for time investment?

Fragmentation of a team occurs when there are multiple specialists with overlapping skill sets caring for the same patient population. For example, an angiofibroma may be treated by a head and neck surgeon, rhinologist, or pediatric otolaryngologist. Internal competition for cases results in dilution of experience.

Logistical problems that need to be considered include

- Clinic
  - Separate or combined?
- Schedules
  - Clinics
  - Operating days
- Location of surgical theater
  - Block times
  - Inclusion of single specialty operations
- Postoperative care during hospitalization
  - Specialty intensive care units
  - Availability of specialists
- Coding and billing
  - Departmental budgets
  - Service lines.

RESOURCES

Does the institution have the necessary resources to support a skull base team? In addition to operating room facilities, equipment, and staff, it is important to have adequate support services. This includes expertise in diagnostic services (radiology, pathology) and clinical services (eg, interventional radiology, critical care).

Equipment for EES

- Endosurgery suite
- Optical system
- Navigation system
- Neurophysiologic monitoring
- Endoscopic instruments
  - Soft tissue dissection
  - Bone dissection
  - Hemostasis
- Doppler probe
- Reconstructive materials.

DYSFUNCTIONAL TEAM

The function of a team greatly depends on the characteristics of the members. Factors that result in a dysfunctional team include

- Age, power disparity
- Inflexible schedules
- Different treatment philosophies
- Disruptive behavior
- Egocentric attitude (see https://youtu.be/THNPmhBI-8I for an example[2]).

Surgeons who differ in age or experience will not be equals in the operating theater. This can limit open communication and surgical innovation. Differing treatment philosophies are not necessarily a problem as long as the team members are receptive to new ideas and willing to reassess their convictions using an evidence-based approach. The most successful teams are those that are able to compromise and are adaptable to change.

FUNCTIONS OF TEAM

The otolaryngologist (rhinologist) and neurosurgeon have different roles in the operating room, as well as in the preoperative and postoperative care of patients. Depending on the type of disease, the preoperative evaluation may be performed by one or the other specialty. For example, the otolaryngologist is the first contact for patients with sinonasal malignancy and completes the preoperative assessment, including imaging and biopsy. In contrast, the neurosurgeon is typically responsible for the preoperative evaluation of patients with chordomas. Although both surgeons share in the surgery, the otolaryngologist will have a bigger role with the removal of extradural tumors, whereas the neurosurgeon will participate more with neoplasms that involve the ventral skull base or extend intracranially. Both surgeons participate in reconstruction. Postoperatively, there is a similar division of labor, depending on the tumor type (adjunctive therapy, tumor surveillance). For EES, the patient will require more visits to the otolaryngologist for postoperative care of the nasal cavity.

TRAINING

Proper training is a key component of building a skull base team. There is a significant learning curve associated with EES of the skull base. Transition from open transcranial surgery to EES requires relearning skull base anatomy from an endoscopic perspective, adapting to 2-dimensional visualization, learning to function as a team, and mastering new surgical techniques. An incremental training program for EES has been proposed based on level of technical difficulty, potential risk of vascular and neural injury, and unfamiliar endoscopic anatomy.[3] Advancement to the higher levels (with intradural dissection) is predicated on a commitment to team surgery, sufficient volume of cases, and adequate resources (**Table 3**).

The volume of surgery necessary to attain proficiency has not been established. In general, the literature suggests that approximately 30 to 50 cases are necessary to build team skills and reduce complications to the baseline level.[4] Mastery of each level of the training program should be achieved before advancing to the next level.

Examination of his or her own learning curve can provide insight for surgeons into areas for improvement. With the treatment of chordomas, a gross total resection (GTR) is the most important factor for prevention of recurrence. Examination of the authors' team experience demonstrated that residual tumor was most likely in the lower clival area, especially deep to the paraclival carotid artery in the petrous apex.[5] With greater team experience came an increased understanding of anatomic relationships and the ability to target this area more effectively. The learning curve demonstrates an increase in GTR with successive quartiles of patients (**Fig. 1**).

FAILURE

Failure to build a successful team is a consequence of multiple factors that have been previously presented. To recapitulate, surgeons fail at EES because

Table 3
Incremental training levels for endoscopic endonasal skull base surgery

Level	Description	Examples
I	Sinus surgery	Endoscopic sphenoethmoidectomy Sphenopalatine artery ligation
II	Advanced sinus surgery Basic skull base surgery	Endoscopic frontal sinusotomy Cerebrospinal fluid leaks Lateral recess sphenoid Sella or pituitary (intrasellar) Medial orbital decompression
III	Extradural skull base	Sella/pituitary (extrasellar) Optic nerve decompression Transodontoid approach (extradural) Transclival approaches (extradural) Petrous apex (medial expansion)
IV	Intradural skull base 1. Cortical cuff 2. No cortical cuff	Petrous apex (exposure of carotid) Transplanum approach (intradural) Craniofacial resection Transclival approaches Transodontoid approach (intradural) Suprapetrous carotid approach
V	Coronal plane Vascular dissection	Infrapetrous carotid approach Parapharyngeal space Aneurysms Vascular malformations Highly vascular tumors

Adapted from Snyderman C, Kassam A, Carrau R, et al. Acquisition of surgical skills for endonasal skull base surgery: a training program. Laryngoscope 2007;117(4):701; with permission.

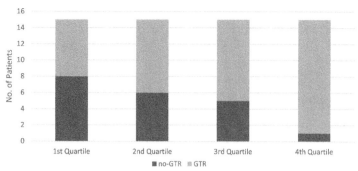

Fig. 1. Resection rates in quartiles of chordoma patients. (*Adapted from* Koutourousiou M, Gardner PA, Tormenti MJ, et al. Endoscopic endonasal approach for resection of skull base chordomas: outcomes and learning curve. Neurosurgery 2012;71(3):620; with permission.)

- They do not work as a team
- Lack of patience with the learning curve
- First case is too difficult
- They do not learn anatomy
- Inadequate instrumentation
- Insufficient volume of cases
  - Rare disease
  - Competition between institutions
  - Competing subspecialties
- Lack of mentoring
- Financial obstacles.

One of the challenges of developing a new skill is a lack of mentoring. The traditional model for acquiring a new surgical skill is to attend a course consisting of anatomic models or laboratory skill sessions. This is followed by a period of observing or assisting a surgeon skilled in the technique. The next stage is to perform cases with supervision. In the absence of such mentorship, patients may be exposed to unnecessary risk and mastery of the surgical technique may not be attained.

Surgical telementoring is the use of telemedicine to provide mentoring without directly controlling the surgery.[6] Surgical telementoring provides the ability to help surgeons develop their surgical skills to a greater level of proficiency for complex surgeries when experienced mentors are not available locally. The technology is reliable and available at most institutions. Perceived benefits of surgical telementoring in EES include improved surgical exposure, increased extent of tumor resection, and decreased duration of surgery. Remote telementoring has the potential to be a cost-effective model for global education in surgical techniques.

The telementoring process includes

- Case selection
  - Review of medical records, scans, pathologic evaluation
  - Discussion of surgical plan
- Schedule session
  - Accommodation for time difference (personnel, facility)
- Technology needs
  - Test connection

- Live session
- Debriefing and evaluation
- Follow-up
  - Outcome
  - Review scans.

CONTINUOUS IMPROVEMENT

Surgeons have an ethical responsibility to monitor their outcomes to determine if variations in care are having a positive or negative impact. Without measurement, there is no baseline for improvement: "You cannot change what you do not measure."

Quality improvement is a repetitive cycle with well-defined steps.[7] Popular tools include the plan, do, study, act (PDSA) or define, measure, analyze, improve, control (DMAIC) cycles (**Fig. 2**).

The first step is to select an appropriate metric for measurement. This may be based on a review of the literature or the surgeon's results. It is important to choose a metric that is personally important, measurable, and subject to change. Types of data include qualitative and quantitative variables, and may include single events (eg, morbidity, mortality, recurrence), almost-never events (eg, nerve or vascular injury), and near-misses (events that could have occurred). It is helpful to visualize the data with graphing of results to detect trends over time. Further analysis will help to identify contributing factors. A common tool is a root cause analysis that asks a series of "why" questions to determine the root causes of an outcome. Root causes that are amenable to change can then be targeted with a quality improvement plan using the PDSA or DMAIC cycle. Once the target has been reached, continuous monitoring maintains the improvement or a new goal is established.

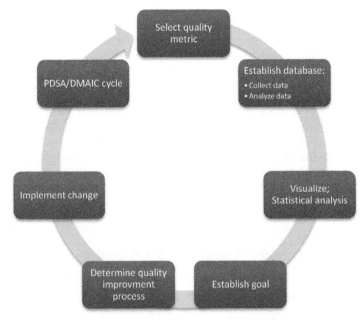

Fig. 2. Quality improvement is a repetitive cycle with well-defined steps.

MARKETING

Marketing of the skull base team provides a service to patients while building the referral base for new patients. Most patient referrals occur by word of mouth; this comes from the provision of excellent patient care and service. Other marketing strategies include a Web presence, community lectures, publications (medical journals and texts), newsletters (patients and physicians), and teaching courses.

CENTERS OF EXCELLENCE

There is a strong association between volume and outcome across many disciplines. Teams that specialize and have a high volume achieve superior results. This is particularly true for rare problems that are high-risk or require complex care. A center of excellence (COE) can be defined as "a cohesive team of specialists who promote collaboration and apply best practices in a specific focus area to improve results and overall outcomes."[8] Through reduction of variation, COEs are thought to improve outcomes while reducing costs. Just as surgical expertise depends on adequate surgical volumes, so does expertise in pathology, radiology, radiation oncology, and other disciplines that are necessary for the care of patients with sinonasal and ventral skull base malignancy. Proposed missions of COE include: (1) provision of superior patient care, (2) education and training, and (3) advancement of the field through research.

REFERENCES

1. Snyderman CH. The art of driving. Available at: www.skullbasecongress.com. Accessed September 25, 2016.
2. Brain Surgeon – That Mitchell and Webb Look, Series 3 – BBC Two. Available at: https://youtu.be/THNPmhBl-8l. Accessed September 25, 2016.
3. Snyderman C, Kassam A, Carrau R, et al. Acquisition of surgical skills for endonasal skull base surgery: a training program. Laryngoscope 2007;117(4):699–705.
4. Smith SJ, Eralil G, Woon K, et al. Light at the end of the tunnel: the learning curve associated with endoscopic transsphenoidal skull base surgery. Skull Base 2010; 20(2):69–74.
5. Koutourousiou M, Gardner PA, Tormenti MJ, et al. Endoscopic endonasal approach for resection of skull base chordomas: outcomes and learning curve. Neurosurgery 2012;71(3):614–25.
6. Snyderman CH, Gardner PA, Lanisnik B, et al. Surgical telementoring: a new model for surgical training. Laryngoscope 2016;126(6):1334–8.
7. Simmonds T, Haraden C, Munch D. Care process improvement. In: Frankel A, Leonard M, Simmonds T, et al, editors. The essential guide for patient safety officers. Oakbrook Terrace (IL): Joint Commission Resources; 2009. p. 103–12.
8. McLaughlin N, Laws ER, Oyesiku NM, et al. Pituitary centers of excellence. Neurosurgery 2012;71:916–26.

Survival, Morbidity, and Quality-of-Life Outcomes for Sinonasal and Ventral Skull Base Malignancies

CrossMark

Suat Kilic, BA[a], Sarah S. Kilic, MA[b], Soly Baredes, MD[a,c],
James K. Liu, MD[a,c,d], Jean Anderson Eloy, MD[a,c,d,e],*

KEYWORDS

- Sinonasal malignancy • Sinonasal cancer • Nasal cavity • Paranasal sinus
- Ventral skull base malignancy • Anterior skull base malignancy • Survival
- Outcomes

KEY POINTS

- Sinonasal and ventral skull base malignancies are rare and this has made it difficult to conduct randomized controlled trials. Much knowledge of the clinical outcomes for these malignancies is based on retrospective chart review studies.
- Overall survival for sinonasal and ventral skull base malignancies remains poor.
- For most histologies, primary treatment with surgical resection with or without adjuvant radiotherapy provides the best survival outcome.

INTRODUCTION

Sinonasal and ventral skull base malignances are uncommon, and this has made it difficult to conduct randomized controlled trials. Much of what is known about the outcomes of these malignancies is based on retrospective, single-institution, or

Financial Disclosure: None.

Conflicts of Interest: None.

[a] Department of Otolaryngology – Head and Neck Surgery, Rutgers New Jersey Medical School, Newark, New Jersey 07103, USA; [b] Department of Radiation Oncology, Rutgers New Jersey Medical School, Newark, New Jersey 07103, USA; [c] Center for Skull Base and Pituitary Surgery, Neurological Institute of New Jersey, Rutgers New Jersey Medical School, Newark, New Jersey 07103, USA; [d] Department of Neurological Surgery, Rutgers New Jersey Medical School, Newark, New Jersey 07103, USA; [e] Department of Ophthalmology and Visual Science, Rutgers New Jersey Medical School, Newark, New Jersey, 07103, USA

* Corresponding author. Endoscopic Skull Base Surgery Program, Department of Otolaryngology – Head and Neck Surgery, Rhinology and Sinus Surgery, Otolaryngology Research, Neurological Institute of New Jersey, Rutgers New Jersey Medical School, 90 Bergen Street, Suite 8100, Newark, NJ 07103.

E-mail address: jean.anderson.eloy@gmail.com

Abbreviations	
AC	Adenocarcinoma
ACC	Adenoid cystic carcinoma
DLBCL	Diffuse large B-cell lymphoma
DSS	Disease-specific survival
ENKTL	Extranodal natural killer/T-cell lymphoma
EP	Extramedullary plasmacytoma
LRC	Locoregional control
MM	Mucosal melanoma
NC	Neuroendocrine carcinoma
ON	Olfactory neuroblastoma
OS	Overall survival
PFS	Progression-free survival
QOL	Quality-of-life
RFS	Recurrence-free survival
RS	Relative survival
SCC	Squamous cell carcinoma

population-based database studies. Population-based databases, such as the Surveillance, Epidemiology, and End Results (SEER) and National Cancer Database (NCDB), allow researchers to pool cases from many institutions to study the behavior of these malignancies. They have significantly expanded the knowledge base on sinonasal and ventral skull base malignancies. However, with regard to outcomes research, these population-database studies have some inherent limitations that necessitate cautious interpretation of their findings.

SEER and NCDB capture approximately 26% and 70% of new cancer diagnoses in the United States, respectively. Therefore, a certain degree of selection bias may exist because cases reported in surveyed areas may not be representative of the entire population. For example, the SEER database collects information primarily from urban areas, where there may be a higher proportion of patients with lower socioeconomic status. Although single-institutional retrospective studies are also susceptible to this bias and many other types of selection bias, population-based studies have additional disadvantages that make it difficult to generalize some of their findings. The information in the databases is derived from the work of many different clinicians and pathologists, and the information is coded into the database by many different people, which may lead to inconsistencies in reporting. In particular, SEER lacks certain details of treatment, such as chemotherapy, the dose of radiotherapy, type of surgical treatment, tumor margins, and complications of treatment. Additionally, the databases do not contain information on the clinical reasoning that may be associated with treatment decisions. For example, in SEER, the intent of radiotherapy is not specified; radiotherapy with curative intent is indistinguishable from palliative radiotherapy. Retrospective chart reviews allow researchers to be able to take such nuances into consideration. Furthermore, death is not the only outcome of significance in oncology. For many of the sinonasal malignancies, recurrence is a key event, causing substantial morbidity even in the absence of mortality. In fact, morbidity is neglected altogether in the SEER database. This may result in studies underestimating the burden of disease for insidious malignancies with devastating local effects.

With regard to survival, the use of these databases presents additional challenges. At tertiary referral centers, the source of most studies not from databases, academic physicians are usually aware of the value of reporting results for rare malignancies and there may be a greater incentive to follow patients for a long period of time. In many population-based survival analyses, a large portion of patients are censored after a short time period. This has the potential to compromise the precision of the reported survival rates.

Another factor to consider is user error. There is a steep learning curve to understanding these databases. Accessing the right data and performing the appropriate analysis can be challenging because there are many subtleties to the use of software used to access the data. For example, SEERStat, the software used for SEER data, has hundreds of selections and settings. Many of these settings, although they may seem minor, can influence the results of a study. Furthermore, the databases undergo frequent changes, and information has to be recoded. This further complicates the coding system; several manuals and appendices may be required to make sense of the database.

Therefore, this article presents a dedicated discussion of outcomes for patients with sinonasal and ventral skull base malignancies organized by histology, without using population-based database study results. It focuses on the outcomes of death and recurrence, using studies in the literature that report survival rates and locoregional control (LRC) rates. Quality-of-life (QOL) outcomes and the side effects of certain treatments are also discussed. Factors that affect these outcome measures are highlighted.

Because there are many ways of calculating survival rates, it is not always possible to perform like-with-like comparisons. For example, some studies report overall survival (OS), whereas others report relative survival (RS) and/or disease-specific survival (DSS). RS takes into account the expected survival rate of people with demographic characteristics similar to the patient. There are several ways of calculating it, and researchers are not always familiar with the complexity of the underlying concepts. Moreover, the methods are not always fully reported in the literature. Articles sometimes fail to mention whether the actuarial or Kaplan-Meier model was used, or whether the Ederer II or Hakulinen method was used to calculate expected cumulative survival. It then becomes difficult to make an analogous comparison of survival outcomes.

In DSS, also known as cancer or carcinoma-specific survival, the outcome event is death from cancer. However, the cause of death is not always so clear. This introduces an interesting quandary, that is, the inability to agree on the definition of death. The term bias of cause-of-death interpretation has been used to describe this significant interobserver variability.[1] There are plenty of conceivable scenarios in which the cause of death may not be clear-cut. Given that patients with head and neck cancer may have an increased risk of suicide compared with the general population,[2] to what is the death of a patient who commits suicide attributed? If a patient with head and neck cancer dies of aspiration pneumonia, should it be assumed that this was a direct consequence of the cancer and, therefore, should be coded as a cancer-related death?

Despite the limitations of these survival metrics, studies can be meaningful when considered in the context of the larger body of literature. Therefore, survival outcomes should be thought of as estimates rather than precise measurements, and clinicians should maintain a healthy level of skepticism until multiple investigations confirm similar results.

OVERALL OUTCOMES

As a whole, malignancy of the sinonasal cavity and ventral skull base portends a poor prognosis. In a report of 220 cases from 2 institutions and meta-analysis of 16,396 cases, a 41% 5-year OS was reported for the meta-analysis group.[3] When cases were broken down by subsite, 5-year OS for the nasal cavity (1960s: 63%; 1970s;

54%; 1980s: 59%; 1990s: 66%) was higher than for the ethmoid (1960s: 27%; 1970s; 37%; 1980s: 56%; 1990s: 51%) and maxillary (1960s: 26%; 1970s; 31%; 1980s: 39%; 1990s: 45%) sinuses.[3] Over these 4 decades, survival for the maxillary and ethmoid sinuses had improved but survival for the nasal cavity remained relatively unchanged.[3]

In the same study, laterality of tumors was also found to affect survival. LRC and DSS at 5-years was highest for tumors with right-sided involvement (70% and 73%, respectively), followed by left-sided involvement (53% and 57%, respectively) and bilateral involvement (25% and 30%, respectively). Increasing tumor stage (T-stage) is associated with decreasing 5-year OS: T1 = 91%, T2 = 64%, T3 = 72%, and T4 = 49%. Demographic determinants of survival were not as clear. The study found that, in the 220 institutional cases, women had better 5-year LRC and DSS when compared with men (69% and 72% vs 53% and 57%, respectively).

Extension of malignancies to the pterygomaxillary fossa, frontal sinus, and sphenoid sinus; erosion of the cribriform plate; and invasion of the dura were factors associated with poor survival outcomes. Although orbital extension may lead to blindness and decrease QOL, it was not clearly found to be associated with decreased survival.

Although the purpose of this article is not to discuss treatment options in detail, treatment-specific survival outcomes are worth examining. In the meta-analysis, the surgery-alone group (70% 5-year DSS) had the highest survival, followed by the surgery and radiotherapy group (56% 5-year DSS), and the radiotherapy-alone group (33% 5-year DSS).[3] Patients receiving chemotherapy, either alone or in combination with other treatment modalities, had 42% 5-year DSS. However, these patients were not randomized into treatment groups. Therefore, patients with localized or smaller lesions may have been more likely to be treated with surgery alone, accounting for the difference in survival seen between the treatment modalities. In the meta-analysis, 13% of patients developed metastasis to the neck lymph nodes and 5% of patients developed lymph node recurrence.[3] Those with primary neck metastasis had a 32% 5-year OS, and those with metastasis to the neck after treatment had a 25% 5-year OS.[3] Treatment of patients with local recurrence was successful 16% of the time.[3] Several studies have expectedly reported decreased survival with increased tumor size and 1 study found that radiological tumor volume may also predict progression-free survival (PFS).[4]

In patients treated with craniofacial surgery (CFS), high rates of postoperative complications have been reported. An international collaborative study of more than 1307 cases treated with CFS has reported any complications in 33%, wound complications in 18%, central nervous system complications in 15%, systemic complications in 4%, orbital complications in 1%, and mortality in 4% of cases.[5] Endoscopic endonasal surgery (EES), which has been promoted as a potentially equally effective treatment option for selected cases, is associated with a shorter hospital stay, although several studies have found no statistically significant difference in complication rates.[6–8]

Intensity-modulated radiation therapy[9] (IMRT) and proton beam therapy[10,11] (PBT) are frequently used to treat sinonasal malignancies, either as primary therapy or adjuvant postoperative therapy. In one study using IMRT, PFS was 47% and LRC was 51% at 5 years. Higher doses of radiation ($\geq$60 Gy) were associated with improved PFS and LRC.[9] One study looking at PBT found an LRC rate of 80%, and an OS rate of 47% at 5 years. In that study, smoking status was found to predict worse LRC; 5-year LRC for current smokers was significantly lower than for nonsmokers (23% vs 83%).[10]

Research on QOL outcomes for patients with sinonasal malignancies has focused on the use of surveys such as the Anterior Skull Base Questionnaire, Sino-Nasal Outcome Test (SNOT), and Rhinosinusitis Outcome Measure.[12] A systematic review has suggested that surgical resection is associated with an increase in QOL.[12] Furthermore, the endoscopic approach seems to be associated with an earlier and greater increase in QOL when compared with open methods.[12] A recent, prospective, SNOT-based study looking at patients with sinonasal cancer undergoing endoscopic resection has reported significant improvement in the psychological and sleep domains of the SNOT scores after 2 years but no significant improvement in rhinologic subdomain and overall SNOT scores.[13]

Another systematic review, focusing on the sinonasal morbidity associated with EES, found that nasal crusting (51%), discharge (40%), airflow blockage, and disturbances in olfaction are the most commonly associated morbidities.[14] Fortunately, most of these symptoms resolve in 3 to 4 months, although symptoms can persist for longer in more complex surgeries.[14] Mucocele formation was seen in 8% of cases but this rate may have been between 14% and 50% in pediatric patients.[14]

HISTOLOGY-SPECIFIC OUTCOMES
Squamous Cell Carcinoma

Most of the available studies not from databases on sinonasal malignancies include multiple histologies. Although several studies focusing exclusively on sinonasal squamous cell carcinoma (SCC) have been published, some of these studies focused on a single subsite and most have small sample sizes. In the meta-analysis previously mentioned, 58% of cases were SCCs. Although survival for all other histologies remained stable from 1950 to 1990, it improved for SCC.[3] Five-year OS for SCCs diagnosed in the 1960s, 1970s, 1980s, and 1990s was 25%, 34%, 45%, and 50%, respectively.[3] In the same study, for the 126 institutional cases of SCC, LRC at 2, 5, and 10 years was 61%, 58%, and 56%, respectively; DSS at 2, 5, and 10 years was 73%, 60%, and 59%, respectively.

In a report of 33 sinonasal SCC cases, at 5-years, DSS and OS were 46% and 40%, respectively.[15] Surgical resection followed by radiotherapy was associated with higher DSS when compared with surgery alone, regardless of stage, suggesting that postoperative radiotherapy may improve 5-year survival.[15] Compared with other histologies, neck lymph node recurrence seems to be more common in SCC. In maxillary sinus SCC, 18.7% of cases have neck lymph node recurrence at 2 years and 20.7% of cases have neck lymph node recurrence at 5 years.[16] In patients with maxillary sinus SCC, involvement of the alveolus and cheek may increase the risk of neck recurrence even further.[17,18]

Histologic variants of sinonasal SCC may have different survival rates. Due to their rarity, few studies have reported specific survival rates for sinonasal SCC variants. However, results from studies on head and neck SCC variants may be used to estimate prognoses for the different variants. Verrucous SCC, a low-grade, human papillomavirus–associated variant, tends to have a more favorable prognosis, whereas basaloid SCC tends to have poorer prognosis.[19] Papillary SCC and sarcomatoid SCC, despite having high locoregional recurrence rates, tend to have higher survival rates.[19] Progression to sinonasal SCC from an inverted papilloma may be another negative prognosticator for SCC.[20] One study of 87 such cases reported a 39.6% 5-year OS and 30.7% 10-year OS.[20] For these tumors, advanced stage, metachronous tumors, and extension to the cranial base or orbit were found to be associated with decreased survival.[20]

Adenocarcinoma

Sinonasal adenocarcinoma (AC), which is thought to be the second or third most common primary sinonasal malignancy, is relatively well-studied. One multicenter study from France has reported on 418 cases.[21] Based on the cell of origin, it may be classified as salivary or nonsalivary type. The nonsalivary type may be classified as either nonintestinal type AC or as intestinal-type AC (ITAC),[22] which has been heavily associated with occupational exposures.[23] ITAC may further be classified into the papillary, colonic, mucinous, solid, or mixed subtypes.

Survival rates for sinonasal AC is thought to be higher than for SCC. According to 1 study, 5-year DSS is 78% for AC, and 60% for SCC.[3] The LRC rate at 5 years is 69% for sinonasal AC.[3] Another study, with 66 cases, reported similar values. Five-year OS and DSS for sinonasal AC were 66% and 79%, respectively.[24] The large, multicenter study previously mentioned also reported a similar rate; 5-year OS was 64%.[21] Several studies have found higher T-stage to predict poor prognosis and, as in SCC, tumor volume was found to be inversely related to survival.[23] Local recurrence, positive surgical margins, female gender, and advanced age (especially when treated with craniofacial resection) have been associated with decreased survival.[23] EES and open surgical methods were found to have comparable outcomes.[24,25]

Histologic subtype also seems to be predictive of survival.[23] Poorly differentiated subtypes, such as the solid and mucinous subtypes of ITAC, have been associated with lower survival compared with the papillary and mucinous subtypes.[23] The cause may also affect survival because cases related to wood-dust exposure have been shown to have higher survival.[23] Immunostaining positive for Ki-67 or CD31, which indicate high tumor growth fraction and microvessel density, respectively, have been associated with lower survival.[23] A more extensive list of histopathologic and molecular or genetic factors that may be associated with decreased survival for sinonasal malignancies can be found in **Table 1**.

Adenoid Cystic Carcinoma

Sinonasal adenoid cystic carcinoma (ACC) is a rare salivary gland malignancy known for its slow growth and high recurrence rates.[26] These tumors are usually locally destructive, often invading the orbit or skull base.[26] Perineural spread is a hallmark of ACC, with the maxillary, mandibular, and vidian nerves being the most commonly affected nerves.[27] For sinonasal ACC, a recent systematic review and meta-analysis reported a 63% 5-year OS, which is lower than survival for salivary gland ACCs.[26] In the same study, local recurrence was seen in 34% of cases.[26] Consequently, despite the favorable survival rate early on (relative to SCC and sinonasal malignancies overall), 10-year OS (32%) is low.[26] Perineural invasion, positive lymph nodes, and positive surgical margins are considered negative prognostic factors.[26] There is no consensus in the literature on the role of histologic appearance. Some studies have found that the solid type was associated with lower survival rates compared with the tubular and cribriform types,[28] whereas others did not.[29] Surgical resection (with negative margins), followed by radiotherapy, may lead to the best survival outcomes.

Mucoepidermoid Carcinoma

Mucoepidermoid carcinoma is a salivary gland malignancy that is rarely found in the sinonasal cavities. Like ACCs, these tumors have a tendency to invade the surrounding bony structures and peripheral nerves. Locoregional recurrence occurs in about

Table 1
Histopathologic and genetic factors associated with decreased survival in various sinonasal malignancies

Factor (Marker)	Effect
↑ Microvessel density (CD31)	↑ Stage, independent prognosticator for ↓ survival (AC and SCC)[62]
↑ Growth fraction (Ki-67)	↑ Stage, ↑ histologic grade, independent prognosticator for ↓ survival (AC and SCC)[62] ↓ Survival for (ACC and MEC)[63,64]
↑ Vascular endothelial growth factor expression	Independent prognosticator for ↓ survival (SCC only)[62]
↓ Annexin A2 expression	↑ Risk of aggressive subtypes (mucinous and solid subtypes) ↓ Survival (ITAC only)[65]
↓ F3 (coagulation factor III, involved in inflammatory and clotting cascades)	↑ Metastasis, ↓ Independent prognosticator for ↓ survival (ITAC only)[66]
↓ BRCA1 (tumor suppressor)	↑ Metastasis, ↓ Independent prognosticator for ↓ survival (ITAC only)[66]
↓ MIF (lymphokine that participates in inflammation, regulates the function of macrophages in the host defense)	↓ Survival (ITAC only)[66]
↑ PIK3CA (oncogene involved in cell survival, migration and intracellular vesicle transit)	↓ Survival (ITAC only)[66]
↑ UTY (minor histocompatibility antigen protein)	↓ Survival (ITAC only)[66]
↑ RELA (proto-oncogene; NF-kB subunit)	↓ Survival (ITAC only)[66]
↑ hTERT (human telomerase reverse transcriptase)	↑ Kadish Stage (ON only)[44]

Abbreviations: ACC, adenoid cystic carcinoma; MEC, mucoepidermoid carcinoma; ON, olfactory neuroblastoma.

one-third of patients and portends a poor prognosis.[30] One study has reported a 5-year recurrence-free survival (RFS) of 41% and OS of 44%.[30]

Mucosal Melanoma

Mucosal melanoma (MM) is one of the most deadly malignancies in the sinonasal cavities. One study with 53 subjects, all of which received at least craniofacial resection, reported a 19% 5-year DSS and RFS, and 18% OS.[31] Another study, which included 61 cases, reported a 5-year DSS of 22%.[32] The location, size, volume, and thickness of sinonasal MM seems to correlate with survival.[32] Tumors in the nasal cavity have been reported to have higher survival rates when compared with tumors in the paranasal sinuses, possibly due to earlier clinical presentation and/or higher chance of achieving negative margins.[33] Within the nasal cavity, tumors on the nasal septum have been shown to have the highest survival rates. One study with 58 cases put this figure at 50% 5-year OS.

Cutaneous melanomas are staged according to thickness (Breslow), thickness and ulceration (American Joint Committee on Cancer), or dermal (Clarke) levels. Due to the large number of available cases of cutaneous melanoma, these staging systems have been shown to have prognostic value. However, due to the rarity of sinonasal MM and the difficulty of obtaining reliable thickness measurements, there is no widely accepted staging system. Although 1 study has demonstrated decreasing survival with increasing T-stage,[34] this has not been confirmed by other studies.[35]

Larger tumor size, volume, and thickness have been associated with lower survival rates in 1 study.[32] Another study also suggests male gender to be a negative prognostic indicator.[33] One study has also shown an inverse correlation between level of pigmentation and survival, as well as decreased LRC in tumors with pseudopapillary architecture.[34] Multiple studies have also shown the presence of more than 10 mitotic figures per high-power field to be an independent prognostic indicator.[34,36,37] A study of 115 cases, the largest single-institution cohort reported to date, has demonstrated significantly higher OS and RFS rates for cases receiving endoscopic treatment.[35] In this series of subjects, almost all of the cases diagnosed since the mid-1990s were treated with EES, suggesting that survival outcomes for EES is at least as good as for open surgery.[35]

Olfactory Neuroblastoma

Olfactory neuroblastoma (ON), also known as esthesioneuroblastoma, is an uncommon malignancy arising from the olfactory epithelium. Despite its rarity, in comparison with most of the other histologies mentioned, it is relatively well-studied. One meta-analysis of 390 cases found that at 5 years, OS was 45% and DSS was 52%.[38] Another meta-analysis of 956 cases found that patients treated with surgery had a 78% 5-year OS and 67% 10-year OS.[39] Adjuvant radiotherapy was not found to significantly affect survival, with these patients having a 75% 5-year OS, and 61% 10-year OS.[39] However, other studies have shown a survival benefit for adjuvant radiotherapy in higher stage (Kadish C) tumors.[40] A more recent retrospective review found 5-year OS and RFS to be 67% and 51%, respectively.[41] Histologic grade has consistently been shown to predict survival. In the same study, tumors with Hyams grade III or IV had 56% 5-year OS and those with grade I or II had 25% 5-year OS (odds ratio = 6.18, 95% CI = 1.3–29.3).

The unique biological behavior of ON has prompted the development of 4 staging systems. Despite this, there is no consensus on the prognostic value of each of the staging systems. Both of the meta-analyses mentioned showed that the Kadish staging classification may have some prognostic value.[38,39] However, 1 study of 124 subjects, the largest cohort reported to date, suggests that neither the Kadish nor Morita staging systems predict survival.[42] This study also found tumors with high Hyams grade to have lower OS and RFS. A study of 109 cases by Van Gompel and colleagues,[40] in 2012, showed a 5-year OS of 63% and 10-year OS of 40%, and that higher modified Kadish stage (D and C), higher Hyams grade (3 and 4), lymph node metastasis, and age 65 years or older were associated with lower survival.

One study found that higher mitotic index and the presence of necrosis to be correlated with lower survival, whereas gland hyperplasia in the absence of spindle features and necrosis correlated with higher survival.[43] Another study found that high levels of human telomerase reverse transcriptase expression are correlated with high Kadish stage.[44] In the future, molecular and cytopathologic tests may be used to predict outcomes for ON.

Undifferentiated Carcinoma

Sinonasal undifferentiated carcinoma is defined by the World Health Organization as a "highly aggressive and clinicopathologically distinct carcinoma of uncertain histogenesis that typically presents with locally extensive disease."[45] It is often considered to be on the spectrum of neuroendocrine carcinomas (NCs) along with ON and sinonasal NC. Due to the rarity of the tumor and its relatively recent (1986) recognition as a distinct clinical entity, reliable survival rates have been hard to come by. However, most of the reported rates have been low, even for a sinonasal malignancy. One study found 5-year and 10-year DSS to be 40% and 24%, respectively. The same study found 5-year and 10-year LRC to be 41% and 33%, respectively.

A more recent study including 23 subjects treated between 1992 and 2010, found 5-year PFS, DSS, and OS to be 42%, 43%, and 32%, respectively.[46] In this study, survival was higher for patients receiving definitive surgery and postoperative radiotherapy with or without chemotherapy when compared with those receiving definitive radiotherapy with or without chemotherapy, suggesting that surgical resection is an indispensable part of multimodality treatment.[46] One meta-analysis of 167 cases has suggested neck disease, even in the absence of distant metastasis, is a poor prognostic indicator.[47]

Neuroendocrine Carcinoma

Sinonasal NC is a group of rare tumors that can be classified as well-differentiated (typical), moderately differentiated (atypical carcinoids), or poorly differentiated (small and non-small cell types). However, due to the similar histopathologic appearance of these tumors, they have not been consistently classified into the different subtypes and there is disagreement on the defining characteristics of some subtypes. One study reported 5-year OS, DSS, and RFS of 67%, 79%, and 44%, whereas another reported 5-year OS and local control of 64% and 29%, respectively.[48] The latter study also found a significantly lower 5-year OS of 29% for sinonasal small cell carcinoma.[49] Other negative prognostic indicators include tumor location other than nasal cavity, foveal involvement, and orbital involvement.[48]

There are few studies on the prognostic role of other subtypes of sinonasal NC. Although 1 study of head and neck NCs has found large differences in survival between the different subtypes,[48] a sinonasal NC-specific study has rejected this claim.[50] The head and neck NC study found a 5-year OS of 100%, 83%, 21.4%, and 20.8%% for typical carcinoid, atypical carcinoid, large cell, and small cell carcinomas, respectively.[48] However, it is important to note that the suspiciously high survival for typical carcinoid could be because, of the 23 total cases, only 2 were typical carcinoid tumors. More research is needed on the survival outcomes for the different subtypes.

Diffuse Large B-cell Lymphoma

Diffuse large B-cell lymphoma (DLBCL) is the most common non-Hodgkin lymphoma and the most common B-cell lymphoma of the sinonasal tract.[51] A wide range of survival rates have been reported for sinonasal DLBCL. One study has reported a 3-year OS of 44% despite a predominantly early-stage cohort. Other studies have reported 10-year OS of 50%,[52] greater than 70%,[53] and 72%.[54] Unlike most of the other histologies discussed here, the role of surgery is limited in the management of sinonasal DLBCL and offers no survival benefit.

A recent study retrospectively looked at the survival outcomes for 80 subjects with sinonasal or nasopharyngeal DLBCL treated with rituximab-cyclophosphamide, doxorubicin, vincristine and prednisone (R-CHOP) with or without adjuvant involved-field radiotherapy (IFRT) reported 5-year OS of 58% in subjects with paranasal sinus involvement and 68% in those without.[55] These rates were not significantly different from each other. Survival was not significantly different between subjects who received adjuvant IFRT and those who did not.

Extranodal Natural Killer/T-cell Lymphoma

In the East (Asia), extranodal natural killer/T-cell lymphoma (ENKTL) is the most common lymphoma of the sinonasal cavities. Due to the necrotizing and invasive lesions it forms in bone, cartilage, and soft tissues, it is also known as lethal midline granuloma.[27] A retrospective, multi-institutional review of 262 cases found 5-year OS to be 50%.[56] However, this value is misleading because 49% of all the deaths occurred in the first 6 months, demonstrating the aggressive nature of these lesions even early on in the disease course.[56]

Independent negative prognosticators were the presence of "B" symptoms (fever, sweats, weight loss), higher Ann Arbor stage, lactate dehydrogenase (LDH) level, and regional lymph nodes.[56] The use of the International Prognostic Index (IPI), which is a risk-stratification scheme validated for many other types of lymphomas, is controversial for sinonasal ENKTL.[56] The Prognostic Index for peripheral T-cell lymphoma unspecified (PTCL-U), which was proposed by Intergruppo Italiano Linfomi for risk stratification has shown more promise than the IPI at predicting prognosis for sinonasal ENKTL.[56] This model is based on age, performance status, LDH level, and bone marrow involvement.[57]

Primary treatment for sinonasal ENKTL is chemotherapy and/or radiotherapy.[58] The National Comprehensive Cancer Network, based on evidence from clinical trials, has recommended several regimens.[58] In a study of 358 subjects, the most common treatment of localized sinonasal ENTK was radiotherapy, dexamethasone, etoposide, ifosfamide, and carboplatin (RT-DeVIC). For more advanced lesions, L-asparaginase–containing chemotherapy regimens were used.[58] At least 1 study has also shown radiotherapy alone to provide the best outcomes for early-stage disease.[59]

Extramedullary Plasmacytoma

Sinonasal extramedullary plasmacytoma (EP) is a rare malignancy that is a subtype of plasmacytoma (monoclonal B-cell neoplasm).[60] One systematic review identified just 175 cases over several decades. Compared with other sinonasal malignancies, the survival rates are high.[60] Radiotherapy is first-line because local control of 80% to 100% has been reported with moderate doses of radiotherapy.[60] One study has reported a 10-year OS of 70%.[60] Although a review by Alexiou and colleagues[61] on head and neck EPs, of which 48% were in the sinonasal cavities, showed that cases treated with surgery and radiotherapy had the best outcomes, studies looking at more recently diagnosed cases suggest that radiotherapy alone may be sufficient. This is likely due to the technological advances in radiotherapy seen in more recent years.

SUMMARY

Sinonasal and ventral skull base malignancies are a rare, heterogeneous group of cancers. Thus, randomized controlled trials of these malignancies, which are the gold standard for medical research, have been difficult to conduct. Much of what is known about outcomes for these tumors comes from retrospective chart reviews in the literature. Stage at presentation, histology, grade, mechanism of carcinogenesis, molecular or genetic properties of tumors, treatment modality, surgical margins, and demographic factors are some of the factors that have been associated with different outcomes. Despite advances in treatment, long-term survival for these tumors remains low.

REFERENCES

1. Machtay M, Glatstein E. Just another statistic. Oncologist 1998;3(3):ii–iv.
2. Kam D, Salib A, Gorgy G, et al. Incidence of suicide in patients with head and neck cancer. JAMA Otolaryngol Head Neck Surg 2015;141(12):1075–81.
3. Dulguerov P, Jacobsen MS, Allal AS, et al. Nasal and paranasal sinus carcinoma: are we making progress? Cancer 2001;92(12):3012–29.
4. Hennersdorf F, Mauz P-S, Adam P, et al. Impact of tumour volume on prediction of progression-free survival in sinonasal cancer. Radiol Oncol 2015;49(3):286–90.
5. Patel SG, Singh B, Polluri A, et al. Craniofacial surgery for malignant skull base tumors. Cancer 2003;98(6):1179–87.
6. Eloy JA, Vivero RJ, Hoang K, et al. Comparison of transnasal endoscopic and open craniofacial resection for malignant tumors of the anterior skull base. Laryngoscope 2009;119(5):834–40.
7. Wood JW, Eloy JA, Vivero RJ, et al. Efficacy of transnasal endoscopic resection for malignant anterior skull-base tumors. Int Forum Allergy Rhinol 2012;2(6):487–95.
8. Dave SP, Bared A, Casiano RR. Surgical outcomes and safety of transnasal endoscopic resection for anterior skull tumors. Otolaryngol Head Neck Surg 2007;136(6):920–7.
9. Askoxylakis V, Hegenbarth P, Timke C, et al. Intensity modulated radiation therapy (IMRT) for sinonasal tumors: a single center long-term clinical analysis. Radiat Oncol 2016;11(1):1.
10. Russo AL, Adams JA, Weyman EA, et al. Long-term outcomes after proton beam therapy for sinonasal squamous cell carcinoma. Int J Radiat Oncol Biol Phys 2016;95(1):368–76.
11. Dagan R, Bryant C, Li Z, et al. Outcomes of sinonasal cancer treated with proton therapy. Int J Radiat Oncol Biol Phys 2016;95(1):377–85.
12. Kirkman MA, Borg A, Al-Mousa A, et al. Quality-of-life after anterior skull base surgery: a systematic review. J Neurol Surg B Skull Base 2014;75(02):73–89.
13. Derousseau T, Manjunath L, Harrow B, et al. Long-term changes in quality of life after endoscopic resection of sinonasal and skull-base tumors. Int Forum Allergy Rhinol 2015;5(12):1129–35.
14. Awad AJ, Mohyeldin A, El-Sayed IH, et al. Sinonasal morbidity following endoscopic endonasal skull base surgery. Clin Neurol Neurosurg 2015;130:162–7.
15. Michel J, Fakhry N, Mancini J, et al. Sinonasal squamous cell carcinomas: clinical outcomes and predictive factors. Int J Oral Maxillofac Surg 2014;43(1):1–6.
16. Cantù G, Bimbi G, Miceli R, et al. Lymph node metastases in malignant tumors of the paranasal sinuses: prognostic value and treatment. Arch Otolaryngol Head Neck Surg 2008;134(2):170–7.
17. Kondo M, Ogawa K, Inuyama Y, et al. Prognostic factors influencing relapse of squamous cell carcinoma of the maxillary sinus. Cancer 1985;55(1):190–6.
18. Kim GE, Chung EJ, Lim JJ, et al. Clinical significance of neck node metastasis in squamous cell carcinoma of the maxillary antrum. Am J Otolaryngol 1999;20(6):383–90.
19. Thompson L. Squamous cell carcinoma variants of the head and neck. Curr Diagn Pathol 2003;9(6):384–96.
20. Liang Q-Z, Li D-Z, Wang X-L, et al. Survival outcome of squamous cell carcinoma arising from sinonasal inverted papilloma. Chin Med J 2015;128(18):2457.
21. Choussy O, Ferron C, Védrine PO, et al. Adenocarcinoma of ethmoid: a GETTEC retrospective multicenter study of 418 cases. Laryngoscope 2008;118(3):437–43.

22. Cantu G, Solero CL, Mariani L, et al. Intestinal type adenocarcinoma of the ethmoid sinus in wood and leather workers: a retrospective study of 153 cases. Head Neck 2011;33(4):535–42.

23. Lund VJ, Chisholm EJ, Takes RP, et al. Evidence for treatment strategies in sinonasal adenocarcinoma. Head Neck 2012;34(8):1168–78.

24. Bhayani MK, Yilmaz T, Sweeney A, et al. Sinonasal adenocarcinoma: a 16-year experience at a single institution. Head Neck 2014;36(10):1490–6.

25. Vergez S, Martin-Dupont N, Lepage B, et al. Endoscopic vs transfacial resection of sinonasal adenocarcinomas. Otolaryngol Head Neck Surg 2012;146(5): 848–53.

26. Husain Q, Kanumuri VV, Svider PF, et al. Sinonasal adenoid cystic carcinoma systematic review of survival and treatment strategies. Otolaryngol Head Neck Surg 2013;148(1):29–39.

27. Kilic S, Shukla PA, Marchiano EJ, et al. Malignant primary neoplasms of the nasal cavity and paranasal sinus. Current Otorhinolaryngology Reports 2016;4(4): 249–58.

28. Wiseman SM, Popat SR, Rigual NR, et al. Adenoid cystic carcinoma of the paranasal sinuses or nasal cavity: a 40-year review of 35 cases. Ear Nose Throat J 2002;81(8):510.

29. Spiro RH, Huvos AG, Strong EW. Adenoid cystic carcinoma: factors influencing survival. Am J Surg 1979;138(4):579–83.

30. Wolfish EB, Nelson BL, Thompson LD. Sinonasal tract mucoepidermoid carcinoma: a clinicopathologic and immunophenotypic study of 19 cases combined with a comprehensive review of the literature. Head Neck Pathol 2012;6(2): 191–207.

31. Ganly I, Patel SG, Singh B, et al. Craniofacial resection for malignant paranasal sinus tumors: report of an International Collaborative Study. Head Neck 2005; 27(7):575–84.

32. Dauer EH, Lewis JE, Rohlinger AL, et al. Sinonasal melanoma: a clinicopathologic review of 61 cases. Otolaryngol Head Neck Surg 2008;138(3):347–52.

33. Lombardi D, Bottazzoli M, Turri–Zanoni M, et al. Sinonasal Adenocarcinoma: a 12-year experience of 58 cases. Head Neck 2016;38(Suppl 1):E1737–45.

34. Moreno MA, Roberts DB, Kupferman ME, et al. Mucosal melanoma of the nose and paranasal sinuses, a contemporary experience from the MD Anderson Cancer Center. Cancer 2010;116(9):2215–23.

35. Lund VJ, Chisholm EJ, Howard DJ, et al. Sinonasal malignant melanoma: an analysis of 115 cases assessing outcomes of surgery, postoperative radiotherapy and endoscopic resection. Rhinology 2012;50(2):203–10.

36. Thompson LD, Wieneke JA, Miettinen M. Sinonasal tract and nasopharyngeal melanomas: a clinicopathologic study of 115 cases with a proposed staging system. Am J Surg Pathol 2003;27(5):594–611.

37. Regauer S, Anderhuber W, Richtig E, et al. Primary mucosal melanomas of the nasal cavity and paranasal sinuses. APMIS 1998;106(1–6):403–10.

38. Dulguerov P, Allal AS, Calcaterra TC. Esthesioneuroblastoma: a meta-analysis and review. Lancet Oncol 2001;2(11):683–90.

39. Kane AJ, Sughrue ME, Rutkowski MJ, et al. Posttreatment prognosis of patients with esthesioneuroblastoma: clinical article. J Neurosurg 2010;113(2):340–51.

40. Van Gompel JJ, Giannini C, Olsen KD, et al. Long-term outcome of esthesioneuroblastoma: hyams grade predicts patient survival. J Neurol Surg B Skull Base 2012;73(Suppl 1):A007.

41. Hwang CS, Seo YW, Park SC, et al. Role of surgical treatment for esthesioneuro-blastomas: 31-year experience at a single institution. J Craniomaxillofac Surg 2016. [Epub ahead of print].
42. Bell D, Saade R, Roberts D, et al. Prognostic utility of Hyams histological grading and Kadish-Morita staging systems for esthesioneuroblastoma outcomes. Head Neck Pathol 2015;9(1):51–9.
43. Gallagher KK, Spector ME, Pepper J-P, et al. Esthesioneuroblastoma updating histologic grading as it relates to prognosis. Ann Otol Rhinol Laryngol 2014; 123(5):353–8.
44. Wang SL, Chen WT, Li SH, et al. Expression of human telomerase reverse tran-scriptase and cyclin-D1 in olfactory neuroblastoma. APMIS 2007;115(1):17–21.
45. Bell D, Hanna EY, Weber RS, et al. Neuroendocrine neoplasms of the sinonasal region. Head Neck 2016;38(Suppl 1):E2259–66.
46. Christopherson K, Werning JW, Malyapa RS, et al. Radiotherapy for sinonasal un-differentiated carcinoma. Am J Otolaryngol 2014;35(2):141–6.
47. Reiersen DA, Pahilan ME, Devaiah AK. Meta-analysis of treatment outcomes for sinonasal undifferentiated carcinoma. Otolaryngol Head Neck Surg 2012;147(1): 7–14.
48. Mitchell EH, Diaz A, Yilmaz T, et al. Multimodality treatment for sinonasal neuro-endocrine carcinoma. Head Neck 2012;34(10):1372–6.
49. Rosenthal DI, Barker JL, El-Naggar AK, et al. Sinonasal malignancies with neuro-endocrine differentiation. Cancer 2004;101(11):2567–73.
50. Likhacheva A, Rosenthal DI, Hanna E, et al. Sinonasal neuroendocrine carci-noma: impact of differentiation status on response and outcome. Head Neck Oncol 2011;3(1):1.
51. Kreisel FH. Hematolymphoid lesions of the sinonasal tract. Head Neck Pathol 2016;10(1):109–17.
52. Hatta C, Ogasawara H, Okita J, et al. Non-Hodgkin's malignant lymphoma of the sinonasal tract—treatment outcome for 53 patients according to REAL classifica-tion. Auris Nasus Larynx 2001;28(1):55–60.
53. Toda H, Sato Y, Takata K, et al. Clinicopathologic analysis of localized nasal/para-nasal diffuse large B-cell lymphoma. PLoS One 2013;8(2):e57677.
54. Proulx GM, Caudra-Garcia I, Ferry J, et al. Lymphoma of the nasal cavity and par-anasal sinuses: treatment and outcome of early-stage disease. Am J Clin Oncol 2003;26(1):6–11.
55. Lee G-W, Go S-I, Kim S-H, et al. Clinical outcome and prognosis of patients with primary sinonasal tract diffuse large B-cell lymphoma treated with rituximab-cyclophosphamide, doxorubicin, vincristine and prednisone chemotherapy: a study by the Consortium for Improving Survival of Lymphoma. Leuk Lymphoma 2015;56(4):1020–6.
56. Lee J, Suh C, Park YH, et al. Extranodal natural killer T-cell lymphoma, nasal-type: a prognostic model from a retrospective multicenter study. J Clin Oncol 2006; 24(4):612–8.
57. Gallamini A, Stelitano C, Calvi R, et al. Peripheral T-cell lymphoma unspecified (PTCL-U): a new prognostic model from a retrospective multicentric clinical study. Blood 2004;103(7):2474–9.
58. Yamaguchi M, Suzuki R, Oguchi M, et al. Treatments and outcomes of patients with extranodal natural killer/T-cell lymphoma diagnosed between 2000 and 2013: a Cooperative Study in Japan. J Clin Oncol 2016;JCO681619.
59. Li Y-X, Yao B, Jin J, et al. Radiotherapy as primary treatment for stage IE and IIE nasal natural killer/T-cell lymphoma. J Clin Oncol 2006;24(1):181–9.

60. D'Aguillo C, Soni RS, Gordhan C, et al. Sinonasal extramedullary plasmacytoma: a systematic review of 175 patients. Int Forum Allergy Rhinol 2014;4(2):156–63.

61. Alexiou C, Kau RJ, Dietzfelbinger H, et al. Extramedullary plasmacytoma. Cancer 1999;85(11):2305–14.

62. Airoldi M, Garzaro M, Valente G, et al. Clinical and biological prognostic factors in 179 cases with sinonasal carcinoma treated in the Italian Piedmont region. Oncology 2009;76(4):262–9.

63. Skalova A, Lehtonen H, von Boguslawsky K, et al. Prognostic significance of cell proliferation in mucoepidermoid carcinomas of the salivary gland: clinicopathological study using MIB 1 antibody in paraffin sections. Hum Pathol 1994;25(9): 929–35.

64. Nordgård S, Franzén G, Boysen M, et al. Ki-67 As a prognostic marker in adenoid cystic carcinoma assessed with the monoclonal antibody MIB1 in Paraffin Sections. Laryngoscope 1997;107(4):531–6.

65. Rodrigo JP, García-Pedrero JM, Llorente JL, et al. Down-regulation of annexin A1 and A2 protein expression in intestinal-type sinonasal adenocarcinomas. Hum Pathol 2011;42(1):88–94.

66. Llorente JL, Aldama P, Álvarez-Marcos C, et al. Nasosinusal adenocarcinoma: molecular and genetic analysis by MLPA. Acta Otorrinolaringol Esp 2008;59(4): 151–8.

Population-Based Results in the Management of Sinonasal and Ventral Skull Base Malignancies

CrossMark

Rami Abdou, MD, Soly Baredes, MD*

KEYWORDS

- Population-based analysis • Registry data • Anterior skull base malignancy
- Ventral skull base malignancy

KEY POINTS

- In the United States, population-based analyses of sinonasal malignancies have relied on the Surveillance, Epidemiology, and End Results (SEER) registry developed and maintained by the National Cancer Institute, representing 17 geographic areas in the United States and accounting for 26.2% of the population.
- Many clinically useful analyses that include epidemiologic and survival information regarding 13 distinct malignant histologies are made possible through the use of registry data.
- Although these analyses are powerful, important limitations, such as selection and confounding bias, omission of chemotherapy data, type of surgical approach used, and timing of radiation treatment, should be considered.

INTRODUCTION TO POPULATION-BASED ANALYSES AND REGISTRY DATA

Population-based cancer registries allow for collection, classification, and consolidation of cases on the scale of populations, outside the limits of any individual institution. This provides a method for measuring and studying patterns of disease over time across state lines, borders, and geographic locations inclusive of a wide spectrum of demographics and genetic compositions.[1]

In the United States, population-based analyses in surgical oncology have relied in part on the use of the Surveillance, Epidemiology, and End Results (SEER) registry developed and maintained by the National Cancer Institute. This database has

Financial Disclosure: None.
Conflicts of Interest: None.
Department of Otolaryngology – Head and Neck Surgery, Neurological Institute of New Jersey, Rutgers New Jersey Medical School, 90 Bergen Street, Suite 8100, Newark, NJ 07103, USA
* Corresponding author.
E-mail address: soly.baredes@rutgers.edu

Otolaryngol Clin N Am 50 (2017) 481–497
http://dx.doi.org/10.1016/j.otc.2016.12.019
0030-6665/17/© 2016 Elsevier Inc. All rights reserved.

oto.theclinics.com

Abbreviations	
AJCC	American Joint Committee on Cancer
API	Asian/Pacific Islander
DLBCL	Diffuse large B-cell lymphoma
DSS	Disease-free Survival
EBV	Epstein-Barr virus
ENB	Esthesioneuroblastoma
EMP	Extramedullary plasmacytoma
ENKTL	Extranodal natural-killer/T-cell lymphoma
NHW	Non-Hispanic white individuals
NPC	Nasopharyngeal carcinoma
OS	Overall survival
RS	Relative survival
RT	Radiation Therapy
SCC	Squamous cell carcinoma
SEER	Surveillance, Epidemiology, and End Results
SNAC	Sinonasal adenocarcinoma
SN-ACC	Sinonasal adenoid cystic carcinoma
SNEC	Sinonasal neuroendocrine tumor
SN-MEC	Sinonasal mucoepidermoid carcinoma
SN-RMS	Sinonasal rhabdomyosarcoma
SNUC	Sinonasal undifferentiated carcinoma

allowed for investigations into the course and treatment outcomes of specific malignancies that are more broadly generalizable than studies from individual institutions. The SEER registry began collecting data in 1973 and currently represents 17 geographic areas in the United States accounting for 26.2% of the population.[2–4] Although the data are considered highly valid, there is a slight overrepresentation of those living below the poverty level, inhabiting urban centers, born in foreign countries, and with education levels below a high-school diploma.[2] Information in the registry includes patient demographics, tumor histology, sites of involvement, extent of disease, use of surgical and/or radiation therapy (RT) modalities of treatment within 4 months of diagnosis, and patient survival, among other parameters.[2] Importantly, however, tumor stage is not always reported, particularly along TNM specifications, and metastases are not specifically defined. Furthermore, preexisting comorbidities, use of chemotherapy, and type of surgical intervention are not reported in the registry.

There are important caveats to consider when assessing applicability of conclusions drawn from population-based analyses as it pertains to the use of registry data. The SEER registry in particular, although clearly a powerful tool, is nonetheless vulnerable to all types of bias, particularly selection and confounding bias.[3,5–7] For instance, the decision-making process leading one patient to receive surgical treatment instead of, or in conjunction with, another treatment modality is not captured by the registry. Similarly, observational studies run the risk of drawing invalid inferences with incomplete control of confounding variables, such as comorbidities, which have a tendency to be undercoded.[2]

An important limitation in the SEER registry is the omission of chemotherapy treatment.[4] The contribution of chemotherapy either as a primary or adjuvant therapy on survival cannot be assessed. For instance, the impact of chemotherapy on lymphoma, which is this entity's treatment of choice, cannot be determined with registry data. Also more subtle comparisons, such as the impact of the BRAF deletion characteristic of mucosal melanoma and its reduced chemo-sensitivity,[8] could not be studied.

Although the use of RT is reported in the registry, 2 important limitations deserve attention. First, the timing of radiation, whether neoadjuvant, adjuvant, or primary, is not consistently reported. Second, the decision making associated with whether to add RT is not included in the registry, resulting in the possibility that radiation treatment is often reserved for refractory or late-stage disease or in patients with difficult surgical approaches. This has the effect of biasing survival analyses, as it would appear that patients treated with RT alone or with combination therapy have worse outcomes, although in reality it is a reflection of more advanced disease that would be expected to have reduced survival.

The conclusions regarding surgical treatments also warrant caution. The SEER registry does not provide information on surgical approaches or extent of surgery, such as gross total, subtotal, debulking, or palliative approaches, making the study of extent of resection difficult. Furthermore, the role of modern day endoscopic resection techniques, popularized over the past 20 years, may be changing the face of overall survival rates. Without this explicitly included in the registry data, conclusions are largely speculative. Finally, but equally important, pathologic data with regard to surgical margin status is not included, making the study of the merits of negative margin resection difficult.

Despite these limitations, in the absence of high-quality randomized controlled trials, the SEER database and other registries offer several advantages in the study of sinonasal and ventral skull base malignancies in particular. As sinonasal malignancies are rare, constituting fewer than 3% of all upper aerodigestive tract malignancies, using a population-based resource to study them allows for access to data from thousands of patients, sufficiently powering the statistical analyses in a way not possible with data from a single institution.[1–3,6] Certain types of bias are reduced, as there is a wide array of geographic areas and institutions represented lending external validity to the studies. Furthermore, active follow-up enables and improves accuracy of survival analyses.[9] As results are more readily generalizable, practitioners are better poised to apply results to individual patients.

GENERAL CONSIDERATIONS IN SINONASAL AND VENTRAL SKULL BASE POPULATION-BASED RESULTS

The SEER registry identified more than 7000 cases of sinonasal malignancies of all types since 1973.[10] Of these patients, 58.3% are of male gender, and 82.2% are white. The tumors are of mainly epithelial origin, including squamous cell carcinoma (SCC) (51.6%), adenocarcinoma (SNAC) (12.6%), esthesioneuroblastoma (ENB) (6.3%), and adenoid cystic carcinoma (SN-ACC) (6.2%), although many others have been studied.

The overall incidence of sinonasal malignancies is 0.556 cases per 100,000, stable over the past 30 years, compared with 1 to 5 per 100,000 for other head and neck sites.[10] There is an overall male-to-female ratio of 1.8:1.0, although incidence among men has trended down over time. With regard to race, incidence among white individuals has been constant, whereas among black individuals and "other" races there has been a decline. In terms of histology, SCC incidence has been declining substantially over time, whereas that of melanoma and ENB has been increasing. Five-year survival for all-comers is 54.5% ± 0.9%, with no significant change over time. Survival is better for white individuals (56.3% ± 1.0%) and "others" (50.3% ± 2.8%) as compared with black individuals (40.0% ± 2.8%). No differences in survival rates over time are noted for gender or for certain pathologies, including SCC, SN-ACC, ENB, melanoma, or sinonasal undifferentiated carcinoma (SNUC). In contrast, 5-year survival for SNAC shows improvement over time and is discussed later in this article.

Recent studies have found the nasal cavity to be the most commonly involved site (43.9%), followed by the maxillary sinuses (35.9%) and ethmoid sinuses (9.5%), although this varies by pathology.[10–12] The frontal and sphenoid sinuses are rarely involved, totaling 3.3% of reported sinonasal cases. Tumors originating in the nasal cavity have significantly better survival than tumors in other sinonasal locations.[11] Tumors are also more likely to present at an advanced stage with concordant poor survival. Reported 5-year relative survival is approximately 80%, 50%, and 30%, with no metastases, regional, and distant metastases respectively.[10]

With respect to 5-year survival, relatively favorable prognosis is seen for ENB (71% ± 2.6%) and SN-ACC (69.5% ± 2.8%), an intermediate prognosis for SCC (53.1% ± 1.1%) and SNAC (63.0% ± 2.1%), and poor prognosis for melanoma (34.7% ± 3.1%) and SNUC (34.7% ± 4%).[10] By site of origin, 5-year survival is best for nasal cavity (71.0% ± 1.3%), followed by ethmoid sinus (45.2% ± 2.8%), sphenoid sinus (40.6% ± 5.2%), maxillary sinus (39.5% ± 1.5%), and frontal sinus (35.3% ± 7.5%). Among those with localized disease, surgery alone offers the best survival, with combination surgery and RT portending a worse survival.[10,11] Patients treated with RT alone trend toward inferior survival (49.4% ± 1.1%) as compared with no RT (64.7% ± 1.5%). In patients with distant disease, those treated with RT have improved survival (31.1% ± 2.9% vs 21% ± 4.2%). Among those with regional disease, surgery, or the combination of surgery and RT (hereby referenced as combination therapy) is superior to RT alone. For those with distant disease, a similar trend is seen, although adding RT to surgery is better than surgery alone.

A query of the Netherlands Cancer Registry, encompassing the entire national population of 16.5 million between 1989 and 2009, found 3329 patients with sinonasal malignancies showing similar histologic trends with SCC as the most common histologic type (48%), followed by SNAC (15%), and melanoma (8%).[13] Consistent with other studies, SCC more commonly involves the nasal cavity and maxillary sinus, whereas SNAC more commonly involves the ethmoid sinus. Incidence among men rose until 1995, but has since seen a decline in both SCC and SN-ACC (11/1,000,000 per year), whereas incidence among woman was stable until 2006 and has since seen a significant increase due to SCC. This is coincident with measures to limit occupational exposure to wood dust in the Netherlands, implemented in 2000.

Multiple studies have concluded that surgery is the single most effective modality for sinonasal malignancy.[10–12,14] Radiation offers limited survival benefit, particularly for early-stage disease. In more advanced lesions, combination therapy consistently failed to demonstrate a significant benefit, although this may represent a selection bias, as more T3/T4 lesions were treated with combination therapy and would be expected to have a reduced survival regardless of therapy.

SPECIFIC SINONASAL MALIGNANCIES
Squamous Cell Carcinoma

As the predominant paranasal sinus solid tumor histologic subtype across all studies, SCC represents approximately half of all cases in the literature.[9] Occupational exposure to nickel, industrial fumes, and textile dust have been identified as risk factors, and SCC is particularly common among men and those of African and Asian (particularly Japanese) descent.[15] Chronic rhinosinusitis, allergies, nasal polyposis, Epstein-Barr virus (EBV), and tobacco are other risk factors. A study by Ansa and colleagues[9] of 2553 patients with SCC in the SEER registry between 1973 and 2009 noted more than half were between ages of 60 to 79, 63.6% were men, 75% were white, and 76% presented with maxillary sinus origin.[16] The overall incidence decreased over time, although incidence was increased among black individuals and other minorities. Of note, presence of "distant" disease decreased from 14.7% to 9.5% over the study period. The more advanced tumors involved the sphenoid and ethmoid sinuses. More than half of all cases were treated surgically with or without RT for all sites except those of the sphenoid sinus that were rarely treated surgically.

The 5-year and 10-year overall survival (OS) is 30.2% and 21.0%, respectively, and noted to be better in men and white individuals than women and black individuals.[9] The benefit of surgery alone versus combination therapy was similar, although both groups were better than RT alone. Factors associated with a higher mortality included advanced-stage disease, older age, and black race, where a 22% increase in mortality was noted with regional and distant disease compared with white individuals, even after control for stage and treatment. No difference in survival by sex or primary tumor site was noted. However, when examined by race, white individuals had the highest long-term survival (30.93% at 20 years), whereas black individuals consistently had the lowest survival rates coupled with the highest incidence rates. Patients with localized disease treated with surgery had the best 5-year survival at 85.71% compared with combination (80.38%) or RT alone (78.47%). Those with regional spread and distant metastases fared significantly worse.[17]

When stratifying SCC by histologic subtype, including conventional SCC, verrucous (V-SCC), papillary (P-SCC), basaloid (B-SCC), sarcomatoid (SCSC), and adenosquamous (ASC), interesting differences are noted.[18] B-SCC is found to have a statistically significant, albeit slightly lower age of diagnosis at 61.8 ± 15.6 years as compared with 66.0 ± 13.3 years for conventional SCC. SCSC is less likely than conventional SCC to arise in the nasal cavity (28.6% vs 46.3%) and possibly more likely to arise in the maxillary sinus (61.2% vs 41.5%, $P = .05$). There is a trend for less maxillary sinus involvement for P-SCC and more maxillary sinus involvement for SCSC relative to conventional SCC. V-SCC, a low-grade variant associated with human papilloma virus regarded as having a favorable prognosis, is more likely to be treated with surgery alone (70.7% vs 31.7%) and less likely to be treated with combination therapy (25.9% vs 40.4%) as compared with conventional SCC. No cases of V-SCC were treated with RT alone. Most cases of SCSC were treated with combination therapy (65.6%) and significantly fewer were treated with RT alone (3.1% vs 20.3%). These patterns are likely predicated on perceptions of each type of tumor's relative aggressiveness.

V-SCC and P-SCC are found to have significantly better 5-year survival as compared with conventional SCC (69.7% and 61.87% vs 45.0%, respectively) possibly related to their predilection for exophytic growth and early detection.[17–19] Sinonasal ASC has a markedly reduced 5-year survival compared with conventional SCC (15%). Although sinonasal V-SCC and P-SCC are found to have favorable prognoses, SCSC and ASC histologies appear to be poor prognostic indicators approaching statistical significance. With respect to advanced-stage disease, V-SCC, P-SCC, and B-SCC all are associated with improved prognoses as compared with conventional SCC. This is particularly interesting as B-SCC is considered by many to be the most aggressive subtype.[20] Among those with early-stage disease, B-SCC and ASC, considered the most deadly subtypes, show significantly worse prognoses, although the confidence interval was wide in this study.[18] Although nodal metastasis is an important prognostic indicator in ASC, scant data limited analysis in this regard.

Sinonasal Adenocarcinoma

Sinonasal adenocarcinoma (SNAC) is the most common primary malignancy of the ethmoid sinuses and associated with wood dust and other occupational exposures thought to afflict men more commonly than women.[21] The SEER registry identified 1270 cases split almost evenly between men and women potentially explained by the decreased role of occupational exposures and by the exclusion of states with the highest concentration of woodworkers reporting to the SEER registry.[22] The cohort is mostly older than 55 (59%), and white (78.0%).

With respect to Disease-free Survival (DSS), survival is 65.2%, 50.9%, 40.9%, and 36.5% at 5, 10, 15, and 20 years, with women having a slightly better, although statistically nonsignificant, survival rate compared with men.[22] Black individuals demonstrate a worse survival than other racial groups, with a DSS of 53.6%, 38.5%, 30.0%, and 30.0% at 5, 10, 15, and 20 years. The best survival is seen among the "other" subgroup, which includes Asian, Native American, and Hispanic individuals, and unknown and mixed races. Survival is reduced with regional and distant spread and 5-year survival drops from 96.0% in patients with stage I disease to 79.6%, 86.2%, and 61.7% in stage II, III, and IV, respectively. The EUROCARE registry, made up of 67 population-based cancer registries in 22 European countries, identified 204 cases of ethmoid sinus adenocarcinoma afflicting mainly men (86%), except Scotland in which men made up a minority of cases (45%).[23] Five-year net survival overall is 46% in this cohort, and is significantly better in those aged 55 to 64 years (60%) and worst among those older than 65 years (33%).

Of note, data on histologic subtype, namely intestinal and nonintestinal, are not available in the SEER registry, so its influence on survival could not be studied. However, nonintestinal SNAC is not thought to be associated with occupational exposures, tends to be localized, and is considered to have a favorable prognosis,[24] although these could not be studied using available population-based registry data.

Esthesioneuroblastoma

Esthesioneuroblastoma (ENB), also known as olfactory neuroblastoma, thought to arise from the olfactory neuroepithelium, is known to have equal sex distribution with wide age distribution, and may affect the cervical lymph nodes.[25] Jethanamest and colleagues[26] used the SEER registry to identify 311 patients, although only 261 could be staged with available information. The mean age of diagnosis is 53 years with most patients between the ages of 40 and 70 years, favoring a unimodal distribution. Most are men (55%), white (83%), and most commonly presented with Kadish B (49.8%) followed by Kadish D (29.1%) disease. The most common site of involvement is the nasal cavity (77%), followed by the ethmoid sinuses (15.6%). The OS is 62.1 at 5 years and 45.6% at 10 years. Overall mean survival time drops from just over 12 years for Kadish A to 4.48 years for Kadish D. OS and DSS drops from 83.4% and 90.0% for Kadish A to 13.3% and 35.6% for Kadish D. Regional nodal involvement is seen in 12.3% of cases and this is associated with a significantly reduced DSS consistent with the existing literature.[25,27–29] In line with current practice, combination therapy is associated with the longest duration of mean survival, followed by surgery alone, although the only statistically significant difference was between RT alone and multimodal therapy.[25,26,29]

Platek and colleagues[30] sought to assess the optimal treatment modality with regard to OS. Among 511 cases, patients received surgery only in 22% of cases, followed by radiation only in 11%, combination in 61%, and no treatment in 6%, with statistically significant difference in 5-year OS among the 4 groups, best for combination (73%) followed by surgery only (68%), radiation only (35%), and no treatment (26%), consistent with currently published protocols.[25,28,29] With regard to pairwise comparisons among the treatment groups, the only significant differences were between combination therapy versus RT only and between surgery only versus RT only. When Cox-regression analysis was performed, the difference between surgery only and RT only was no longer significant, although all the differences were no longer statistically significant at 10 years. Importantly, comparisons by stage were not performed, and surgical treatment details are not available. Selection bias with respect to treatment planning is an obvious limitation, as the rationale behind treatment decisions are not captured by the information contained in the SEER database.

Histologic grade of ENB has been reliably reported in the SEER database only over the past 20 years, with grades I and II representing low-grade ENB and grades III and IV as high-grade ENB, although these do not necessarily correlate with a true Hyams grade. Tajudeen and colleagues[31] analyzed a total of 281 patients in whom both grade and stage were reported. Low-grade tumors made up 48% of the cohort, with 52% having high-grade tumors. Advanced age, tumor grade, and modified Kadish stage are independent negative prognostic indicators of OS, whereas female sex independently predicts better OS. With respect to DSS, advanced tumor grade and modified Kadish stage are negative prognostic indicators, whereas radiation predicts better DSS. When looking at low-grade tumors, only surgery is predictive of DSS (hazard ratio [HR] 0.0135, $P<.004$) with no effect by RT on DSS or OS. With respect to high-grade tumors, neck disease, RT, surgery, and Kadish grade predict DSS. Multivariate analysis reveals modified Kadish stage (HR 2.025, $P<.001$), and RT (HR 0.433, $P<.01$) as independent predictors of DSS. Advanced tumor stage and modified Kadish stage are associated with worse DSS, whereas RT independently predicts better DSS with no influence of age or sex on DSS. These results suggest that for high-grade tumors, combination therapy is warranted, whereas for low-grade tumors, surgery with negative margins may be sufficient treatment.[28,32] However, the role and timing of RT for local control requires further study.

Sinonasal Adenoid Cystic Carcinoma

Adenoid cystic carcinoma, known for its long clinical course and perineural invasion, is of particular clinical interest in the sinonasal tract given the potential for skull base invasion along neural pathways.[33,34] A SEER registry study involving 412 cases of SN-ACC found both a female predilection and higher incidence among women, accounting for 57.52% of cases, in contrast to most other sinonasal malignancies, although this is consistent with ACC at other locations.[35] SN-ACC occurs predominantly in patients older than 55 years and most are white (77.43%), followed by black individuals (11.41%), and primarily involves the paranasal sinuses (63.35%), followed by the nasal cavity and nasopharynx (19.66% and 16.99%, respectively). There has been a significant decline in incidence over the past 30 years among women. Incidence rates are significantly decreasing among all races, particularly among black individuals and "others" as compared with white individuals, which may reflect changing socioeconomic standards among minorities. OS at 20 years is 22.39%, with a trend for higher survival among women, although this is not statistically significant at 5, 10, and 20 years (69.29%, 50.43%, and 28.84% vs 67.87%, 44.97%, and 28.14% for men). Survival rates at 10 years are significantly lower in this study than prior population-based analyses that reported 10-year survival of 79.88%.[36] White individuals have a significantly better survival rate as compared with black individuals, which is a trend previously reported for ACC at other head and neck sites.[37] Unfortunately, data on histologic subtype, type of treatment, and surgical margin status are not available, limiting a population-based analysis of various treatment paradigms.

Sinonasal Mucoepidermoid Carcinoma

Mucoepidermoid carcinoma, the second most common sinonasal malignancy of salivary gland origin after adenoid cystic carcinoma, is still very rare, accounting for fewer than 0.1% of sinonasal neoplasms.[38] A comparative analysis between sinonasal mucoepidermoid carcinoma (SN-MEC) and common salivary gland MEC (SG-MEC) using the SEER registry identified 4383 cases, of whom 149 were SN-MEC.[39] Both SN-MEC and SG-MEC are similar with respect to sex ratio and racial distribution. Of the SN-MEC, 51% are men, mean age of diagnosis is 58.6 years, and mostly affects whites (78.5%). The most common sites of involvement are the maxillary sinus (51.7%), followed by nasal cavity (32.9%) and ethmoid sinus (11.4%). With respect to histology, SN-MEC is more likely to present with high histologic grade (42.3%) as compared with SG-MEC (25.5%), possibly reflecting a delay in diagnosis or differences in tumor biology. Better 5-year survival is seen with SG-MEC (84.1% vs 61.7%). Survival for high-grade SN-MEC is significantly lower than for low-grade histology (43.6% vs 78%). There is also a significantly higher survival rate in SG-MEC for low-grade and high-grade histology compared with similarly graded SN-MEC tumors. With respect to treatment, survival is best for SN-MEC treated with surgery alone (81.3%), followed by combination therapy (64.4%) and RT alone (25.6%). Although this trend is seen for SG-MEC also, survival was significantly better among the SG-MEC as compared with SN-MEC for each treatment modality. Only MEC in the submandibular gland fails to show a significantly higher survival as compared with SN-MEC. High-grade lesions involving the parotid gland demonstrate a significantly better survival compared with high-grade SN-MEC (60.7 vs 43.6, $P = .026$), consistent with previously reported prognostic value of tumor grade. Parotid and sublingual gland MEC demonstrated better survival for equivalent treatment as compared with SN-MEC.

Female gender has a lower hazard of death from SN-MEC compared with men, similar to SNAC and SN-ACC, whereas older age, involvement of the ethmoid sinus, and high-grade histology are associated with a greater hazard of death. Primary RT treatment and tumor size larger than 4 cm are associated with markedly increased hazards of death (HR 6.65 and 8.36, respectively) and corroborate surgery as the treatment of choice for this entity.

Nasopharyngeal Carcinoma

Nasopharyngeal carcinoma (NPC), although rare in nonendemic areas and linked to various food preservatives and EBV, often presents at an advanced stage due to subclinical growth.[40] A SEER analysis of 1234 cases of nonkeratinizing (NK-NPC) and keratinizing (K-NPC) subtypes between 2004 and 2009 reveals a male predominance that is more pronounced for NK-NPC.[41] A significantly lower age of diagnosis is seen for NK-NPC (54.2 years vs 60.8 years). Affected persons are mostly white individuals in K-NPC (72.8%), whereas Asian/Pacific Islander (API) individuals make up most K-NPC cases (48.7%). APIs constitute only 15.6% of the K-NPC cases. Incidence is noted to be increasing over the noted period for NK-NPC but not for K-NPC, possibly representing immigration trends. NK-NPC is more likely to present with grade III (poorly differentiated) histology as compared with K-NPC (62.7% vs 28.5%), with most K-NPC cases either well (12.1%) or moderately (35.4%) differentiated. Both subtypes present at an advanced stage (stage III and IV) and most patients have "regional" disease. The 5-year DSS for NK-NPC was significantly higher at 60.2% compared with 46.0% for K-NPC, which has a nearly twofold increased hazard of death. Female gender is associated with a higher 5-year relative survival (RS) for NK-NPC and significantly lower 5-year RS for K-NPC, whereas API is associated with a higher 5-year RS for both subtypes. However, the influence of EBV status, a known positive prognostic indicator,[42] could not be determined in this study. Interestingly, survival difference by histologic grade is noted only for K-NPC, with grades III and IV demonstrating improved RS compared with grade I. For both cohorts, stage IV disease is a significantly poor prognostic indicator with markedly increased hazards of death. Consistent with prior studies, NK-NPC proved to be more radiosensitive and RT is associated with increased 5-year RS, although in both groups omission of RT is associated with worse outcomes.[43,44] Importantly, the role of chemotherapy could not be determined, although consensus exists for treating advanced disease with combination therapy.[45]

Sinonasal Undifferentiated Carcinoma

SNUC is a rare and aggressive malignancy of the small round blue-cell variety.[46] A study of 318 cases from the SEER database shows a male preponderance at 62%, afflicting mainly whites (82.7%), with mean age of diagnosis at almost 58 years, although distribution between the ages of 20 to 80 is fairly even.[47] Most patients are treated with radiation (79.6%) with 44.7% treated with combination therapy. Median survival for the entire cohort is 22.1 months, with 3 to 5 and 10- year survival at 44.3%, 34.9%, 31.3%, which has increased significantly over the study period. Those diagnosed after age 60 have significantly worse survival than all other age groups, with a 2.67 greater rate of mortality by age 80. Although survival improves after treatment with both RT and surgery alone, combination therapy is associated with a 42% reduction in mortality compared with those with single modality or no therapy. Importantly, both extent of surgery and treatment with chemotherapy are not assessed and SNUC is deemed sensitive to both induction and concurrent chemotherapy regimens.

Kuan and colleagues[48] extrapolated staging by the modified Kadish system from the SEER registry and is the first population-based analysis to detect a difference in survival by tumor stage. A total of 328 cases were identified, with the most common subsites being the nasal cavity (29.3%), and maxillary (27.4%) and ethmoid sinuses (21.0%). Most present with modified Kadish stage C (51.2%) with regional and/or distant metastases identified in 18.9% of cases. The greatest number are treated with combination therapy (45.7%) and 42.7% are treated with either surgery or radiation. Median DSS is 2.9 years with 2-year, 5-year, and 10-year OS of 43%, 30%, and 25%, respectively. Older age, advanced Kadish stage, and larger tumor size are associated with worse OS and DSS. Treatment with combination therapy is associated with improved OS and DSS achieving a fourfold increase in survival.

In a subset analyses, improved DSS and OS are noted among Asian individuals as compared with white individuals and black individuals. There is also improved OS for tumors in the nasal cavity as compared with the maxillary sinus. Both OS and DSS were reduced with advanced tumor stages. Kadish A is not significantly different from other stages with respect to survival, although this is probably due to the low number of cases. Younger age, RT (and not surgery), and lower Kadish stage are independent positive prognostic indicators with respect to OS. This study, in contrast to prior case series, did not detect an association between nodal disease and survival, although this is possibly due to underreporting of nodal status in the SEER database (an overall incidence of 9.7% is reported).[49]

Sinonasal Neuroendocrine Tumor

Sinonasal neuroendocrine carcinoma (SNEC) is a rare sinonasal malignancy accounting for fewer than 5% of tumors at this site.[50] A total of 201 cases are identified using the SEER registry with a mean age at diagnosis of 55.8 years, mostly men (59.2%), and white (83.6%), followed by black individuals (8.0%).[51] The most common location involved is the nasal cavity (40.8%), followed by the ethmoid sinuses (20.4%), maxillary sinuses (18.4%), and sphenoid sinuses (12.9%), consistent with prior studies.[52,53]

The middle turbinate is commonly cited as the most common site of origin, although at least 1 study notes the ethmoid sinus as the most common location.[54] Most cases are grade III and IV (poorly differentiated, undifferentiated and anaplastic types), accounting for 62.7% of cases, although grade is missing in approximately 30% of cases. Staging information is available for 30% of cases and, of these, 70% were stage IV at diagnosis. The most common treatment is combination therapy (45.3%) followed by RT alone (14.9%) and surgery alone (14.9%).

There is a trend toward both increased incidence and survival rate over time, although these are not statistically significant. Overall 5-year survival was 50.8% with no difference with respect to sex or race. Involvement of the sphenoid sinus is associated with highest DSS at 5 years of 80.7% for unclear reasons, followed by the nasal cavity (59.2%), maxillary sinus (34.5%), and ethmoid sinus (33.3%). RS demonstrates the same trend being the highest for the sphenoid sinus (71.7%) followed by the nasal cavity (61.8%). Involvement of the maxillary and ethmoid sinus is associated with a greater hazard of death compared with nasal cavity involvement. The frontal sinus is not included in the analysis due to low numbers. As expected, survival is best for low-grade SNEC (5-year DSS 92.3%) compared with high-grade (5-year DSS 37%), although this was no longer significant after Bonferroni correction. Interestingly, those treated with surgery alone had the highest DSS at 69.0% compared with combination therapy (59.4%) and RT alone (39.9%).

Sinonasal Mucosal Melanoma

Sinonasal mucosal melanoma, comprising 4% of all head and neck melanomas, has frequently been combined with oral cavity melanoma in previously published case reports and single-institution retrospective studies to increase numbers at the expense of potentially obscuring important differences in survival.[55,56] Gal and colleagues[57] identified 304 patients using the SEER registry between 2000 and 2007, mostly women (56.3%) and whites (90.8%). The mean age of diagnosis was 71.2 years and the nasal cavity was the most commonly affected site (65.5%), followed by the maxillary sinus (15.1%). The primary treatment modality was surgery (81.6%) with or without postoperative RT. Overall 5-year survival was 24.2% with median survival 18 months for both sixth or seventh American Joint Committee on Cancer (AJCC) staging systems. The sixth and seventh editions upgraded mucosal melanoma T staging automatically to T3, eliminating T1 and T2 classifications, to emphasize depth of invasion as an important prognostic indicator as opposed to invasion of a specific anatomic site, as with other histologies.[58] Each additional 10 years of age is associated with a 20% increased risk of death. With respect to treatment, there is a significant increase in survival with combination treatment and surgery alone as compared with radiation alone. However, no significant differences are detected between combination treatment and surgery alone, supporting the idea of mucosal melanoma as a surgical disease. Nodal disease is uncommon in this cohort (only 2 had neck disease), although this information was missing in almost 28% of patients. With respect to the AJCC staging changes, the seventh edition staging system did detect a slightly improved survival profile for stage IVA as compared with IVB or IVC that may represent a more accurate disease profile compared with the sixth edition staging.

Survival based on location reveals a higher DSS and RS for nasal cavity tumors at both 1 year (81.06%) and 5 years (36.66%). The lowest survival is seen in patients with multiple sinus involvement (1 year DSS 54.55%).[59] Relative to nasal cavity tumors, there is a greater hazard of death for maxillary sinus (HR 1.34), ethmoid sinus (HR 1.60), and overlapping sinuses (HR 2.30), explained in part by tumors extending above "Ohngren's line," which pose a challenge to complete surgical resection. The sample sizes for frontal and sphenoid sinus disease are small and not included in the analysis, although all these patients died within a year of diagnosis. There are significantly more T4 tumors (44.13% vs 80.56%, $P<.001$) and TNM stage IV malignancies (51.05% vs 82.86%, $P<.05$) in the maxillary sinus compared with the nasal cavity, suggesting late diagnosis relative to nasal cavity tumors. With respect to treatment, those with maxillary sinus disease are more likely to receive RT. In patients with nasal cavity disease, patients treated with surgery alone and combination therapy have similar 5-year survival, although those treated with RT alone had significantly reduced 5-year survival. Interestingly, patients with maxillary sinus disease witness the best 5-year survival with surgical resection alone, and reduced survival with combination therapy (46.75% vs 19.63%), although this may be due to advanced disease, positive margins, and/or difficult surgical approaches in those who receive RT. These findings are consistent with current data supporting surgical resection with negative margins for optimal survival, with no established benefit of RT on survival.[60]

Diffuse Large B-Cell Lymphoma

Diffuse large B-cell lymphoma (DLBCL) is one of the most common sinonasal lymphomas, presenting with nonspecific signs and symptoms across a wide age range.[61] A SEER analysis of 852 patients between 1973 to 2009 shows a mean age at diagnosis of 65.8 years, slightly more men than women (54.5%), mostly white individuals (80.9%), and no significant change in incidence during the time period of study.[62] The most common site of tumor involvement is the maxillary sinus (36.9%), consistent with prior studies, followed by the nasal cavity (34.0%), ethmoid sinus (8.7%), sphenoid sinus (4.1%), and frontal sinus (2.3%), with overlapping lesions in 4.3% of cases. Overall 1-year and 5-year survival is 83.7% and 68.7%, with no significant differences by age or sex. There are no statistically significant differences in survival between DLBCL of the sinonasal tract as compared with other head and neck sites. Only overlapping sinus involvement shows a significantly worse survival compared with tumors in the nasal cavity (HR 1.8, $P<.05$), although the literature suggests a worse prognosis for nasal cavity tumors, not seen in the SEER study. RT is associated with increased DSS and is noted to be a positive prognostic factor. The role of chemotherapy, considered a mainstay of treatment,[63] on survival could not be assessed.

Extranodal Natural-Killer/T-cell Lymphoma

Extranodal natural-killer (NK)/T-cell lymphoma (ENKTL) nasal type is a rare form of non-Hodgkin's lymphoma associated with EBV, more common in Asia and Latin America with less known about the clinical behavior of this entity in Western, non-Asian, and non-Hispanic populations.[64] The California Cancer Registry identified 213 non-Hispanic white individuals (NHW) and API patients between 2001 and 2008.[65] ENKTL has a higher incidence among APIs than NHWs but is still lower than rates seen in Asian countries. There is a significant increase in incidence among Hispanic men, possibly due to immigration patterns or environmental and lifestyle exposures unique to this population, such as pesticides or solvents. OS is uniformly poor for all racial groups with no association with age, sex, socioeconomic status, or human immunodeficiency virus status.

In a comparative study of sinonasal (SN-ENKTL) and extranasal (EN-ENKTL) disease, the investigators identified 241 cases of SN-ENKTL and 287 cases of EN-ENKTL in the SEER registry.[66] There is a significantly greater male preponderance in cases of EN-ENKTL (72.47% vs 59.75%) with a slightly younger age of diagnosis for SN-ENKTL (49.9 years vs 53.8 years). White individuals make up the most among both types (more than 70%), followed by others (20%–25%) and black individuals

(4%–6%). With respect to location, SN-ENKTL commonly involves the nasal cavity (80.50%), followed by the maxillary sinus (6.22%). B symptoms are more common at diagnosis among those patients with EN-ENKTL (38.41% vs 22.86%). SN-ENKTL more commonly presents at stage IE as compared with EN-ENKTL, which presents at stage IIIE/IV. EN-ENKTL has a lower DSS at 1 year and 5 years (41.72% and 28.33% vs 62.34% and 39.13%), possibly due to late diagnosis, and there is no association with gender, race, or histology. With respect to stage, SN-ENKTL has better 1-year and 5-year DSS with stage IE disease (76.59% and 53.99% vs 51.79% and 33.33%) and patients with advanced EN-ENKTL fare worse at 1 year and 5 years (26.48% and 14.63% vs 32.45% and 24.34%). Of note, patients with SN-ENKTL presenting at stage IIE have a nearly threefold increase in mortality than those with stage IE disease, with 5-year DSS dropping to 27.79%. Presence of B-symptoms impacts survival only in the EN-ENKTL group and is associated with a greater hazard of death (HR 1.66, $P<.05$). Both groups see improved survival with RT, although regression analysis finds withholding radiation only impacts prognosis in the SN-ENKTL group. However, when looking at early-stage disease, both groups have improved prognosis with RT.

Extramedullary Plasmacytoma

Extramedullary plasmacytomas (EMP) are monoclonal B-cell neoplasms that may arise in the head and neck in up to 80% of cases, with nearly two-thirds in the sinonasal tract.[67] A recent SEER registry analysis compared sinonasal (SN-EMP) with other head and neck (HN-EMP) sites between 1973 and 2011.[68] A total of 778 cases were identified, with 411 cases of SN-EMP. SN-EMP presents at a slightly later age than HN-EMP (61.3 years compared with 59.9 years), although there is a male predilection for both locations, which is stronger for SN-EMP (3.65:1 vs 1.87:1). Whites are more commonly afflicted in both types, comprising more than 80% of cases. The B-cell precursor type is the most common histologic type for both groups, followed by differentiated type and most are localized at time of diagnosis. For SN-EMP, the nasal cavity is the most commonly affected region (40.6%), followed by nasopharynx (31.6%) and maxillary sinus (15.5%). Most patients in both groups are most commonly treated with surgery and adjuvant RT, and next most commonly by RT alone. Survival outcomes are excellent in both groups, demonstrating comparable RS and DSS (88.2% at 5 years, 83.3% at 10 years for SN-EMP). Maxillary sinus involvement is associated with worse RS and DSS compared with nasal cavity and nasopharyngeal tumors. Of note, all 3 treatment modalities (surgery alone, RT alone, and combination therapy) have excellent and comparable 10-year DSS consistent with prior studies.[69,70]

Sinonasal Sarcoma

As a whole, sinonasal sarcomas make up fewer than 10% to 15% of tumors in this location and historically have portended a poor prognosis and high mortality.[71] The standard of treatment in other locations is wide resection, a luxury not often afforded in the sinonasal region.[72] Between 1973 and 2008, a total of 352 patients were identified using the SEER database, mostly men (55%) with a mean age at diagnosis of 44 years, although there was even distribution among all age groups.[71] Patients were predominately white (78%) with disease located in the maxillary sinus (58%). Sinonasal rhabdomyosarcoma (SN-RMS) is the most common histology (34%). Median survival time is 50 months, with 1-year, 5-year, and 10-year RS of 78.8%, 47.4%, and 38.1%, respectively. Men have significantly lower survival relative to women (42.5% vs 53.1% 5-year survival), with women having 30% lower hazard of death. Of the histologic subtypes, chondrosarcoma is associated with the lowest mortality rate with a 5-year survival of 64.4%. Relative to this group, the hazard of death from rhabdomyosarcoma and Kaposi sarcoma is more than 3 and 5 times greater, respectively. Sphenoid sinus involvement has the lowest mortality rate, whereas frontal sinus involvement has the highest. Fibrosarcoma, incredibly rare in the head and neck, and not explicitly studied in the previously referenced analysis, has an overall higher survival rate compared with other histologies at 5 years (OS 71.7%), with worse outcomes in patients receiving RT only.[73] Sinonasal carcinosarcoma, also exceedingly rare, has a female predilection and poor 5-year OS of 48.5%, which is significantly lower than carcinosarcoma at other head and neck sites, excluding the salivary glands.[74]

With regard to SN-RMS, common in the young pediatric population, more than 55% of cases are female, and involve the nasopharynx and nasal cavity most commonly.[75] Interestingly, incidence among men and white individuals has increased over the past 20 years, whereas that of women and black individuals has decreased over this period. Survival, however, is consistently higher at 5 and 10 years in women at 54.88% and 52.83%, respectively, compared with men, at 36.9% and 36.9%, although this is markedly lower than RMS at other head and neck sites.[10] White individuals also have higher survival rates compared with black individuals. Embryonal SN-RMS demonstrated the highest survival rates up to 20 years as compared with other histologic subtypes, although this was not statically significant.

SUMMARY

Population-based analyses offer a means of obtaining key epidemiologic and prognostic information for rare pathologies that would be difficult to obtain from a single institution. In the United States, the SEER registry has been an invaluable resource for studying incidence, epidemiology, and survival of sinonasal and ventral skull base malignancies. Overall, sinonasal malignancies are rare, tend to affect whites, have a male preponderance, and are managed surgically in most cases. As these studies rely on registry data, there are important limitations, including selection and confounding bias, that warrant caution.

REFERENCES

1. Thygesen LC, Ersboll AK. When the entire population is the sample: strengths and limitations in register-based epidemiology. Eur J Epidemiol 2014;29:551–8.

2. Nathan H, Pawlik TM. Limitations of claims and registry data in surgical oncology research. Ann Surg Oncol 2008;15:415–23.

3. Warren JL, Klabunde CN, Schrag D, et al. Overview of the SEER-Medicare data: content, research applications, and generalizability to the United States elderly population. Med Care 2002;40:Iv-3-18.

4. Yu JB, Gross CP, Wilson LD, et al. NCI SEER public-use data: applications and limitations in oncology research. Oncology (Williston Park) 2009;23:288–95.

5. Izquierdo JN, Schoenbach VJ. The potential and limitations of data from population-based state cancer registries. Am J Public Health 2000;90:695–8.

6. Kent EE, Malinoff R, Rozjabek HM, et al. Revisiting the Surveillance Epidemiology and End Results Cancer Registry and Medicare Health Outcomes Survey (SEER-MHOS) linked data resource for patient-reported outcomes research in older adults with cancer. J Am Geriatr Soc 2016;64:186–92.

7. Clegg LX, Reichman ME, Hankey BF, et al. Quality of race, Hispanic ethnicity, and immigrant status in population-based cancer registry data: implications for health disparity studies. Cancer Causes Control 2007;18:177–87.

8. Algazi AP, Cha E, Ortiz-Urda SM, et al. The combination of axitinib followed by paclitaxel/carboplatin yields extended survival in advanced BRAF wild-type melanoma: results of a clinical/correlative prospective phase II clinical trial. Br J Cancer 2015;112:1326–31.

9. Ansa B, Goodman M, Ward K, et al. Paranasal sinus squamous cell carcinoma incidence and survival based on Surveillance, Epidemiology, and End Results data, 1973 to 2009. Cancer 2013;119:2602–10.

10. Turner JH, Reh DD. Incidence and survival in patients with sinonasal cancer: a historical analysis of population-based data. Head Neck 2012;34:877–85.

11. Dutta R, Dubal PM, Svider PF, et al. Sinonasal malignancies: a population-based analysis of site-specific incidence and survival. Laryngoscope 2015;125:2491–7.

12. Grau C, Jakobsen MH, Harbo G, et al. Sino-nasal cancer in Denmark 1982-1991– a nationwide survey. Acta Oncol 2001;40:19–23.

13. Kuijpens JH, Louwman MW, Peters R, et al. Trends in sinonasal cancer in The Netherlands: more squamous cell cancer, less adenocarcinoma. A population-based study 1973-2009. Eur J Cancer 2012;48:2369–74.

14. Blanch JL, Ruiz AM, Alos L, et al. Treatment of 125 sinonasal tumors: prognostic factors, outcome, and follow-up. Otolaryngol Head Neck Surg 2004;131:973–6.

15. Dubal PM, Bhojwani A, Patel TD, et al. Squamous cell carcinoma of the maxillary sinus: a population-based analysis. Laryngoscope 2016;126:399–404.

16. Unsal AA, Dubal PM, Patel TD, et al. Squamous cell carcinoma of the nasal cavity: a population-based analysis. Laryngoscope 2016;126:560–5.

17. Sanghvi S, Khan MN, Patel NR, et al. Epidemiology of sinonasal squamous cell carcinoma: a comprehensive analysis of 4994 patients. Laryngoscope 2014; 124:76–83.

18. Vazquez A, Khan MN, Blake DM, et al. Sinonasal squamous cell carcinoma and the prognostic implications of its histologic variants: a population-based study. Int Forum Allergy Rhinol 2015;5:85–91.

19. Shah AA, Jeffus SK, Stelow EB. Squamous cell carcinoma variants of the upper aerodigestive tract: a comprehensive review with a focus on genetic alterations. Arch Pathol Lab Med 2014;138:731–44.

20. Kuan EC, Peng KA, Bhuta S, et al. Basaloid squamous cell carcinoma of the maxilla: report of a case and literature review. Am J Otolaryngol 2015;36:402–7.

21. Bhayani MK, Yilmaz T, Sweeney A, et al. Sinonasal adenocarcinoma: a 16-year experience at a single institution. Head Neck 2014;36:1490–6.

22. D'Aguillo CM, Kanumuri VV, Khan MN, et al. Demographics and survival trends of sinonasal adenocarcinoma from 1973 to 2009. Int Forum Allergy Rhinol 2014;4: 771–6.

23. Gatta G, Bimbi G, Ciccolallo L, et al. Survival for ethmoid sinus adenocarcinoma in European populations. Acta Oncol 2009;48:992–8.

24. Leivo I. Sinonasal adenocarcinoma: update on classification, immunophenotype and molecular features. Head Neck Pathol 2016;10:68–74.

25. Bradley PJ, Jones NS, Robertson I. Diagnosis and management of esthesioneuroblastoma. Curr Opin Otolaryngol Head Neck Surg 2003;11:112–8.

26. Jethanamest D, Morris LG, Sikora AG, et al. Esthesioneuroblastoma: a population-based analysis of survival and prognostic factors. Arch Otolaryngol Head Neck Surg 2007;133:276–80.

27. Herr MW, Sethi RK, Meier JC, et al. Esthesioneuroblastoma: an update on the Massachusetts Eye and Ear Infirmary and Massachusetts General Hospital experience with craniofacial resection, proton beam radiation, and chemotherapy. J Neurol Surg B Skull Base 2014;75:58–64.
28. Tajudeen BA, Arshi A, Suh JD, et al. Esthesioneuroblastoma: an update on the UCLA experience, 2002-2013. J Neurol Surg B Skull Base 2015;76:43–9.
29. Diaz EM Jr, Johnigan RH 3rd, Pero C, et al. Olfactory neuroblastoma: the 22-year experience at one comprehensive cancer center. Head Neck 2005;27:138–49.
30. Platek ME, Merzianu M, Mashtare TL, et al. Improved survival following surgery and radiation therapy for olfactory neuroblastoma: analysis of the SEER database. Radiat Oncol 2011;6:41.
31. Tajudeen BA, Arshi A, Suh JD, et al. Importance of tumor grade in esthesioneuroblastoma survival: a population-based analysis. JAMA Otolaryngol Head Neck Surg 2014;140:1124–9.
32. Biller HF, Lawson W, Sachdev VP, et al. Esthesioneuroblastoma: surgical treatment without radiation. Laryngoscope 1990;100:1199–201.
33. Kim KH, Sung MW, Chung PS, et al. Adenoid cystic carcinoma of the head and neck. Arch Otolaryngol Head Neck Surg 1994;120:721–6.
34. Rhee CS, Won TB, Lee CH, et al. Adenoid cystic carcinoma of the sinonasal tract: treatment results. Laryngoscope 2006;116:982–6.
35. Sanghvi S, Patel NR, Patel CR, et al. Sinonasal adenoid cystic carcinoma: comprehensive analysis of incidence and survival from 1973 to 2009. Laryngoscope 2013;123:1592–7.
36. Ellington CL, Goodman M, Kono SA, et al. Adenoid cystic carcinoma of the head and neck: incidence and survival trends based on 1973-2007 Surveillance, Epidemiology, and End Results data. Cancer 2012;118:4444–51.
37. Lloyd S, Yu JB, Wilson LD, et al. Determinants and patterns of survival in adenoid cystic carcinoma of the head and neck, including an analysis of adjuvant radiation therapy. Am J Clin Oncol 2011;34:76–81.
38. Wolfish EB, Nelson BL, Thompson LD. Sinonasal tract mucoepidermoid carcinoma: a clinicopathologic and immunophenotypic study of 19 cases combined with a comprehensive review of the literature. Head Neck Pathol 2012;6:191–207.
39. Patel TD, Vazquez A, Patel DM, et al. A comparative analysis of sinonasal and salivary gland mucoepidermoid carcinoma using population-based data. Int Forum Allergy Rhinol 2015;5:78–84.
40. Yu MC. Nasopharyngeal carcinoma: epidemiology and dietary factors. IARC Sci Publ 1991;(105):39–47.
41. Vazquez A, Khan MN, Govindaraj S, et al. Nasopharyngeal squamous cell carcinoma: a comparative analysis of keratinizing and nonkeratinizing subtypes. Int Forum Allergy Rhinol 2014;4:675–83.
42. Yip KW, Shi W, Pintilie M, et al. Prognostic significance of the Epstein-Barr virus, p53, Bcl-2, and survivin in nasopharyngeal cancer. Clin Cancer Res 2006;12:5726–32.
43. Erkal HS, Serin M, Cakmak A. Nasopharyngeal carcinomas: analysis of patient, tumor and treatment characteristics determining outcome. Radiother Oncol 2001;61:247–56.
44. Cheung F, Chan O, Ng WT, et al. The prognostic value of histological typing in nasopharyngeal carcinoma. Oral Oncol 2012;48:429–33.
45. Serin M, Erkal HS, Cakmak A. Radiation therapy and concurrent cisplatin in management of locoregionally advanced nasopharyngeal carcinomas. Acta Oncol 1999;38:1031–5.

46. Frierson HF Jr, Mills SE, Fechner RE, et al. Sinonasal undifferentiated carcinoma. An aggressive neoplasm derived from Schneiderian epithelium and distinct from olfactory neuroblastoma. Am J Surg Pathol 1986;10:771–9.

47. Chambers KJ, Lehmann AE, Remenschneider A, et al. Incidence and survival patterns of sinonasal undifferentiated carcinoma in the United States. J Neurol Surg B Skull Base 2015;76:94–100.

48. Kuan EC, Arshi A, Mallen-St Clair J. Significance of tumor stage in sinonasal undifferentiated carcinoma survival: a population-based analysis. Otolaryngol Head Neck Surg 2016;154:667–73.

49. Pitman KT, Costantino PD, Lassen LF. Sinonasal undifferentiated carcinoma: current trends in treatment. Skull Base Surg 1995;5:269–72.

50. Mills SE. Neuroectodermal neoplasms of the head and neck with emphasis on neuroendocrine carcinomas. Mod Pathol 2002;15:264–78.

51. Patel TD, Vazquez A, Dubal PM, et al. Sinonasal neuroendocrine carcinoma: a population-based analysis of incidence and survival. Int Forum Allergy Rhinol 2015;5:448–53.

52. Smith SR, Som P, Fahmy A, et al. A clinicopathological study of sinonasal neuroendocrine carcinoma and sinonasal undifferentiated carcinoma. Laryngoscope 2000;110:1617–22.

53. Menon S, Pai P, Sengar M, et al. Sinonasal malignancies with neuroendocrine differentiation: case series and review of literature. Indian J Pathol Microbiol 2010; 53:28–34.

54. Mitchell EH, Diaz A, Yilmaz T, et al. Multimodality treatment for sinonasal neuroendocrine carcinoma. Head Neck 2012;34:1372–6.

55. Medina JE, Ferlito A, Pellitteri PK, et al. Current management of mucosal melanoma of the head and neck. J Surg Oncol 2003;83:116–22.

56. Conley JJ. Melanomas of the mucous membrane of the head and neck. Laryngoscope 1989;99:1248–54.

57. Gal TJ, Silver N, Huang B. Demographics and treatment trends in sinonasal mucosal melanoma. Laryngoscope 2011;121:2026–33.

58. Luna-Ortiz K, Aguilar-Romero M, Villavicencio-Valencia V, et al. Comparative study between two different staging systems (AJCC TNM VS BALLANTYNE'S) for mucosal melanomas of the head & neck. Med Oral Patol Oral Cir Bucal 2016;21(4):e425–30.

59. Khan MN, Kanumuri VV, Raikundalia MD, et al. Sinonasal melanoma: survival and prognostic implications based on site of involvement. Int Forum Allergy Rhinol 2014;4:151–5.

60. Moreno MA, Roberts DB, Kupferman ME, et al. Mucosal melanoma of the nose and paranasal sinuses, a contemporary experience from the M. D. Anderson Cancer Center. Cancer 2010;116:2215–23.

61. Yen TT, Wang RC, Jiang RS, et al. The diagnosis of sinonasal lymphoma: a challenge for rhinologists. Eur Arch Otorhinolaryngol 2012;269:1463–9.

62. Kanumuri VV, Khan MN, Vazquez A, et al. Diffuse large B-cell lymphoma of the sinonasal tract: analysis of survival in 852 cases. Am J Otolaryngol 2014;35: 154–8.

63. Sehn LH. Chemotherapy alone for localized diffuse large B-cell lymphoma. Cancer J 2012;18:421–6.

64. Aozasa K, Takakuwa T, Hongyo T, et al. Nasal NK/T-cell lymphoma: epidemiology and pathogenesis. Int J Hematol 2008;87:110–7.

65. Ai WZ, Chang ET, Fish K, et al. Racial patterns of extranodal natural killer/T-cell lymphoma, nasal type, in California: a population-based study. Br J Haematol 2012;156:626–32.
66. Vazquez A, Khan MN, Blake DM, et al. Extranodal natural killer/T-cell lymphoma: a population-based comparison of sinonasal and extranasal disease. Laryngoscope 2014;124:888–95.
67. Bachar G, Goldstein D, Brown D, et al. Solitary extramedullary plasmacytoma of the head and neck–long-term outcome analysis of 68 cases. Head Neck 2008;30: 1012–9.
68. Patel TD, Vazquez A, Choudhary MM, et al. Sinonasal extramedullary plasmacytoma: a population-based incidence and survival analysis. Int Forum Allergy Rhinol 2015;5:862–9.
69. Sasaki R, Yasuda K, Abe E, et al. Multi-institutional analysis of solitary extramedullary plasmacytoma of the head and neck treated with curative radiotherapy. Int J Radiat Oncol Biol Phys 2012;82:626–34.
70. D'Aguillo C, Soni RS, Gordhan C, et al. Sinonasal extramedullary plasmacytoma: a systematic review of 175 patients. Int Forum Allergy Rhinol 2014;4:156–63.
71. Wu AW, Suh JD, Metson R, et al. Prognostic factors in sinonasal sarcomas: analysis of the surveillance, epidemiology and end result database. Laryngoscope 2012;122:2137–42.
72. Sercarz JA, Mark RJ, Tran L, et al. Sarcomas of the nasal cavity and paranasal sinuses. Ann Otol Rhinol Laryngol 1994;103:699–704.
73. Patel TD, Carniol ET, Vazquez A, et al. Sinonasal fibrosarcoma: analysis of the Surveillance, Epidemiology, and End Results database. Int Forum Allergy Rhinol 2016;6:201–5.
74. Patel TD, Vazquez A, Plitt MA, et al. A case-control analysis of survival outcomes in sinonasal carcinosarcoma. Am J Otolaryngol 2015;36:200–4.
75. Sanghvi S, Misra P, Patel NR, et al. Incidence trends and long-term survival analysis of sinonasal rhabdomyosarcoma. Am J Otolaryngol 2013;34:682–9.

Index

Note: Page numbers of article titles are in **boldface** type.

A

Adenocarcinoma, chemotherapy in, 437
   intestinal-type, 451
   sinonasal, 232–236, 485–486
     survival outcomes of, 472
   subtypes of, 237
Adenoid cystic carcinoma, 232–236, 237, 451–452, 487–488
   grading system for, 235
   radiation therapy in, 427–428
   survival outcomes of, 472

C

Cavernous sinus, in malignancies, aggressive transcranial approaches to, 370–371
     anterlateral transcavernous approach to, 372–373
     anteromedial transcavernous approach to, 371–372
     cerebral revascularization in, 379–380
     endoscopic endonasal transsphenoidal approaches to, 375
     endoscopic transfacial approaches to, 369–370, 373
     endoscopic transptergoid approach to, 375–376
     needle biopsy via foramen ovale in, 369
     radical en bloc oncological resection of, 376–379
     surgical management of, **365–383**
     transcavernous biopsy of, 367–369
   involvement in sinonasal malignancies, 213–214
Cavernous sinus meningioma resection-decompression technique, 374–375
Chondrosarcoma, clival, 317
   radiotherapy for, 428–429
Chordoma(s), 236–237, 238
   clival, 316–317
   radiotherapy for, 428–429
Clival lesions, differential diagnosis of, 316–322
   radiologic characteristics of, 316, 317, 318, 319, 320
Clival malignancies, 214
   endoscopic resection of, **315–329**
     intraoperative approach for, 324–325
     postoperative care in, 326
     preoperative considerations for, 322–323
     reconstruction after, 325–326
Clivus, anatomy of, 249–251
   metastasis to, 321–322

Otolaryngol Clin N Am 50 (2017) 499–504
http://dx.doi.org/10.1016/S0030-6665(17)30025-7
0030-6665/17

Moving?

Make sure your subscription moves with you!

To notify us of your new address, find your **Clinics Account Number** (located on your mailing label above your name), and contact customer service at:

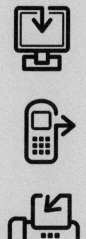

Email: journalscustomerservice-usa@elsevier.com

800-654-2452 (subscribers in the U.S. & Canada)
314-447-8871 (subscribers outside of the U.S. & Canada)

Fax number: 314-447-8029

Elsevier Health Sciences Division
Subscription Customer Service
3251 Riverport Lane
Maryland Heights, MO 63043

ELSEVIER

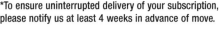

Printed and bound by CPI Group (UK) Ltd, Croydon, CR0 4YY

03/10/2024

01040392-0014